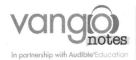

Hear it. Get It.

In partnership with **Audible** Education

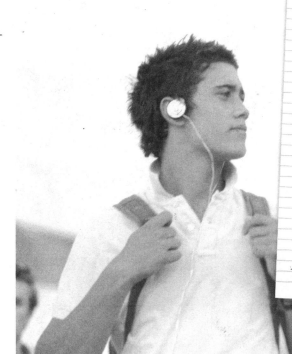

Study on the go with VangoNotes.

Just download chapter reviews from your text and listen to them on any mp3 player. Now wherever you are--whatever you're doing--you can study by listening to the following for each chapter of your textbook:

Big Ideas: Your "need to know" for each chapter

Practice Test: A gut check for the Big Ideas-- tells you if you need to keep studying

Key Terms: Audio "flashcards" to help you review key concepts and terms

Rapid Review: A quick drill session -- use it right before your test

VangoNotes.com

Pearson Nursing Reviews & Rationales

Fluids, Electrolytes, & Acid–Base Balance

Third Edition

SERIES EDITOR

MaryAnn Hogan, MSN, RN

Clinical Assistant Professor
School of Nursing
University of Massachusetts–Amherst
Amherst, Massachusetts

CONSULTING EDITORS

Margaret M. Gingrich, RN, MSN

Professor
Harrisburg Area Community College
Harrisburg, Pennsylvania

Edward Nichols, RN, MSN

Professor
San Jacinto College–Central
Houston, Texas

PEARSON

Boston   Columbus   Indianapolis   New York   San Francisco   Upper Saddle River
Amsterdam   Cape Town   Dubai   London   Madrid   Milan   Munich   Paris   Montréal   Toronto
Delhi   Mexico City   São Paulo   Sydney   Hong Kong   Seoul   Singapore   Taipei   Tokyo

Cataloging-in-Publication Data on File with the Library of Congress

Director of Readypoint™: Maura Connor
Executive Editor: Jennifer Farthing
Developmental Editor: Elisa Rogers
Editorial Assistant: Deirdre MacKnight
Director, Digital Product Development: Alex Marciante
Media Product Manager: Travis Moses-Westphal
Vice President, Director Sales & Marketing: David Gesell
Senior Marketing Manager: Phoenix Harvey
Marketing Coordinator: Michael Sirinides

Director of Media Production: Allyson Graesser
Media Project Manager: Rachel Collett
Managing Editor, Production: Patrick Walsh
Production Editor: GEX Publishing Services
Manufacturing Manager: Ilene Sanford
Art Director/Cover Designer: Mary Siener
Composition: GEX Publishing Services
Printer/Binder: Edwards Brothers
Cover Printer: Lehigh/Phoenix Color Hagerstown

10 9 8 7 6 5 4 3 2 1

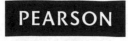

ISBN 10: 0-13-295855-4
ISBN 13: 978-0-13-295855-4

Contents

Welcome to the Pearson Nursing Reviews & Rationales Series!

This series has been specifically designed to provide a clear and concentrated review of important nursing knowledge in the following content areas:

- Anatomy & Physiology
- Nursing Fundamentals
- Nutrition & Diet Therapy
- Fluids, Electrolytes, & Acid–Base Balance
- Medical-Surgical Nursing
- Pathophysiology
- Pharmacology
- Maternal-Newborn Nursing
- Child Health Nursing
- Mental Health Nursing
- Health & Physical Assessment
- Community Health Nursing
- Leadership & Management

The books in this series are designed for use either by current nursing students as a study aid for nursing course work, for NCLEX-RN® exam preparation, or by practicing nurses seeking a comprehensive yet concise review of a nursing specialty or subject area.

This series is truly unique. One of its most special features is that it has been developed and reviewed by a large team of nurse educators from across the United States and Canada to ensure that each chapter is edited by a nurse expert in the content area under study. The series editor, MaryAnn Hogan, designed the overall series in collaboration with a core Pearson team to take full advantage of Pearson's cutting edge technology. The consulting editors for each book, also experts in that specialty area, then reviewed all chapters and test questions submitted for comprehensiveness and accuracy. Finally, MaryAnn Hogan reviewed the chapters in each book for consistency, accuracy, and applicability to the NCLEX-RN® Test Plan.

All books in the series are identical in their overall design for your convenience. As an added value, each book comes with a comprehensive support package, including access to additional questions online, complete eText, and a tear-out *NursingNotes* card for clinical reference and quick review.

Study Tips

Use of this book should help simplify your review. To make the most of your valuable study time, also follow these simple but important suggestions:

1. Use a weekly calendar to schedule study sessions.
   - Outline the time frames for all of your activities (home, school, appointments, etc.) on a weekly calendar.
   - Find the "holes" in your calendar, which are the times when you can plan to study. Add study sessions to the calendar at times when you can expect to be mentally alert and follow your plan!
2. Create the optimal study environment.
   - Eliminate external sources of distraction, such as television, telephone, etc.
   - Eliminate internal sources of distraction, such as hunger, thirst, or dwelling on items or problems that cannot be worked on at the moment.
   - Take a break for 10 minutes or so after each hour of concentrated study, both as a reward and as an incentive to keep studying.
3. Use prereading strategies to increase comprehension of chapter material.
   - Skim the headings in the chapter (because they identify chapter content).
   - Read the definitions of key terms, which will help you learn new words to comprehend chapter information.
   - Review all graphic aids (figures, tables, boxes) because they are often used to explain important points in the chapter.

4. Read the chapter thoroughly but at a reasonable speed.
   - Comprehension and retention are actually enhanced by not reading too slowly.
   - Do take the time to reread any section that is unclear to you.
5. Summarize what you have learned.
   - Use the accompanying online resource, NursingReviewsandRationales.com, to test yourself with hundreds of NCLEX-RN®-style practice questions.
   - Review again any sections that correspond to questions you answered incorrectly or incompletely.

Test-Taking Strategies

Test-taking strategies accompany the rationales for every question in the series. These strategies will assist you to select the correct answer by breaking down the question, even if you don't know the correct response. Use the following strategies to increase your success on nursing tests or examinations:

- Get sufficient sleep and have something to eat before taking a test. Avoid eating concentrated sweets, though, to prevent rapid upward and then downward surges in your blood glucose. Avoid also high-fat foods that will make you sleepy.
- Take deep breaths during the test as needed. Remember, the brain requires both oxygen and glucose as fuel.
- Read the question carefully, identifying the stem, all the options, and any critical words or phrases in either the stem or options.
  - Critical words in the stem such as *most important* indicate the need to set priorities, because more than one option is likely to contain a statement that is technically correct.
  - Remember that the presence of absolute words such as *never* or *only* in an answer option is more likely to make that option incorrect.
- Determine who is the client in the question; often this is the person with the health problem, but it may also be a significant other, relative, friend, or another nurse.
- Decide whether the stem is a true response stem or a false response stem. With a true response stem, the correct answer will be a true statement, and vice-versa.

- Determine what the question is really asking, sometimes referred to as the core issue of the question. Evaluate all answer options in relation to this issue, and not strictly to the "correctness" of the statement in each individual option.
- Eliminate options that are obviously incorrect, then go back and reread the stem. Evaluate those remaining options against the stem once more to make a final selection.
- If two answers seem similar and correct, try to decide whether one of them is more global or comprehensive. If one option includes the alternative option within it, it is likely that the more global option is the correct answer.

The NCLEX-RN® Licensing Examination

Upon graduation from a nursing program, successful completion of the NCLEX-RN® licensing examination is required to begin professional nursing practice. The NCLEX-RN® examination is a Computer Adaptive Test (CAT) that ranges in length from 75 to 265 individual (stand-alone) test items, depending on your performance during the examination. The blueprint for the exam is reviewed and revised every three years by the National Council of State Boards of Nursing using the results of a job analysis study of new graduate nurses practicing within the first six months after graduation. Each question on the exam is coded to a *Client Need Category* and an *Integrated Process*.

Client Need Categories   There are four categories of client needs, and each exam will contain a minimum and maximum percent of questions from each category. Each major category has subcategories within it. The *Client Needs* categories according to the NCLEX-RN® Test Plan effective April 2010 are as follows:

- Safe Effective Care Environment
  - Management of Care (16–22%)
  - Safety and Infection Control (8–14%)
- Health Promotion and Maintenance (6–12%)
- Psychosocial Integrity (6–12%)
- Physiological Integrity
  - Basic Care and Comfort (6–12%)
  - Pharmacological and Parenteral Therapies (13–19%)
  - Reduction of Risk Potential (10–16%)
  - Physiological Adaptation (11–17%)

Integrated Processes The integrated processes identified on the NCLEX-RN® Test Plan effective April 2010, with condensed definitions, are as follows:

- Nursing Process: a scientific problem solving approach used in nursing practice; consisting of assessment, analysis, planning, implementation, and evaluation.
- Caring: client–nurse interaction(s) characterized by mutual respect and trust and that are directed toward achieving desired client outcomes.
- Communication and Documentation: verbal and/or non-verbal interactions between nurse and others (client, family, health care team); a written or electronic recording of activities or events that occur during client care.
- Teaching and Learning: facilitating client's acquisition of knowledge, skills, and attitudes that lead to behavior change.

More detailed information about this examination may be obtained by visiting the National Council of State Boards of Nursing website at http://www.ncsbn.org and viewing the *2010 NCLEX-RN® Detailed Test Plan.*[1]

---

[1]Reference: National Council of State Boards of Nursing, Inc. *2010 NCLEX-RN® Test Plan.* Effective April, 2010. Retrieved from http://www.ncsbn.org/2010_NCLEX_RN_TestPlan.pdf.

HOW TO GET THE MOST OUT OF THIS BOOK

Each chapter has the following elements to guide you during review and study:

Chapter Objectives describe what you will be able to know or do after learning the material covered in the chapter.

Objectives

➤ Review the basic physiology of acid–base balance.

➤ Identify potential acid–base imbalances.

➤ Identify priority nursing diagnoses for acid–base imbalances.

➤ Describe the therapeutic management of acid–base imbalances.

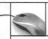

NCLEX-RN® Test Prep

Use the accompanying online resource, NursingReviewsandRationales, to test yourself with hundreds of NCLEX®-style practice questions.

Review at a Glance contains a glossary of key terms used in the chapter, with definitions provided up-front and available at your fingertips, to help you stay focused and make the best use of your study time.

Review at a Glance

hyperkalemia serum potassium level above the laboratory normal value (usually 5.1 mEq/L)

hypokalemia serum level of potassium falls below 3.5 mEq/L

relative hyperkalemia movement of potassium from the intracellular fluid to the extracellular fluid, leading to elevated serum potassium levels without a true body increase of potassium, such as occurs with acidosis

relative hypokalemia movement of potassium from the extracellular fluid to the intracellular fluid, leading to lowered serum potassium levels without a true decrease of potassium in the body, such as occurs with insulin therapy

sodium-potassium pump controls the concentration of potassium by removing three sodium ions from the cell for every two potassium ions that return to the cell; fueled by the breakdown of ATP and responsible for causing muscle cells to generate action potentials and transmit impulses

Pretest provides a 10-question quiz as a sample overview of the material covered in the chapter and helps you decide in what areas you need the most—or the least—review.

PRETEST

❶ The nurse would expect a client to have a high serum level of magnesium after seeing which health problem listed in the medical history?

1. Malabsorption
2. Anemia
3. Overuse of laxatives
4. Alcoholism

Practice to Pass questions are open-ended, stimulate critical thinking, and reinforce mastery of the chapter information.

Practice to Pass

In caring for a client with hypernatremia, what should the nurse do to help ensure client safety?

NCLEX Alert identifies concepts that are likely to be tested on the NCLEX-RN® examination. Be sure to learn the information highlighted wherever you see this icon.

Case Study, found at the end of the chapter, provides an opportunity for you to use your critical thinking and clinical reasoning skills to "put it all together." It describes a true-to-life client case situation and asks you open-ended questions about how you would provide care for that client and/or family.

Case Study

A 69-year-old client with chronic obstructive pulmonary disease (COPD) is admitted with an acute respiratory infection. You are the nurse assigned to the care of this client.

1. What would this client's ABGs look like?
2. What will you do to help improve the client's respiratory status?
3. Why is a client with COPD given oxygen at a low flow rate?
4. Why is this client's $PaCO_2$ different than a client who does not have COPD?
5. What teaching does this client require in order to prevent development of metabolic alkalosis?

For suggested responses, see page 205.

Posttest provides an additional 10-question quiz at the end of the chapter. It provides you with feedback about mastery of the chapter material following review and study. All pretest and posttest questions contain comprehensive rationales for the correct and incorrect answers, and are coded according to cognitive level of difficulty, and the NCLEX-RN® Test Plan category of client need and integrated process.

POSTTEST

1 When assessing a client with diabetes insipidus (DI), the nurse expects to find which of the following?

1. Nausea and vomiting
2. Polyuria and polydipsia
3. Dysuria
4. Confusion

NCLEX-RN® Test Prep: NursingReviewsandRationales.com

For those who want to prepare for the NCLEX-RN®, practicing online will help you become more familiar with the computer-based testing experience, especially for the new alternate item formats such as audio, media-enhanced, hot spot, and exhibit questions. With this new edition, use the code printed inside the front cover of the book to access Nursing Reviews & Rationales, which offers 450 practice questions using all NCLEX®-style formats. This includes the practice questions found in all chapters of the book as well as 30 additional questions per chapter. Nursing Reviews & Rationales allows you to choose two ways to prepare for the NCLEX-RN®. Both approaches personalize your practice experience according to what stage you are at in your NCLEX® preparation.

Nursing Reviews & Rationales includes the eText version of *Pearson Nursing Fluids, Electrolytes, & Acid–Base Balance*, Third Edition. This eText is fully searchable and includes features like note-taking, highlighting, and more. The eText allows you to take your review with you anywhere you have an internet connection to NursingReviewsandRationales.com.

Pearson NursingNotes Card

This tear-out card provides a reference for frequently used facts and information related to the subject matter of the book. These are designed to be useful in the clinical setting, when quick and easy access to information is so important!

About the Fluids, Electrolytes, and Acid–Base Balance Book

Chapters in this book cover "need-to-know" information about principles of fluids, electrolytes, and acid–base balance, including focused assessments and how they affect entire body systems. Individual chapters focus on specific electrolytes (sodium, potassium, calcium, magnesium, chloride, and phosphorus), acid–base disturbances, and replacement therapies for common fluid and electrolyte imbalances. Each chapter includes definitions, etiologies, clinical manifestations, and therapeutic management of fluids, electrolytes, and acid–base problems in the context of the nursing process.

Acknowledgments

This book is a monumental effort of collaboration. Without the contributions of many individuals, this edition of *Fluids, Electrolytes, & Acid–Base Balance: Reviews & Rationales* would not have been possible. Thank you to all the contributors and reviewers who devoted their time and talents to the third edition. The contributors for this edition are Margaret M. Gingrich, RN, MSN, Harrisburg Area Community College, Harrisburg, Pennsylvania and Edward Nichols, RN, MSN, San Jacinto College Central, Houston, Texas. The reviewers for this edition are Faisal Aboul-Enein, DrPH, RN, NP, Texas Women's University, Houston, Texas; Susan J. Brillhart, DNS(c), RN, PNP-BC, Borough of Manhattan Community College, New York, New York; Patricia Boyle Egland, MSN, RN, CPNP-PC, The City University of New York, Borough of Manhattan Community College, New York, New York; Andrea R. Mann, MSN, RN, CNE, Aria Health School of Nursing, Philadelphia, Pennsylvania.

Thanks also to the contributors and reviewers who assisted with the previous editions of this book: Daryle Wane, APRN, BC, MS, Pasco-Hernando Community College, New Port Richey, Florida; Julie A. Adkins, RN, MSN, FNP, Family Nurse Practitioner, West Frankfort, Illinois; Linda Wilson Covington, PhD, RN, Middle Tennessee State University, Murfreesboro, Tennessee; June S. Goyne, RN, MSN, EdD(C), CEN, Columbus State University, Columbus, Georgia; Ann Putnam Johnson, EdD, RN, Western Carolina University, Cullowhee, North Carolina; Kristy A. Nielson, BSN, CCRN, BS, Western Wyoming Community College, Memorial Hospital of Sweetwater County, Rock Springs, Wyoming; Mary Catherine Rawls, Castleton State College, Castleton, Vermont; Lynn Rhyne, MN, RN, Coastal Georgia Community College, Brunswick, Georgia; Bernadette VanDeusen, MSN, RN, Ohlone College, Fremont, California; Kathy M. Ketchum, RN, PhD, Southern Illinois University Edwardsville, Edwardsville, Illinois; Karen Whitman, RN, MS CCPN, Walter Reed Army Medical Center, Washington DC. Their work will surely assist both students and practicing nurses alike to extend their knowledge in the area of fluids, electrolytes, and acid–base balance.

I owe a special debt of gratitude to the wonderful team at Pearson Nursing for their enthusiasm for this project, as well as their good humor, expertise, and encouragement as the series developed. Maura Connor, Director of Readypoint™ was unending in her creativity, support, encouragement, and belief in the need for this series. Jennifer Farthing, Executive Editor, Readypoint™ organized this revision with insight, talent, and zeal, and fostered a culture of true collaboration and teamwork. Elisa Rogers, Developmental Editor, devoted many long hours to coordinating different facets of this project. Her high standards and attention to detail contributed greatly to the final "look" of this book. Editorial Assistant, Deirdre MacKnight, helped to keep the project moving forward on a day-to-day basis, and I am grateful for her efforts as well. A very special thank you goes to the designers of the book and the production team, led by Patrick Walsh, Managing Editor, who brought the ideas and manuscript into final form.

Thank you to the team at GEX Publishing Services, led by Michelle Durgerian, Project Coordinator, for the detail-oriented work of creating this book. I greatly appreciate their hard work, attention to detail, and spirit of collaboration.

Finally, I would like to acknowledge and gratefully thank my children, Michael Jr., Kathryn, Kristen, and William, who sacrificed precious hours of family time so this book could be revised. I would also like to thank my students, past and present, for continuing to inspire me with their quest for knowledge and passion for nursing. You are the future!

–MaryAnn Hogan

Fluid Balance and Imbalances

1

Chapter Outline

Overview of Fluid Movement   Fluid Volume Deficit (FVD)   Fluid Volume Excess (FVE)

Objectives

➤ Review concepts related to fluid movement.
➤ Review assessment data and diagnostic testing indicated to determine fluid volume deficit (dehydration) and fluid volume excess (overload).
➤ Identify clinical presentations of clients exhibiting fluid volume deficit or fluid volume excess.
➤ Identify priority nursing diagnoses for clients experiencing fluid imbalance.
➤ Describe the therapeutic management of clients exhibiting fluid volume deficit and fluid volume excess.
➤ Describe the nursing management of clients exhibiting fluid imbalances.

NCLEX-RN® Test Prep

Use the accompanying online resource, NursingReviewsandRationales, to test yourself with hundreds of NCLEX®-style practice questions.

Review at a Glance

albumin a major plasma protein produced by the liver

aldosterone adrenal gland hormone that causes the kidneys to reabsorb sodium into the blood (causing more water to be reabsorbed by osmosis) and excrete potassium into urine, resulting in concentrated urine and lower urine output

anasarca generalized edema in the body

antidiuretic hormone (ADH) hormone produced by hypothalamus and stored/released by posterior pituitary that causes the kidneys to retain more water in the blood, thus increasing body water, resulting in concentrated urine and lower urine output

colloids large solute particles, such as protein, in solution that exert a pulling force for water

colloid osmotic pressure (COP) pulling force for water created by colloids in solution

diffusion movement of particles in a solution from an area of higher

concentration to an area of lower concentration in order to equalize the concentration

electrolyte a substance that, when dissolved in water, separates into charged particles (ions)

extracellular fluid (ECF) fluid space that lies outside of cells; composed of two spaces, the interstitial (tissue) spaces around cells and the vascular space inside blood vessels

filtration movement of fluid and solute through a semipermeable membrane due to hydrostatic and osmotic forces

free water a hypotonic solution that provides more water than electrolytes, diluting the ECF, making it hypotonic; water then shifts by osmosis from the ECF to the ICF until osmotic equilibrium is reached in both spaces; this rehydrates the ICF as well as the ECF

hemoconcentration condition in which the plasma is more concentrated than normal (higher osmolality than normal)

hemodilution condition in which the plasma is more dilute than normal (lower osmolality than normal)

hydrostatic pressure pushing force of a fluid against the walls of the space it occupies

hypertonic having an osmolality higher than normal plasma

hypervolemia a state of fluid volume excess or overload in the bloodstream

hypotonic having an osmolality lower than normal plasma

hypovolemia a state of insufficient fluid volume circulating in the bloodstream

interstitial fluid fluid space that lies around the cells (cells "float" in interstitial fluid); the interstitial space and vascular space make up the extracellular fluid (ECF)

intracellular fluid (ICF) fluid space that lies inside of the cells

isotonic having the same osmolality as normal plasma

PRETEST

oncotic pressure pulling force a solution has for water due to its protein content

osmolality concentration of solute (particles) per kilogram of water, which creates the pulling power of that solution for water

osmolarity concentration of solute (particles) per liter of solution, which creates the pulling power of that solution for water

osmosis the pulling of water through a semipermeable membrane from an area of lower concentration (fewer particles, more water) to an area of higher concentration (more particles, less water) in order to equalize concentration on both sides

osmotic pressure pulling force a solution has for water; a solution's osmotic pressure is determined by its osmolality (concentration)—the higher the osmolality, the higher the osmotic pressure (force with which it will pull water in from other areas)

semipermeable membrane a membrane that allows some particles to pass through freely and not others (e.g., cell walls and capillary membranes)

specific gravity a measure of the concentration of a solution using solute–solvent ratio; specific gravity of water (no solute) is 1.000; urine specific gravity is normally 1.010–1.030, and is used to indirectly reflect serum osmolality

vascular space space within the blood vessels, usually discussed in terms of blood volume carrying capacity

PRETEST

1 The nurse determines that which client is at highest risk for developing a fluid volume deficit (FVD)?

1. A 76-year-old client who has a nasogastric (NG) tube to low suction following surgery for colon cancer
2. A thin 55-year-old client who smokes and takes glucocorticoids for chronic lung disease
3. A one-year-old child being treated in the clinic for a runny nose and ear infection
4. A 30-year-old client jogging in 50-degree weather

2 The nurse is assisting in a health fair at a senior citizen center. Which instruction should the nurse include when giving an older adult guidelines about remaining hydrated in hot weather?

1. "If your urine is clear yellow, you are drinking adequate fluids."
2. "Drink only water to keep yourself properly hydrated."
3. "Popsicles, gelatin, and ice cream provide fluid intake as well as liquids you drink."
4. "Use your thirst as a guide to the amount of fluid you should be drinking."

3 An adult client in the clinic reports a cough, fever, feeling weak and dizzy, and having nausea and vomiting for three days. Examination reveals dry tongue and oral mucosa, and concentrated urine. To best assess the client's fluid status, the nurse checks which assessment parameters?

1. Core and body temperature
2. Respiratory rate and depth
3. BP and pulse in lying and standing positions
4. Pulse oximetry reading at rest

4 The nurse evaluates the hydration status of a client who has been receiving intravenous (IV) fluids at 150 mL/hour. The nurse identifies that the client has fluid volume excess (FVE) after assessing which of the following? Select all that apply.

1. Neck veins are distended when head of the bed is elevated 45 degrees
2. Hand veins empty when hand is raised above the heart
3. Peripheral pulses are rapid and weak
4. Client becomes short of breath when ambulating
5. Pitting edema is present over tibia

5 A client hospitalized for gastrointestinal (GI) bleeding has orders for nasogastric tube (NGT) placement with irrigations until the returns are clear. Which prescribed solution should the nurse plan on using?

1. 10% dextrose in water ($D_{10}W$)
2. 5% dextrose in water (D_5W)
3. 0.9% sodium chloride (NaCl)
4. 0.45% sodium chloride (½ NaCl)

6 A 70-year-old client with a past medical history of hypertension and myocardial infarction is postoperative after stomach surgery. Vital signs have been stable with an IV of $D_5\frac{1}{2}NS$ infusing at 100 mL/hour. The client now reports dyspnea, has a moist cough, and oxygen saturation has fallen to 92%. What action should the nurse take first?

1. Measure blood pressure (BP) and heart rate
2. Assess legs and arms for pitting edema
3. Telephone and notify the physician
4. Slow the intravenous rate to 10 to 20 mL/hour

7 A 45-year-old client with fluid volume excess (FVE) because of acute kidney dysfunction is placed on a 1000 mL fluid restriction per 24-hour period. The client asks the nurse, "Why is there such a severe fluid restriction when I already have dry lips and mouth?" Which response by the nurse is best?

1. "The doctor ordered the fluid restriction, so it is important to comply with those orders."
2. "Your kidneys cannot eliminate extra fluid right now, so intake must be limited to protect your heart and lungs from being overloaded with fluid."
3. "You probably drank too much fluid before you got sick, so you can't compare your usual intake to your limitations now that your kidneys are not working."
4. "Too much fluid will cause your heart to fail and your lungs to fill with water, which could be fatal."

8 A 45-year-old client is receiving a loop diuretic for treatment of edema. The nurse determines the client is experiencing an excessive response to the treatment when the client demonstrates which of the following?

1. Blood urea nitrogen (BUN) 28 mg/dL, hematocrit (Hct) 45%, and an 8-pound weight loss in 24 hours
2. BUN 21 mg/dL, Hct 29%, and an 8-pound weight gain in 24 hours
3. BUN 16 mg/dL, Hct 31%, and an 8-pound weight loss in 24 hours
4. BUN 25 mg/dL, Hct 33%, and an 8-pound weight gain in 24 hours

9 A client is receiving an intravenous (IV) infusion of 0.0225% sodium chloride at 50 mL/hour. It is most important for the nurse to monitor which of the following to detect complications of therapy?

1. Urine output and concentration
2. Legs and arms for edema
3. Tongue and mouth for dryness
4. Mental status and orientation

10 When caring for an adult receiving an intravenous (IV) infusion of 3% sodium chloride (NaCl), the nurse places priority on monitoring which of the following to detect complications of therapy? Select all that apply.

1. Neurological status
2. Urine specific gravity
3. Serum glucose levels
4. Lung sounds
5. Serum sodium level

➤ *See pages 29–30 for Answers and Rationales.*

I. OVERVIEW OF FLUID MOVEMENT

A. Fluid transport issues

1. Body fluid spaces (see Figure 1-1)
    a. **Intracellular fluid (ICF)**: fluid within the cells; two-thirds of body fluid is ICF
    b. **Extracellular fluid (ECF)**: fluid outside of the cells; made up of two components, the **interstitial fluid** (fluid surrounding the cells) and fluid within the **vascular space** (the blood vessels)
    c. Fluid constantly moves among the intracellular, interstitial, and vascular spaces to maintain body fluid balance

Figure 1-1

Body fluid spaces

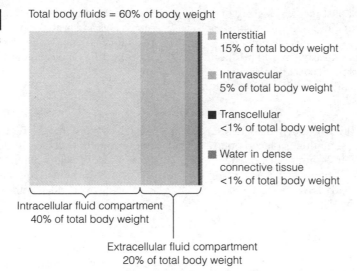

Total body fluids = 60% of body weight

Interstitial
15% of total body weight

Intravascular
5% of total body weight

Transcellular
<1% of total body weight

Water in dense
connective tissue
<1% of total body weight

Intracellular fluid compartment
40% of total body weight

Extracellular fluid compartment
20% of total body weight

1) ICF is the most stable and is fairly resistant to major fluid shifts
2) Vascular fluid is the least stable; it is quickly lost or gained in response to fluid intake or losses
3) Interstitial fluid is the reserve fluid, replacing fluid either in the blood vessels or cells, depending on the need

2. **Osmosis** (see Figure 1-2)
    a. Water moves through a **semipermeable membrane** (membrane that allows water and small particles, but not large particles, to easily pass through) from an area of lower concentration (fewer particles, more water) to an area of higher concentration (more particles, less water) until concentrations are equalized on both sides of the membrane
    b. Osmosis is a major force in body fluid movement and intravenous (IV) fluid therapy
        1) Cell membranes and capillary membranes are semipermeable
        2) Water moves into and out of the cells and capillaries by osmosis

3. Osmolality and osmotic pressure
    a. Osmolality and osmolarity are both terms that refer to the concentration of a solution, which creates its **osmotic pressure** (the pulling power of a solution for water)

Figure 1-2

Osmosis

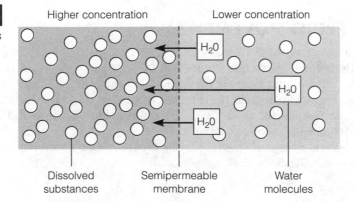

Higher concentration   Lower concentration

H_2O

H_2O

H_2O

Dissolved
substances

Semipermeable
membrane

Water
molecules

1) **Osmolality** is the concentration of solute (particles) per kilogram of water, while **osmolarity** is the concentration of solute (particles) per liter of a solution (the solvent does not have to be water)

2) Because body fluid solvent is water and 1 liter of water weighs 1 kilogram, the terms can be used interchangeably in discussing human fluid physiology; the term osmolality will be used here

3) The higher the osmolality (concentration) of a solution, the greater its pulling power for water

b. Serum osmolality is the concentration of particles (major particles are sodium and protein) in the plasma

   1) Normal serum osmolality is 275 to 295 milliosmoles/liter (mOsm/L)

   2) Serum osmolality can be estimated

      a) Sodium is the major solute in plasma contributing to its osmolality (estimated serum osmolality = 2 times the serum sodium level)

      b) Urea (BUN) and glucose are both large particles that increase serum osmolality when present in excess amounts in the blood

      c) When either or both are elevated, the serum osmolality will be higher than 2 times the sodium level, so the following formula will be more accurate:

$$\text{Serum osmolality} = 2 \times \text{serum sodium} + \frac{\text{BUN}}{3} + \frac{\text{glucose}}{18}$$

c. The term **isotonic** is defined as having the same osmolality as normal plasma

   1) Isotonic IV fluids have the same osmolality as normal plasma; no osmotic pressure difference is created, so the fluids remain primarily in the ECF

   2) Isotonic IV fluids are used to replace extracellular fluid and electrolyte losses and to expand vascular volume quickly

   3) Isotonic IV fluids (see Table 1-1)

      a) Normal saline (NS; 0.9% NaCl): sodium and chloride in water with same osmolality as normal plasma; NS provides no calories or **free water** (water without solute)

      b) Ringer's solution: contains sodium, potassium, calcium, and potassium in similar concentrations to plasma, but no dextrose, magnesium, or bicarbonate; Ringer's solution provides no calories or free water

      c) Lactated Ringer's solution (LR): contains sodium, chloride, potassium, calcium, and lactate in concentrations similar to normal plasma; LR provides no dextrose, magnesium, or free water

d. The term **hypotonic** is defined as having a lower osmolality than normal plasma

   1) Hypotonic IV fluids have a lower osmolality than normal plasma (< 290 mOsm/L)

   2) Water is pulled out of vessels into the cells, resulting in decreased vascular volume and increased cell water

   3) Hypotonic IV fluids are used to prevent and treat cellular dehydration by providing free water to the cells or to restore renal functioning

   4) Clients requiring hypotonic IV fluids require frequent monitoring of vital signs, level of consciousness, and circulation to detect depletion of vascular volume and cerebral cellular edema

   5) Hypotonic IV fluids are contraindicated in acute brain injuries because cerebral cells are very sensitive to free water, absorbing it rapidly and leading to cellular edema

   6) Hypotonic intravenous fluids (see Table 1-1 again)

Table 1-1   Hydrating Solutions

Solution	Uses	Nursing Implications
Isotonic 0.9% sodium chloride (normal saline or NS) Lactated Ringer's (LR) 5% dextrose in water (D_5W)	Has same concentration of solutes as plasma, so it remains in vascular compartment, expanding vascular volume NS and LR are crystalloid solutions that ↑ fluid volume in both intravascular and interstitial spaces with minimal fluid volume expansion NS is the only solution to be administered with blood products D_5W is isotonic on initial administration but provides free water when metabolized, expanding intra- and extracellular fluid volumes	Assess for signs of hypervolemia • Bounding pulse • Shortness of breath • Distended neck veins Assess for signs of hypovolemia • Urine output < 30 mL/hr • Weak, thready pulse • Subnormal temperature • Flat neck veins
Hypotonic 0.45% sodium chloride (½ NS) 0.225% sodium chloride (¼ NS)	Has lesser concentration of solutes than plasma, so treats cellular dehydration through fluid shifting out of blood vessels into cells; promotes elimination by kidneys	Do not administer to clients at risk for third-space fluid shift or fluid sequestration in a body space (results in circulating volume loss and ↑ risk for organ failure or ↑ intracranial pressure)
Hypertonic 5% dextrose in normal saline (D_5NS) 5% dextrose in 0.45% sodium chloride (D_5½NS) 5% dextrose in lactated Ringer's (D_5LR) 10% dextrose in water ($D_{10}W$) 20% dextrose in water ($D_{20}W$) 50% dextrose in water ($D_{50}W$)	Has higher concentration of solutes than plasma, thus causing fluid to shift from cells into vascular compartment, expanding vascular volume 10% dextrose—stand-by solution for clients receiving TPN 50% dextrose—used for hypoglycemia	Do not administer to clients with kidney or heart disease or clients who are dehydrated; monitor for signs of hypervolemia
Volume Expanders (colloid solutions) Albumin 5% (Buminate 5%) Albumin 25% (Buminate 25%) Dextran 40 (Gentran 40) Hetastarch (Hespan [HESI]) Plasma protein fraction (Plasmanate, others)	Colloid solutions contain substances that cannot diffuse through capillary walls, resulting in ↑ plasma volume and ↑ osmotic pressure, causing fluids to move into vascular compartment; used to treat hypovolemic shock	Establish baseline vital signs, lung and heart sounds, and central venous pressure; repeat per agency protocols Administer with a large-gauge (18–19 gauge) needle Monitor intake and output Monitor for signs of hypervolemia
Nutrient 5% dextrose (D_5W) 5% dextrose in 0.45% sodium chloride (D_5½NS)	Contain some form of carbohydrate (e.g., dextrose, glucose) and water D_5W provides 170 calories per liter	Useful in preventing dehydration but does not provide sufficient calories to promote wound healing, weight gain, or normal growth in children
Electrolyte 0.9% sodium chloride (NS) Ringer's solution (has sodium, chloride, potassium, calcium) 5% dextrose in 0.45% sodium chloride (D_5 ½NS)	Saline and electrolytes restore vascular volume and replace electrolytes LR is also an alkalinizing solution that treats metabolic acidosis (D_5½NS) is an acidifying solution to treat metabolic alkalosis	Monitor fluid and electrolytes Monitor arterial blood gases Monitor intake and output

Source: Hogan, Mary Ann; Skrabal, Julie, *Pearson Reviews & Rationales: Comprehensive Review For Nclex-Pn® — Instant Access*, 2nd Ed., ©2012. Reprinted and Electronically Reproduced by permission of Pearson Education Inc., Upper Saddle River, New Jersey.

a) 5% dextrose in water (D_5W): *although D_5W is isotonic in the IV bag, it has a hypotonic effect in the body*; the dextrose is quickly metabolized once infused intravenously, leaving free water that shifts by osmosis from vessels into cells; for each liter of D_5W, roughly ⅔ enters cells and ⅓ remains in extracellular space

    b) 0.45% saline (½NS) and 0.225 saline (¼NS): provide free water to cells as well as small amounts of sodium and chloride; approximately ½ of each liter infused moves into cells and ½ remains in extracellular space

    c) Maintenance fluids: saline mixed with dextrose and water

      i. 5% dextrose in 0.45 saline (D_5½NS) and 5% dextrose in 0.225% saline (D_5¼NS): both are hypertonic in the IV bag, but because of rapid dextrose metabolism, both also have a degree of hypotonic effect, providing some water to cells; provide calories and are often used as maintenance fluids; the dextrose content does not meet daily nutritional caloric requirements, but it does help prevent ketosis associated with starvation

      ii. 5% dextrose in 0.9% saline (D_5NS) is also hypertonic in the bag, but provides some free water and calories to cells; dextrose is mixed with NS and provides less free water and more extracellular water than D_5½NS or D_5¼NS

e. The term **hypertonic** is defined as having a higher osmolality than normal plasma

  1) Hypertonic IV fluids have a higher osmolality than normal plasma, causing water to be pulled from the cells into the vessels, resulting in increased vascular volume and decreased cell water

  2) Hypertonic solutions are used to treat very specific problems and are administered in carefully controlled, limited doses in order to avoid vascular volume overload and cellular dehydration; they are also used to pull excess fluid from cells and to promote osmotic diuresis

  3) Hypertonic IV solutions (see Table 1-1 again)

    a) Include saline solutions greater than 0.9% (3% saline and 5% saline); used infrequently

    b) Are clinically indicated when the serum sodium is dangerously low (115 mg/dL or less); it is given with great caution in carefully controlled, limited doses using an IV infusion pump

    c) Note: Clients receiving hypertonic saline solutions require frequent monitoring of vital signs, neurological status, lung sounds, urine output, and serum sodium levels to avoid hypernatremia and vascular volume overload

    d) Dextrose solutions greater than 5% (such as 10% dextrose and 50% dextrose) are also considered hypertonic; these are used on a limited basis to treat clients with hypoglycemia

    e) Hypertonic dextrose solutions are given in controlled settings by IV push or IV infusion pump; 50% dextrose is used as part of a hypoglycemic treatment protocol; a 10% dextrose solution is used to treat newborns as part of a hypoglycemic treatment protocol

    f) **Colloid** volume expanders (Albumin, Dextran, Hetastarch)

      i. A colloid is a large solute particle, such as protein in solution, that normally does not pass through cell and capillary membranes (semipermeable membranes)

      ii. Increasing colloids (proteins within a space) results in an increase in osmolality, thus the pulling power for water

      iii. Colloid volume expanders pull fluid from tissue into the vessels by osmosis, increasing vascular volume

    g) Osmotic diuretics (such as mannitol [Osmitrol]) pull fluid from third spaces, tissues, and cells into blood vessels for elimination by kidneys

4. Diffusion (see Figure 1-3)

  a. Particles move from an area of higher concentration (more particles, less water) to an area of lower concentration (fewer particles, more water) until concentrations are equalized; some particles easily diffuse through semipermeable membranes and other do not

Figure 1-3

Diffusion

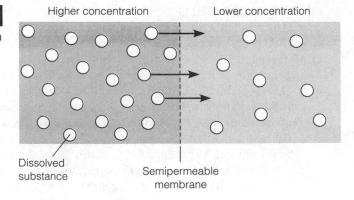

Higher concentration   Lower concentration

Dissolved substance   Semipermeable membrane

    b. Electrolytes (e.g., sodium, potassium, chloride, calcium, magnesium, and phosphate) are small particles that tend to move through semipermeable membranes easily

    c. Urea, glucose, and **albumin** (a plasma protein produced by the liver) are large particles that do not pass through semipermeable membranes easily

B. Capillary fluid movement (see Figure 1-4)

  1. Hydrostatic pressure

    a. Hydrostatic pressure is the pushing force of a fluid against the walls of the space it occupies

    b. Hydrostatic pressure in blood vessels is generated by the heart's pumping action and varies within the vascular system

  2. Oncotic pressure

    a. Oncotic pressure (also called **colloid osmotic pressure** or **COP**) is the pulling force exerted by colloids in a solution (the pulling force of proteins within the vascular space)

    b. Albumin is important in maintaining normal serum oncotic pressure (pulling force for water) and adequate vascular fluid volume

    c. Since plasma proteins do not normally cross the blood vessel wall, plasma protein concentration remains the same in arteries, veins, and the capillaries

  3. Starling's Law of the Capillaries

    a. Filtration (net fluid movement into or out of the capillary) is determined by the difference between the forces favoring filtration and those opposing it (like a tug of war—pushing and pulling)

    b. Interstitial hydrostatic pressure (pushing water into capillary) and interstitial oncotic pressure (pulling water out of capillary) are very low and are essentially equal, thus normally exert little influence on fluid movement into or out of capillaries

Figure 1-4

Capillary filtration dynamics

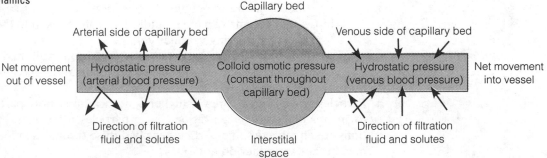

Capillary bed

Arterial side of capillary bed   Venous side of capillary bed

Net movement out of vessel   Hydrostatic pressure (arterial blood pressure)   Colloid osmotic pressure (constant throughout capillary bed)   Hydrostatic pressure (venous blood pressure)   Net movement into vessel

Direction of filtration fluid and solutes   Interstitial space   Direction of filtration fluid and solutes

    c. Capillary hydrostatic pressure (pushing water out of capillary) and capillary oncotic pressure (pulling water into capillary) are not the same, and fluid movement is seen in the capillary bed

        1) At the arterial end of the capillary, capillary hydrostatic pressure (pushing water out of capillary) exceeds capillary oncotic pressure (pulling water into capillary), thus net fluid movement is from the capillary into tissue, carrying nutrients with it

        2) At the venous end of the capillary, capillary hydrostatic pressure (pushing water out of capillary) is less than capillary oncotic pressure (pulling water into capillary), thus net fluid movement is into the capillary from the tissue, carrying wastes with it

C. Chemical regulation of fluid balance

    1. Antidiuretic hormone (ADH) (see Figure 1-5)

        a. ADH is a hormone synthesized by the hypothalamus and secreted by the posterior pituitary, which regulates water by acting on the distal tubules of the kidneys

        b. ADH is released and inhibited in a feedback loop

            1) ADH release is triggered by a drop in BP or blood volume or by a rise in blood osmolality (increased concentration), causing the kidneys to reabsorb more water (resulting in higher vascular volume and low output of concentrated urine)

            2) ADH release is inhibited by a rise in BP or blood volume or by a drop in blood osmolality (decreased concentration), causing the kidneys to excrete more water in the urine (resulting in lower vascular volume and high output of dilute urine)

    2. Aldosterone (see Figure 1-6)

        a. Aldosterone is an adrenal gland hormone that conserves sodium in the body by causing the kidneys to retain sodium and excrete potassium in its place

        b. Water follows sodium due to osmosis, thus aldosterone has an indirect effect on water

        c. Aldosterone is released and inhibited in a feedback loop as part of the renin-angiotensin-aldosterone system (refer again to Figure 1-6)

            1) Aldosterone release is triggered by a drop in BP, blood volume, or serum sodium, or a rise in serum potassium

                a) Aldosterone causes the kidneys to reabsorb more sodium into the blood, increasing serum sodium levels; water follows sodium into the blood by osmosis, raising vascular volume

                b) As more sodium is retained in the blood, the kidneys must excrete more potassium in the urine to maintain a balance of positive ions in the blood; this mechanism lowers serum potassium levels

            2) Aldosterone release is inhibited by a rise in BP, blood volume, or serum sodium, or a drop in serum potassium

                a) Decreasing aldosterone levels cause the kidneys to excrete more sodium in the urine, decreasing serum sodium levels; water follows sodium, thereby lowering vascular volume

                b) As more sodium is excreted in the urine, the kidneys must retain more potassium in the blood to maintain positive ion balance in the blood; this mechanism raises serum potassium levels

    3. Glucocorticoids (cortisol)

        a. Cortisol is a glucocorticoid hormone produced and released by the adrenal gland when the body is stressed

        b. Glucocorticoids promote renal retention of sodium and water

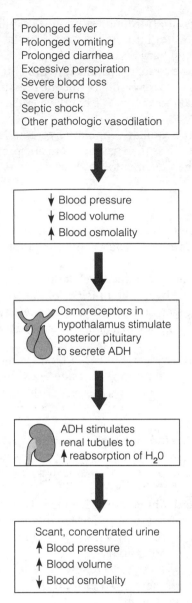

Figure 1-5
ADH regulation of water

Prolonged fever
Prolonged vomiting
Prolonged diarrhea
Excessive perspiration
Severe blood loss
Severe burns
Septic shock
Other pathologic vasodilation

⬇ Blood pressure
⬇ Blood volume
⬆ Blood osmolality

Osmoreceptors in hypothalamus stimulate posterior pituitary to secrete ADH

ADH stimulates renal tubules to ⬆ reabsorption of H_2O

Scant, concentrated urine
⬆ Blood pressure
⬆ Blood volume
⬇ Blood osmolality

Figure 1-6
Aldosterone regulation of sodium and water

⬆ K^+
⬇ Na^+
⬇ Blood volume
⬇ Cardiac output
⬇ Arterial blood pressure

⬇ Renal perfusion

⬇ Glomerular filtration rate

⬆ Renin

Conversion of angiotensin I to angiotensin II in the lungs

Secretion of aldosterone in the adrenal cortex

⬆ Absorption of Na^+
⬆ Absorption of H_2O
⬆ Excretion of K^+
⬆ Excretion of H ions

4. Atrial natriuretic peptide (ANP)
  a. ANP is a cardiac hormone found in the atria of the heart that is released when atria are stretched by high blood volume or high BP
  b. ANP lowers blood volume and BP by the following:
    1) Causing vasodilation by direct effect on blood vessels and suppression of renin-angiotensin system

2) Decreasing aldosterone release by adrenal glands, causing increased urinary excretion of sodium and water

3) Decreasing ADH release by pituitary gland, causing increased urinary excretion of water

4) Increasing glomerular filtration rate, increasing rate of urine production and water excretion

5. Brain natriuretic peptide (BNP)

a. BNP is a cardiac hormone found within ventricles that is released with increased blood volume and pressure when ventricles are stretched

b. BNP works to decrease blood volume and pressure through the following mechanisms:

1) Vasodilates arteries and veins

2) Decreases release of aldosterone

3) Causes diuresis with excretion of both sodium and water

6. Thirst mechanism

Practice to Pass

An adult client has 3% saline infusing intravenously. What nursing observations and measures should be implemented to protect client safety? Why?

a. Thirst normally occurs with even small fluid losses or small increases in serum osmolality; it is stimulated by thirst receptors in the hypothalamus that can detect as little as 1 mOsm/L change in plasma concentration

b. Thirst also stimulates ADH and aldosterone release, which promotes reabsorption of water

c. The thirst mechanism is depressed in older people (> 60 years old), including healthy older adults living in the community and people living with debilitating illnesses

II. FLUID VOLUME DEFICIT (FVD)

A. Etiology and pathophysiology

1. Isotonic fluid loss

a. Fluid and solute are lost in proportional amounts, thus serum osmolality remains normal and no osmotic force is created

b. Intracellular water is not disturbed and fluid losses are primarily ECF (especially the vascular volume), which can quickly lead to shock

c. Causes

1) Hemorrhage results in loss of fluid, electrolytes, proteins, and blood cells in proportional amounts, often resulting in inadequate vascular volume (**hypovolemia**)

2) Gastrointestinal losses (vomiting, continuous NG suction, diarrhea, drainage from fistulas and tubes and ostomies) contain abundant electrolytes; thus GI fluid and electrolytes tend to be lost in fairly proportional amounts

3) Large amounts of wound drainage or wound suctioning can lead to both fluid and electrolyte losses

4) Fever, environmental heat, diaphoresis, and shock can result in profuse sweating, which causes water and sodium loss from the skin in fairly equal proportions

5) Burns (especially large burns) initially damage skin and capillary membranes, allowing fluid, electrolytes, and proteins to escape into the burned tissue area, which often results in inadequate vascular volume

6) Diuretics can cause excessive loss of fluid and electrolytes in fairly proportional amounts

7) Third space fluid shifts occur when fluid moves from the vascular space into physiologically useless extracellular spaces (where it is unavailable as reserve fluid or to transport nutrients)

d. Isotonic fluid loss is primarily an extracellular fluid loss that requires extracellular fluid replacement, with emphasis on the vascular volume

2. Hypertonic dehydration
    a. More water is lost than solute (primarily sodium), creating a fluid volume deficit and a relative solute excess
    b. Solute (sodium or glucose more commonly) can also be gained in excess of water, creating a similar imbalance
    c. Serum osmolality is elevated, resulting in hypertonic extracellular fluid that pulls fluid into vessels from cells by osmosis and causes the cells to shrink and become dehydrated
    d. Causes of hypertonic dehydration
        1) Inadequate fluid intake
            a) Clients who are unable to respond to thirst independently (infants, older adults, disabled, and bedridden), who have nausea, anorexia, or dysphagia, or who are NPO (nothing by mouth) without IV fluid replacement, are at risk to develop fluid volume deficit
            b) Decreased water intake results in increased ECF solute concentration, which leads to cellular dehydration
            c) A client can go several weeks to months without food, but only two to three days without water
        2) Severe or prolonged isotonic fluid losses
            a) May occur in conditions such as vomiting and diarrhea and eventually result in loss of more water than solute
            b) ECF becomes hypertonic as compensatory mechanisms are exhausted, and the body has no more water to conserve through the kidneys
            c) The hypertonic ECF then begins to draw water from the cells, dehydrating them as well
        3) Watery diarrhea causes loss of more water than electrolytes
        4) Diabetes insipidus (DI) is caused by insufficient ADH production or release, which leads to massive, uncontrolled diuresis of very dilute urine (as much as 30 liters per day) and can quickly lead to shock and death
            a) Brain injury that damages or puts pressure on the hypothalamus or pituitary often causes DI
            b) Once acute DI develops, parenteral administration of vasopressin (Pitressin), a pharmacologic form of ADH, is indicated to stop the massive fluid loss
        5) Increased solute intake (e.g., salt, sugar, protein) without a proportional intake of water increases plasma osmolality, resulting in water being pulled from cells, increasing ECF, and causing cellular dehydration; increasing ECF is dangerous for clients with heart or kidney problems, and the resulting osmotic diuresis actually makes the cellular dehydration worse; conditions that can cause hypertonic dehydration include the following:
            a) Highly concentrated enteral or parenteral feedings (increased glucose)
            b) Improperly prepared infant formulas (too concentrated)
            c) Hyperglycemia and/or diabetic ketoacidosis (excess glucose and ketones in the blood)
            d) Increased sodium ingestion (e.g., seawater ingestion, salt tablets)
            e) Excess osmotic diuretic use
    e. Fluid loss is both extracellular and intracellular
3. Third spacing
    a. Third spaces are extracellular body spaces in which fluid is not normally present in large amounts, but in which fluid can accumulate
    b. Fluid that accumulates in third spaces is physiologically useless because it is not available for use as reserve fluid or to transport nutrients

      c. Common locations for third space fluid to accumulate include the following:
        1) Tissue spaces (edema)
        2) Abdomen (ascites)
        3) Pleural spaces (pleural effusion)
        4) Pericardial space (pericardial effusion)
      d. Causes of third spacing
        1) Injury or inflammation (e.g., massive trauma, crush injuries, burns, sepsis, cancer, intestinal obstruction, abdominal surgery) increase capillary permeability, allowing fluid, electrolytes, and proteins to leak from vessels
        2) Malnutrition or liver dysfunction (e.g., starvation, cirrhosis, chronic alcoholism) prevent the liver from producing albumin, thus lowering capillary oncotic pressure
        3) High vascular hydrostatic pressure (e.g., heart failure, renal failure, or other forms of vascular fluid overload) pushes abnormal volumes of fluid from vessels

B. Dehydration concepts
  1. Isotonic dehydration involves equal losses of all fluid components and is the most commonly seen type of fluid volume deficit
  2. Hypotonic dehydration involves greater losses of electrolytes, leading to a decreased plasma osmolality; fluid shifting occurs as ECF volume decreases
  3. Hypertonic dehydration involves greater losses of ECF volume than electrolytes, leading to an increased plasma osmolality; fluid shifting occurs as the body tries to compensate to restore balance

C. Assessment
  1. Clinical manifestations of dehydration
      a. Thirst (an early sign), unreliable as an indicator in older adults and in the young who cannot express needs
      b. Concentrated urine and low urine volume
        1) Minimum normal urine output in children is 1 to 2 mL/kg/hour
        2) Minimum normal urine output in the average adult is 0.5 mL/kg/hr or 30 mL/hour (240 mL/8 hours)
        3) Concentrated, dark urine with high **specific gravity** greater than 1.030 (concentration of a solution, for urine normally 1.010 to 1.030)
        4) Note: If diabetes insipidus is causing the fluid volume deficit, urine will be pale, dilute, and high in volume
      c. Dry skin with decreased turgor and elasticity and dry mucous membranes
        1) Skin "tenting" occurs as tissues stick together because of interstitial fluid loss
        2) Skin of older clients loses elasticity with aging (elastin decreases), so tenting is not a reliable sign in older adults
        3) Test skin of older adults on sternum, forehead, inner thigh, or top of hip bone rather than arms or legs
        4) Skin of infant is very elastic, even when there is a fluid volume deficit, thus tenting is not a reliable sign in infants
        5) Check tenting in infants over abdomen or inner thighs, but rely on other signs (heart rate, tongue and mucous membranes, urine output, mental status, behavior, and presence vs. absence of tears when crying)
        6) Breathing and environmental conditions can cause dry lips when oral mucosa is actually moist; keep this in mind when assessing mucous membranes
        7) Dry tongue with longitudinal furrows is a reliable sign in all age groups
        8) Decreased tearing and dry conjunctiva
      d. Sunken eyeballs; sunken or depressed fontanels in infants < 18 months old

e. Flat neck veins and poor peripheral vein filling
    1) Flat neck veins even with head of bed < 45 degrees (normally some distention seen due to gravity when lying down flat; however, this is not seen in infants or young children)

 f. Hypotension (late sign in infants and young children)
    1) Postural hypotension
      a) Rise in pulse rate > 10 to 15 beats per minute and/or fall in systolic BP > 10 to 15 mm Hg after rising from lying to standing position
      b) Indicates vascular volume has fallen enough that the body cannot maintain adequate BP when standing; the greater the fall in BP and/or rise in heart rate, the greater the fluid volume deficit
    2) Frank hypotension (low BP even when lying down)
    3) Complaints of weakness, dizziness, light-headedness
    4) Syncope when rising from lying position

g. Other signs of decreased cardiac output
    1) Tachycardia (*early sign*, especially in infants and young children)
    2) Weak, thready pulses
    3) Cool extremities with delayed capillary refill

h. Tachypnea (usually without shortness of breath) related to the body's perceived loss of blood volume

i. Low grade fever (higher fever can occur in severe dehydration) as the body's perceived loss of fluid volume results in blood vessel constriction, which decreases heat loss

j. Mental status changes (e.g., irritability, restlessness, lethargy, confusion, drowsiness)
    1) This is often the first sign noticed in older adults and is often the first sign causing alarm in parents of infants and small children
    2) Changes in mental status are a serious sign of significant fluid loss; if the fluid loss if severe, the client can progress to seizures and coma

k. Acute weight loss (an important sign in infants and young children)
    1) 1L water = 1 kg (2.2 pounds)
    2) Considered a more accurate reflection of fluid balance than I&O (intake and output) because of the difficulty in keeping accurate records
    3) Note: Exception occurs in weight changes with significant third space fluid shifts as weight gain is often seen; clients with third spacing may initially have signs/symptoms of **hypervolemia** but the primary problem is fluid volume deficit
    4) 2% body weight loss = mild fluid deficit (may only see thirst; ~1 to 2 L fluid loss in adult)
    5) 5% body weight loss = moderate fluid deficit (signs and symptoms appear; ~3 to 5 L fluid loss in adult)
    6) 8% body weight loss = severe fluid deficit (frank hypotension and delirium; ~5 to 10 L fluid loss in adult)
    7) > 15% body weight loss can be fatal (anuria, coma; > 10 L fluid loss in adult)

2. Diagnostic and laboratory findings

a. Normal or high hematocrit (Hct) and blood urea nitrogen (BUN) because of **hemoconcentration** (plasma is more concentrated than normal, increasing the number of red blood cells and urea particles per liter of plasma); *note*: if hemorrhage is the cause of the fluid volume deficit, red blood cells are being lost in proportion to plasma, thus Hct will be low

b. High urine specific gravity (> 1.030) as kidneys conserve water while continuing to excrete solute (unless the cause is diabetes insipidus, in which specific gravity will be low [< 1.010])

    c. Urine osmolality measures particle numbers in solution and reflects ability of kidneys to concentrate urine; reflects hydration status

    d. Urine osmolality (normal 500–800 mOsm/kg) is a more precise indicator of hydration

    e. In hypertonic dehydration, lab values will also reflect increased plasma concentration

        1) Serum osmolality elevated > 300 mOsm/kg

        2) Serum sodium elevated (hypernatremia) > 150 milliequivalents/liter (mEq/L)

        3) Serum glucose elevated (if that is the cause of the dehydration) > 120 mg/dL

3. Identification of risk factors (predisposing to fluid volume deficit)

    a. Age, gender, and body fat

        1) Infants and young children

            a) Total body water percentage is higher (infant 80%, premature infant 90%, adult 60%); thus infants require more water for size than older children and adults

            b) ECF, which is more easily lost, equals 40% of an infant's body water (compared to 20% of an adult's); infants may exchange 50% of their ECF daily, compared to 18% in an adult

            c) Kidneys are immature up to age two years, thus cannot conserve or excrete water or sodium in response to imbalances as efficiently as adults, making them less able to handle large amounts of solute-free water or concentrated fluids

            d) Body surface area is relatively larger, thus infants lose more fluid through the skin for their size than adults

            e) Higher metabolic rate of infants requires more water for size than adults and produces more heat, which results in more water loss

            f) Fever tends to be higher and last longer in acute illnesses of infants and children, which increases fluid loss with acute illness

            g) Children 2 to 12 years of age have less stable regulatory responses to fluid imbalances than adults

        2) Older adults

            a) After age 60, only 45 to 50% of body weight is water (compared to 60% in younger adult), thus small water losses have a greater impact

            b) Skeletal muscle mass (which holds more water than fat) declines and percentage of body fat rises with aging

            c) Kidneys lose function and cannot concentrate or dilute urine as efficiently, thus cannot compensate as well for imbalance or excrete heavy solute loads (such as those from tube feedings)

            d) Diminished thirst mechanism is seen with aging

            e) Decreased pancreatic functioning and glucose tolerance with aging increases risk of hyperglycemia and resulting osmotic diuresis

        3) Women and obese individuals have a higher percentage of body fat, which holds less water than muscle; thus they have a lower percentage of body water for their weight

    b. Acute illness

        1) Surgery can result in blood and fluid loss

        2) Gastroenteritis causing nausea, vomiting, and/or diarrhea or nasogastric suctioning lead to fluid and electrolyte loss

        3) Burns: the larger the burn surface area, the greater the fluid loss

        4) Brain injury from stroke, trauma, or tumor can cause cerebral edema, which can put pressure on the hypothalamus and/or pituitary, altering ADH release; problems with ADH regulation can lead to the client developing syndrome of inappropriate ADH secretion (SIADH) or diabetes insipidus (DI), which is more commonly seen

        5) Large draining wounds and wound suctioning lead to fluid loss by interruption of skin barrier

   c. Chronic illness

        1) Liver disease reduces the production of albumin, which affects the ability to maintain adequate circulating vascular volume

        2) Renal disease limits ability to regulate fluid or electrolytes via urine output

        3) Diabetes mellitus increases risk for hyperglycemia and hypertonic dehydration

        4) Cancer can predispose to fluid shifts; chemotherapy often causes nausea and vomiting with loss of fluid and lack of intake

   d. Environmental factors

        1) Vigorous exercise increases metabolism, ventilation, and sweating, causing both an increased demand for fluid as well as increased fluid losses

        2) Heat injuries: Exposure to hot, humid environments can increase sweat production to as much as 2 L/hour; body fluid weight loss > 7% is associated with failure of body cooling mechanisms, leading to heat injuries

   e. Diet and lifestyle

        1) Difficulty chewing or swallowing can lead to inadequate intake of oral fluids and food (which is also a major source of fluid intake)

        2) Malnutrition, starvation, and low protein intake will affect volume status

        3) Excess alcohol consumption causes liver damage and/or malnutrition leading to altered volume status

   f. Medications

        1) Diuretics and laxatives can predispose the client to excess fluid loss

        2) Chemotherapy can cause nausea, vomiting, and poor oral intake of fluids and food

D. Priority nursing diagnoses

  1. Deficient Fluid Volume related to excessive fluid losses and/or decreased fluid intake

  2. Risk for Hypovolemic Shock related to fluid loss

  3. Risk for Injury related to altered sensorium and/or dizziness

  4. Altered Comfort related to signs and symptoms of fluid deficit

  5. Risk for Impaired Skin Integrity related to skin and mucous membrane dryness

  6. Deficient Knowledge related to risk factors and therapeutic interventions

E. Therapeutic management

  1. Oral replacement therapies

   a. Fluids can be replaced orally if the deficit is mild, thirst is intact, and client can drink

        1) Commercial oral rehydration solutions (ORSs) provide fluids, glucose, and electrolytes in a concentration that is quickly absorbed even if vomiting and diarrhea are present; these include such brand names as Pedialyte, Gastrolyte, Oralyte, Rehydralyte, and Resol; client should drink small amounts frequently

        2) Infants and young children may only tolerate a few teaspoonfuls every few minutes, but will absorb a significant amount each hour, even if vomiting; for small children, freeze fluids into flavored ice pops, which are often better received than liquids; as fluids are replaced, begin alternating with low-sodium fluids such as water, breast milk, lactose-free formula, or half-strength lactose formula

        3) Adults should sip frequent, small amounts of ORS, progressing to a variety of oral fluids

   b. During initial rehydration, avoid fluids such as sodas, fruit juice, and sports drinks because their high sugar content (hypertonic) can worsen diarrhea and promote fluid loss; avoid salty fluids that can make diarrhea worse; avoid caffeine because it is a mild diuretic and may worsen fluid loss

Practice to Pass

A 23-year-old client is admitted to the emergency department with multiple fractures of the legs and pelvis. BP is 86/40, heart rate 120, respirations 30, skin is cool and pale, and peripheral pulses are weak and thready. What intravenous fluids should be given immediately? Why?

   c. Early reintroduction of regular diet has been shown to decrease the number of diarrhea stools and shorten the duration of gastroenteritis; BRAT diet (bananas, rice, applesauce, and toast) may be utilized briefly during the acute phase, although it provides inadequate electrolytes, protein, or calories for the long term

2. Parenteral replacement therapies

  a. Parenteral therapy for isotonic fluid losses

    1) Initially, expand ECF volume with isotonic IV fluids until adequate circulating blood volume and renal perfusion are achieved

      a) Fluid challenges (large amounts of IV fluids infused rapidly, often in 30 minutes or less) may be used

      b) Infuse a 1 to 2 liter bolus of isotonic fluid (e.g., NS) for adults, with up to two or three additional boluses to achieve response to therapy (improving urine output, blood pressure, heart rate, and mental status)

      c) Infuse a 20–30 mL/kg bolus of isotonic fluid (e.g., NS) for infants and young children, with up to two or three further boluses to achieve response to therapy (improving urine output, heart rate, respiratory rate, and mental status)

      d) Blood transfusion should be considered to replace lost red blood cells for clients experiencing severe hypovolemia due to hemorrhage

    2) Once initial parenteral rehydration is accomplished for mild to moderate fluid losses, oral rehydration can be continued at home

    3) If dehydration is severe, IV rehydration may continue with maintenance IV fluids (usually saline and dextrose combination fluids such as $D_5\frac{1}{2}NS$ or D_5NS)

    4) If the cause of the fluid volume deficit is third spacing, osmotic diuretics can be used to mobilize some of the fluid back into the blood vessels for elimination by the kidneys; however, due to the nature of the disease processes that often cause third space fluid shifts, this is usually only a temporary measure; large third space fluid collections may need to be physically removed (paracentesis for ascites; thoracentesis for pleural effusion) and the vascular space rehydrated with IV fluids

  b. Parenteral therapy for hypertonic dehydration

    1) If hypovolemia and impending shock are present, isotonic fluids are given first to achieve adequate circulation and renal perfusion

    2) Cellular dehydration is corrected with IV solutions having a hypotonic effect (provide free water to cells); be alert—hypotonic fluids must be given slowly to prevent rehydrating brain cells too rapidly, which could result in cerebral edema and brain injury

    3) If hypervolemia is present (as with excess sodium intake), a diuretic may be given with hypotonic fluid infusions (to provide free water to cells while preventing vascular volume overload)

3. Monitoring of client during therapy

  a. Vital signs for changes in heart rate, BP, respiratory rate; breath sounds and mucous membranes

  b. Mental status and behavior for improvement in mentation (less lethargic, more alert, less confused, appropriate behavior for situation); lack of improvement or worsening mental status could indicate too rapid infusion of hypotonic fluids

  c. Monitor urine concentration and output for improvement; adequate urine output of normal color and concentration (in healthy kidneys) is a good indicator of adequate vascular volume

  d. Monitor IV infusion rate to avoid administration of excess fluid, especially in those with cardiac or renal dysfunction, older adults, infants, and young children (who are all at increased risk for fluid volume overload); use infusion pumps in this population to prevent fluid overload

   e. Monitor intake, output, and daily weights (same scale, same time of day, same clothing for consistency)

   f. Auscultate breath sounds for crackles, which could indicate fluid accumulation in alveoli of lungs

F. Planning and implementation

1. Monitor specific assessment parameters related to the management of FVD

2. Assist with rehydration and promote return to adequate oral intake

   a. Provide indicated oral fluids in frequent, small amounts; keep fluids fresh and place within easy reach

   b. Remind older adults to drink something each hour due to decreased thirst mechanism

   c. Chill, warm, or freeze the indicated fluids to enhance intake based on client's preference

   d. Clients with altered mobility may require assistance in drinking fluids

   e. When using an infusion pump, check it frequently to ensure it is delivering fluid according to programmed settings

3. Provide comfort measures

   a. Provide oral hygiene frequently, including brushing teeth and rinsing mouth, to promote comfort

   1) A rinse of equal parts peroxide and water can help deodorize the mouth

   2) Avoid glycerin and lemon or alcohol-based commercial mouthwash, which can be drying

   3) Avoid sucking on hard candy or chewing gum, both of which can further dry oral mucous membranes

   b. Apply a lip moisturizer

   c. Apply skin moisturizer to dry skin to prevent cracking and breakdown

4. Listen to client's concerns, answer questions, and implement teaching

   a. Explain and answer questions in simple terms that foster client understanding

   b. Focus on client's concerns and demonstrate respect for client's feelings

   c. Offer reassurance and emotional support

5. Provide measures to prevent fluid volume deficits and dehydration; provide additional plain water boluses periodically during enteral feedings

   a. Note: 1 mL of water is recommended for each kCal of formula

   b. If one can of formula has 380 kCal in 240 mL of fluid, an additional 140 mL of fluid is needed to achieve the recommended total fluid intake

   c. However, watch for signs of water toxicity and hyponatremia, which can result if water boluses are excessive; check serum sodium levels periodically

6. Implement measures to control nausea, vomiting, diarrhea, and high fever as these may cause further complications

7. Recognize acutely ill clients at risk for inadequate fluid intake and initiate measures to provide adequate fluids by the oral, enteral, or parenteral routes

G. Medication therapy

1. Antiemetics are used to prevent fluid losses due to nausea and vomiting (e.g., promethazine [Phenergan])

2. Antidiarrheals are used to prevent fluid losses from the GI tract (e.g., loperamide [Imodium])

3. ADH: Vasopressin (Pitressin) is used to correct diabetes insipidus

4. Antipyretics are used to control fever and minimize fluid losses (e.g., acetaminophen [Tylenol] or ibuprofen [Motrin])

H. Client education

1. Awareness of predisposing factors

   a. Explain the nature of the client's condition and the causes for it

Practice to Pass

An 80-year-old client is admitted to the hospital for treatment of urinary tract infection and dehydration. While in the emergency department, one liter of NS has infused and now $D_5\frac{1}{4}$ NS is infusing at 80 mL/hour. What monitoring is important during therapy and why?

       b. Explain risk factors and help identify those relevant to client (e.g., age, gender, body size, physical activities, illnesses, medications, diet, and lifestyle)

       c. Explain early signs of impending fluid volume deficit and importance of initiating ORS in small, frequent amounts early to decrease nausea and replace electrolytes

       d. Explain importance of contacting a physician if illness lasts more than 24 hours, if client is an older adult or very young, or if client has a chronic illness (such as diabetes, heart disease, kidney disease, or liver problems)

  2. Explain measures to help prevent fluid deficit and dehydration

       a. Older adults should drink a variety of fluids frequently throughout the day even if not thirsty, especially in hot, humid weather, since thirst is not a reliable indicator because of diminished thirst mechanism

       b. Foods that are liquid at room temperature provide fluid intake (frozen ice pops, ice cream, gelatin) for those at risk

       c. Drink cool water prior to exercise, 5–6 oz every 15 minutes during exercise, and following exercise

          1) If exercise is prolonged (> 1 hour for average person) or vigorous or if it occurs in a hot, humid climate, drink solutions for hydration that contain both water, carbohydrates, and electrolytes (e.g., sports drinks)

          2) Avoid highly salty fluids or salt tablets, which can raise sodium levels and draw fluid from cells, worsening dehydration

  3. Provide dietary education

       a. Commercial oral rehydration solutions are recommended for vomiting and diarrhea, especially in children; they do not contain large amounts of sugar that can make diarrhea and dehydration worse but do contain needed electrolytes

       b. During diarrhea, avoid ingesting salty fluids (e.g., salty broth) as well as those high in sugar (gelatin, soda, and fruit juice) because the high solute content can worsen diarrhea and dehydration

       c. Avoid caffeine because it acts as a mild diuretic, increasing fluid loss

       d. Recommend early progression to a soft, easily digestible, regular diet; limiting intake to a BRAT diet exclusively has fallen out of favor, especially in acute diarrhea, because it contains few electrolytes and is low in energy and protein; recommend use of ORSs that are rich in electrolytes to provide needed nutritional value

I. Evaluation

  1. Adequate fluid volume reflected by the following:

       a. Adequate urine output and concentration

       b. Stable heart rate and blood pressure (lying and standing) within individual norms

       c. Skin and mucous membranes moist with normal turgor and elasticity; fontanels soft

       d. Return to usual mental state and behavior

       e. Hct, BUN, serum osmolality, and serum electrolytes within normal range during first 48 to 72 hours

  2. Free of injury

       a. No signs of injury from falls (e.g., bruises, abrasions, bumps)

       b. No reported episodes of falls with injury

  3. Skin and mucous membranes intact

       a. Absence of cracks, fissures, or ulcers

       b. Mouth and oral mucosa moist

  4. Verbalizes adequate knowledge of condition as well as therapeutic and preventive measures

       a. Verbalizes understanding of risk factors and preventive measures

       b. Verbalizes understanding of follow-up care

Practice to Pass

A young mother phones the clinic and reports that her eight-month-old infant awakened about six hours ago with fever, vomiting, and diarrhea. She has taken him off food and formula and has been giving him plain water to drink. What advice should you give her and why?

III. FLUID VOLUME EXCESS (FVE)

A. Etiology and pathophysiology

1. Isotonic fluid excess (hypervolemia and edema)

    a. Fluid and solute (primarily sodium) are gained or retained in proportional amounts, leading to an overall gain in extracellular fluid volume without a change in serum osmolality

    b. Excess vascular fluid volume results in the development of hypervolemia

    c. Excess tissue (interstitial) fluid volume results in the development of edema, which can occur throughout the body or can be situated in a specific body tissue or organ

    d. Causes of isotonic FVE (see Types of FVE, Table 1-2)

2. Hypotonic fluid excess (water intoxication) (see Table 1-2)

    a. More fluid is gained than solute (primarily sodium), creating FVE and a relative deficit of sodium

    b. Serum osmolality falls, resulting in hypotonic ECF that gets pulled into the cells by osmosis, causing cells to swell; cerebral cells absorb free water more readily than other cells, thus are very sensitive to hypotonic ECF

B. Mechanisms of edema formation

1. Increased capillary hydrostatic pressure disrupts the normal filtration of fluid into and out of capillaries (refer back to Figure 1-4)

    a. The increased pushing pressure within the capillary (blood pressure) forces more fluid out of the arterial end of the capillary and draws less fluid back into the venous end, resulting in excess fluid accumulation (edema) in the tissues

    b. Hypertension and vascular fluid volume overload (hypervolemia) are causes of edema

2. Decreased capillary oncotic pressure also disrupts the normal movement of fluid into and out of capillaries

    a. Weaker pulling pressure within the capillary (because of decreased albumin, plasma proteins) allows more fluid to be pushed out of the arterial end of the capillary and draws less fluid back into the venous end, resulting in excess fluid accumulation (edema) in the tissues

    b. Causes of low capillary oncotic pressure

      1) Injury or inflammation (e.g., trauma, burns, sepsis, bacterial infections, allergic reactions, cancer, intestinal obstruction), which increases capillary permeability, allowing fluid and proteins to leak from vessels

      2) Malnutrition or liver dysfunction (e.g., starvation, cirrhosis, chronic alcoholism) prevents the liver from producing albumin, decreasing capillary oncotic pressure (which normally helps keep adequate fluid inside vessels)

      3) Lymphatic obstruction or surgical removal of lymph nodes impairs lymph drainage and the normal flow of lymph fluid from body tissues to the venous system, creating local edema distal to the obstruction or node removal

      4) Sodium excess (e.g., due to renal failure, decreased renal perfusion, or excess aldosterone or corticosteroids) causes water retention that elevates blood pressure, increasing hydrostatic pressure within capillaries; this forces more fluid into tissues, resulting in edema

C. Assessment

1. Clinical manifestations of FVE

    a. Peripheral edema

      1) Edema tends to follow gravity; thus it is often seen in the legs, ankles, feet, and hands of ambulatory clients and on the sacrum and back of clients confined to bed

Table 1-2 Types of Fluid Volume Excess (FVE)

Type	Causes	Related Physiology
Isotonic	1. Renal failure 2. Heart failure 3. Excess fluid intake 4. High corticosteroid levels due to therapy, stress, or disease 5. High aldosterone levels due to stress response, adrenal dysfunction, liver damage, or metabolic problems	1. Decreased excretion of water and sodium. 2. Stasis of blood in circulation, venous congestion, and decreased renal blood flow lead to decreased renal excretion of fluid and sodium. 3. Rapid infusion or excessive infusion of isotonic fluid exceeds heart and kidney's ability to compensate. 4. Sodium and water are retained. 5. Sodium and water are retained.
Hypotonic	1. Repeated administration of plain water enemas, NG irrigation, or bladder irrigation 2. Excess use or rapid infusion of hypotonic IV fluids, such as D_5W, 0.025% saline and 0.045% saline 3. Excessive intake of free water without electrolyte replacement 4. Inappropriate prepared infant formula and/or excess water; frequent use of a water bottle as a pacifier 5. SIADH, Syndrome of Inappropriate Antidiuretic Hormone; excessive release of ADH can be precipitated by stress, surgery, anesthesia, opioid analgesics, pain, and lung and brain tumors 6. Psychogenic polydipsia, a compulsive drinking of excess water associated with psychiatric disorders	1. The free water can be drawn into and expelled water takes electrolytes with it. 2. Excess free water is taken into cells too quickly. When D_5W is infused, the dextrose is quickly metabolized, leaving free water. 3. If isotonic fluids and/or electrolytes are lost, they need to be replaced with water and electrolytes, especially sodium. 4. Parents may dilute infant formula or give excessive free water in effort to stretch formula. Both result in excess ingestion of free water. 5. Excessive ADH causes kidneys to retain large amounts of water without sodium. In turn, the excessive hypotonic extracellular fluid is drawn into cells by osmosis. 6. Excessive intake of free water leads to water intoxication.
Interstitial	1. Increased blood hydrostatic pressure 2. Decreased blood colloid osmotic pressure secondary to low plasma proteins; associated with liver failure, malnutrition, nephritic syndrome 3. Increased capillary permeability, caused by damage to capillaries; associated with trauma, burns, and crushing injuries 4. Impaired lymphatic drainage associated with lymphedema and tumors *Note: Some causes are the same as those associated with hypotonic excess.*	1. Extracellular fluid excess increases fluid volume in vascular space leading in increased pressure against capillary walls with movement of fluid into interstitial spaces. 2. Plasma proteins hold fluid in the capillary spaces. When low, the pulling force is lost and fluid seeps into interstitial spaces. 3. The capillaries become permeable to protein, which leaks into interstitial spaces, carrying fluid with it. 4. Lymph vessels normally return small proteins and excess fluid to the vascular compartment; when blocked, the fluid remains in the interstitial space.

2) Edema can develop from local obstruction of veins, as when legs and feet swell after sitting for long periods; this usually resolves with walking and/or leg elevation

3) Edema that is present in the legs and feet even after elevating them for a period of time (e.g., upon awakening in the morning) and in the face as puffiness, especially around the eyes (periorbital edema and puffy eyelids), is more

Practice to Pass

A young mother who comes to the clinic with her two-month-old infant for a well-baby visit tells the nurse that she has been mixing the formula half-strength because it is so expensive. What fluid imbalance does this predispose the infant to develop? Why? How should the nurse respond to the mother?

indicative of generalized edema (**anasarca**) related to fluid overload associated with a heart or kidney problem

    4) Edematous skin is often tight and shiny due to decreased circulation in swollen tissue

    5) Edema severity can be estimated on a scale from 1+ (minimal) to 4+ (severe)

    6) Pitting edema occurs when a finger pressed into the edematous area leaves an imprint that does not resolve immediately when the finger is removed

    7) In infants, edema is often generalized

    8) Edema in children occurs in dependent parts and may be evident in sacral areas if the child is supine in bed; the scrotum or labia may also be edematous

b. Tense or bulging fontanels in children under 18 months old

c. High central venous pressure with venous engorgement

    1) Distended neck veins when head of bed is elevated to 45 degrees or higher (normally veins are flat due the effect of gravity); infants often do not display distended neck veins

    2) Delayed or absent hand vein emptying when hand is raised above heart (normally three to five seconds); engorged veins are evident

    3) Gallop heart rhythm in adults (S_3 heart sound) is evident when ventricles become overdistended due to venous congestion

    4) Hepatomegaly and splenomegaly are signs of venous congestion

d. Pulmonary edema because of increasing extravascular fluid retention

    1) Tachypnea and dyspnea, irritated cough (often early sign of fluid in alveoli)

    2) Hacking cough that eventually becomes moist and productive (clear to white sputum); a late sign of fluid in the alveoli and larger airways

    3) Labored breathing (seen as intercostal and substernal retractions, nasal flaring, and expiratory grunting in infants)

    4) Wet lung sounds (moist crackles) on auscultation (first appear in bases bilaterally and progress upward as the lung water increases when the client is sitting upright in semi-Fowler's position)

    5) Decreased O_2 saturation due to inadequate or mismatched ventilation and perfusion as a result of FVE

    6) Wet lung sounds (moist crackles) on auscultation

    7) Cyanosis (a late sign of hypoxemia)

    8) Note: Acute pulmonary edema is a life-threatening medical emergency caused by large amounts of fluid pooling in the alveoli and airways; respiratory signs and symptoms will be severe and immediate action is required to prevent death

e. Vital signs (reflect normal or increased cardiac output)

    1) Normal heart rate

    2) Full or bounding peripheral pulses

    3) Warm extremities

    4) Capillary refill less than three seconds

f. Third space fluid accumulations: may be present as fluid is forced from vessels into spaces that normally do not contain much fluid (ascites, pleural effusion, pericardial effusion)

g. Acute, rapid weight gain

h. Urine output and concentration

    1) In the client with functioning heart and kidneys, the body will maintain homeostasis by increasing urine output, leading to polyuria

    2) Decreased urine output associated with fluid retention is seen in clients with impaired cardiac or renal function

    i. A weight gain of three pounds or more can occur over two to five days in adults
        1) 2% body weight gain = mild fluid excess
        2) 5% body weight gain = moderate fluid excess
        3) 8% body weight gain = severe fluid excess
        4) Note: infants and children are more susceptible to complications of fluid gains and may exhibit more severe symptoms with a mild fluid excess

2. Diagnostic and laboratory findings

    a. Hct and BUN are decreased due to **hemodilution** (plasma has more water than normal, thus is more dilute); the percentage of RBCs and urea particles per liter of plasma is lower than normal in dilute plasma even though the actual number of cells and particles has not dropped; once extra fluid is removed, Hct and BUN return to normal

    b. In hypotonic fluid volume excess (water intoxication):
        1) Serum osmolality (concentration) is low (< 275 mOsm/kg)
        2) Serum sodium is very low (< 125 mEq/L)

    c. Chest x-ray may show pleural effusions

    d. Arterial blood gases
        1) Low pO_2 indicates hypoxemia, which usually occurs before pCO_2 is affected (carbon dioxide diffuses more easily than oxygen)
        2) Low pCO_2 (hyperventilation) is often present in early phases of compensation but will be low (hypoventilation) in later phases when compensation is failing
        3) As pulmonary edema progresses to hypoventilation and respiratory failure, respiratory acidosis causes the pH to drop

3. Identification of risk factors predisposing to fluid volume excess

    a. Age
        1) Because of decreased heart and kidney function, older adult clients are not able to compensate as easily for fluid volume excess
        2) Infants (up to age two years) have immature kidneys and cannot dilute urine well to eliminate excess fluid as efficiently as adults
        3) Children 2 to 12 years of age have less stable regulatory responses to fluid imbalances

    b. Acute illness
        1) Surgery stimulates the stress response, which increases release of cortisol, ADH, and aldosterone, promoting water and sodium retention
        2) Clients with medical problems (acute or preexisting) receiving IV fluids are prone to develop fluid imbalances leading to FVE

    c. Chronic illness
        1) Cardiovascular disease reduces the pumping strength of the heart and results in diminished blood flow to the kidneys, which causes sodium and water retention, leading to fluid volume excess
        2) Renal disease can lead to the abnormal retention of water, sodium, potassium, and other electrolytes

    d. Medications: Long-term glucocorticoid therapy predisposes to sodium and fluid retention

    e. See Table 1-3 for specific examples of age-related concerns with fluid volume excess

D. Priority nursing diagnoses

    1. Excess Fluid Volume related to excessive fluid or sodium intake and/or retention
    2. Risk for Pulmonary Edema related to hypervolemia
    3. Altered Comfort related to signs and symptoms of fluid excess
    4. Risk for Impaired Skin Integrity related to edema

    5. Knowledge Deficit related to risk factors and therapeutic interventions

---

Practice to Pass

A 62-year-old client with coronary artery disease is receiving D5½NS at 150 mL/hour after surgery. The client reports trouble breathing, and sits up in bed and coughs up small amounts of clear mucus. What priority nursing action and follow-up actions are needed and why?

Table 1-3 Lifespan Considerations for Health Maintenance

Lifespan Considerations	Common Risk Factors for Imbalances	Nursing Implications
Infants	**FVE** Dilution of infant formula Use of free water in bottles	Instruct parents to follow directions for formula dilution closely. Explain dangers of "stretching the formula" by adding excessive water. Discourage the excessive use of free water in bottles as pacifiers.
Pediatrics	**FVE** Excessive use of free water when treating flu and diarrhea Nephrotic syndrome	Instruct parents to replace electrolytes using an electrolyte solution such as Pedialyte Impaired kidney function leads to fluid retention. Monitor child closely for signs of FVE. Instruct parents on sodium restriction.
Adults	**FVE** Psychogenic polydipsia SIADH Excessive use of hypotonic solutions Excessive intake of water without electrolyte replacement Heart failure	Supervise clients with psychiatric disorders closely for excessive intake of fluids. Monitor clients at risk for SIADH for decreased urine output and fluid retention. Monitor clients receiving hypotonic solutions for signs of FVE. Educate clients of the need to replace electrolytes along with water when engaging in activities that produce excessive sweating and diuresis. Monitor clients with a history of HF for signs of FVE.

Source: London, Marcia L.; Ladewig, Patricia W.; Ball, Jane W.; Bindler, Ruth C.; Cowen, Kay J., *Maternal & Child Nursing Care.*, 3rd Ed. © 2011. Reprinted and Electronically reproduced by permission of Pearson Education, Inc., Upper Saddle River, New Jersey.

E. Therapeutic management

1. Restrict fluid intake
   a. Fluid intake by all routes my may be limited, sometimes as low as 1000 to 1500 mL per 24-hour period
      1) Sodium-restricted diets help decrease water retention
      2) Level of sodium restriction commonly varies from mild (4 to 5 grams sodium per day) to moderate (2 grams per day) to enhance compliance
      3) Stricter (0.5 gram sodium per day) restrictions are reserved for very severe conditions
   b. IV access is often maintained with a "saline lock" device to avoid administering any excess IV fluids

2. Promote excretion

   a. Diuretics promote the excretion of water through urine
      1) Loop diuretics are commonly used (e.g., furosemide [Lasix])
      2) Potassium-sparing diuretics may also be used (e.g., spironolactone [Aldactone])
      3) Thiazide diuretics may also be used (e.g., thiazide [Diuril])
   b. Human B-type natriuretic peptide (hBNP) such as nesiritide (Natrecor) may be administered in acute heart failure to facilitate smooth muscle relaxation, renal perfusion, and thus urinary elimination
   c. Medications such as digoxin (Lanoxin), low-dose beta blocking agents, and angiotensin-converting enzyme (ACE) inhibitors used to treat congestive heart failure may be beneficial in promoting urinary excretion by improving cardiac efficiency

      d. Protein intake may be increased in clients who are malnourished and have low serum proteins to increase capillary oncotic pressure, thus pulling fluid out of tissues into vessels where it can be eliminated by the kidneys

3. Monitoring during therapy

      a. Monitor respiratory status, assessing for signs of worsening gas exchange, such as increased respiratory effort, falling O_2, saturation (SaO_2), and lung crackles

      b. Note: Pulse oximetry values below 95% are considered low in people with healthy lungs; trend the ABG results, assessing for decreasing PaO_2 and increasing $PaCO_2$

      c. Assess for improving or worsening venous engorgement

      d. Assess fluid I&O carefully, looking for improved urine output in response to therapy

      e. Monitor daily weights (same time, same clothing, same scale) looking for acute weight gain

      f. Assess for peripheral edema, especially in the mornings before the client arises or after client has been reclining with feet elevated for some time (to differentiate dependent, or stasis, edema from the more generalized edema related to heart, kidney, or liver problems)

      g. Observe for signs of developing or worsening water intoxication (hypotonic fluid volume excess), often associated with neurological changes

      h. Evaluate for overcorrection, in which signs of fluid volume deficit begin to appear

      i. Monitor lab values for normalizing BUN, Hct, serum sodium, and arterial blood gases; watch for electrolyte imbalances (low sodium, low or high potassium) due to drug therapy

F. Planning and implementation

1. Monitor assessment parameters, observe response to therapy, note any sign of improvement, and watch for signs of hypovolemia due to overcorrection

2. Restrict fluids as ordered

      a. Teach clients to measure items that are liquid at room temperature and include them in fluid intake totals

      b. Involve client in dividing fluid allowances over 24-hour period; plan for more fluids during times for meals and taking oral medications

      c. Use an infusion pump to help prevent inadvertent administration of excess fluid

      d. Provide mouth care and use measures to moisten mouth regularly to decrease thirst; ice chips can be soothing, but count as fluid intake (1 cup ice chips = ½ cup water), so calculate them into the allowed fluid intake

      e. Encourage cold fluids, which tend to decrease thirst better than warm ones; avoid or limit sweet or salty foods to minimize thirst

3. Measure fluid losses/gains

      a. Measure I&O, noting color and concentration of urine

      b. Weigh daily and monitor patterns of weight loss/gain (remember: a change of 2.2 lbs [1 Kg] is equivalent to a 1 L water loss or gain)

4. Institute measures to prevent fluid volume excess

      a. Irrigate NG tube and bladder with normal saline rather than plain water

      b. Avoid repeated plain tap water enemas

      c. Mix infant formula according to package directions; do not use a water bottle as a pacifier for infants

      d. Monitor infusion rates closely; use a volume control device and pump and use only small bags (250–500 mL) for infants and young children

5. Remain alert for acute pulmonary edema, an emergency requiring prompt action

      a. Anxious client with labored breathing

      b. Moist crackles on auscultation, bilaterally from bases into upper lung fields

      c. Productive cough with frothy, clear sputum

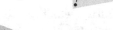

Practice to Pass

A two-month-old infant is being treated for gastroenteritis and dehydration. The infant has received normal saline boluses and has just been switched to D_5¼NS at 40 mL/hour. What monitoring and nursing measures should be implemented at this time? Why?

        d. SaO$_2$ below 95%; blood gases likely reveal low pO$_2$ (hypoxia); if impending respiratory failure, high pCO$_2$ (hypercarbia and respiratory acidosis)

        e. Prompt action: Stop or limit any ongoing fluid intake; assess client (e.g., vital signs, lung sounds, pulse oximetry, mental status); implement actions to increase gas exchange (e.g., high-Fowler's position, supplemental oxygen); and notify physician as soon as possible

      6. Skin care

        a. If edema is present, provide skin care and protection to prevent tissue trauma and skin breakdown.

G. Medication therapy

      1. Diuretic therapy

        a. Loop diuretics and thiazide diuretics cause potassium and sodium loss while potassium sparing diuretics can cause hyperkalemia

        b. Monitor electrolytes during diuretic therapy

        c. Give diuretics in the morning to avoid sleep disruption; if ordered twice per day, administer second dose by midafternoon

      2. Treat underlying disease processes that place client at risk for developing FVE, such as congestive heart failure, or treatment with low-dose beta blocking agents and/or ACE inhibitors

      3. Evaluate client for potential fluid and electrolyte imbalances as a consequence of corrective therapy

H. Client education

      1. Teach clients risk factors for development of FVE

      2. Teach adults to weigh themselves daily and report a gain of more than two pounds per week

      3. Teach clients with peripheral edema to elevate extremities and change position frequently

      4. Dietary education

        a. Teach clients about sodium-restricted diet, including rationale, limitations, and dietary choices (see Table 1-4)

          1) Suggest use of alternative seasonings, such as natural sodium-free herbs and spices

          2) Clients taking potassium-sparing diuretics and/or ACE inhibitors (which cause potassium retention) should not use salt substitutes because most contain potassium

        b. Teach clients to avoid adding salt while cooking or at the table

Table 1-4   Sodium-Restricted Diets

High-Sodium Foods	Low-Sodium Foods
Canned, processed, and pickled foods are *higher* in sodium content.	Fresh foods are *lower* in sodium content.
• Foods prepared in brine (e.g., pickles, olives, sauerkraut) • Salty or smoked meats (e.g., bologna, hotdogs, ham, lunch meats, sausage) • Salty or smoked fish (e.g., anchovies, herring, sardines, smoked salmon) • Salty snacks (e.g., potato chips, popcorn, nuts, crackers, pretzels) • Salty seasonings (e.g., seasoned salts, soy sauce, Worcestershire sauce, barbecue sauces) • Processed cheeses • Canned and instant soups • Canned vegetables and fruits	• Fresh meat and fish • "No added salt" snack items • Sodium-free spices and flavorings • Soups made with fresh items • Fresh fruits and vegetables • Low-sodium canned products

c. Teach clients to assess sodium content by reading food/OTC drug labels

d. Consult dietitian for more detailed dietary information regarding sodium and fluid restrictions

I. **Evaluation**

1. The client will regain fluid volume balance

a. Peripheral edema is resolved; in the pediatric client fontanels are soft and non-bulging

b. Unlabored breathing; lungs clear to auscultation; chest x-ray shows no infiltrates or effusion

c. Vital signs return to baseline

d. Level of consciousness and orientation return to baseline

e. Hct, BUN, serum osmolality, and serum electrolytes return to client's baseline

f. Weight returns to baseline

2. Resolution of underlying cause of fluid volume excess

3. Client/family verbalize understanding of risk factors, prevention, and follow-up care for fluid volume excess

Case Study

A nine-month-old infant enters the emergency department. The mother reports fever, vomiting, and diarrhea for the past two days. You are the nurse caring for them.

1. What questions will you ask the mother about the child initially?

2. What assessment findings will alert you to a serious fluid imbalance?

3. If intravenous fluids are ordered, what are the priorities of care and monitoring during the intravenous infusion?

4. What rehydration instructions should be given to the mother in preparation for discharge?

5. When the mother asks about the BRAT diet her friends have told her to follow until the diarrhea is gone, how would you respond?

For suggested responses, see page 202.

For suggested responses, see page 202.

POSTTEST

1 A 78-year-old client is admitted with dehydration and urinary tract infection. After IV infusion of 750 mL normal saline, the client begins to cough and asks for the head of the bed to be raised to ease breathing. The nurse assesses jugular vein distention (JVD) and increased respiratory rate. How should the nurse interpret this data?

1. The fluid volume deficit is worsening.
2. Hypervolemia is developing.
3. Hypotonic water intoxication is beginning.
4. Ascites is causing respiratory compromise.

2 The nurse is helping a client who was recently placed on a low-sodium diet to reduce fluid retention to choose foods for lunch. The nurse recommends which lunch menu that would be most beneficial for this client?

1. Grilled chicken sandwich on white bread, apple, salad, and iced tea
2. Tuna salad sandwich on wheat bread, canned fruit cocktail, salad, and a soda
3. Ham and bean soup, fresh fruit salad, low-sodium crackers, and a diet soda
4. Cheeseburger, grapes, fresh pineapple, and tomato juice

POSTTEST

3 A 28-year-old client is admitted with severe bleeding from a fractured femur. Which intravenous (IV) fluid does the nurse anticipate as the most appropriate for use to replace potential fluid losses?

1. 0.9% sodium chloride (0.9% NaCl)
2. 3% sodium chloride (3%NaCl)
3. 5% dextrose in water (D_5W)
4. 5% dextrose in 0.22% sodium chloride ($D_5¼NS$)

4 The nurse is preparing to administer 25 mg furosemide (Lasix) intravenously to a client with peripheral edema and lung crackles. The 2 mL vial is labeled 20 mg/mL. How many mL of solution should the nurse draw up? Record your answer rounding to two decimal places.

Fill in your answer below:
_____ mL of solution

5 The nurse caring for the following group of clients considers which client to be at highest risk for developing deficient fluid volume?

1. A thin, 52-year-old female receiving corticosteroid therapy for bronchitis
2. A 60-year-old male who had a left inguinal herniorrhaphy 12 hours ago
3. A 76-year-old male who has a nasogastric (NG) tube to intermittent suction following colon resection
4. A 68-year-old female who is NPO for a flexible sigmoidoscopy procedure

6 A 17-year-old client who sustained a head injury in a motorcycle collision two days ago is responsive only to pain. Which intravenous (IV) fluid order would the nurse question because it could increase the risk of complications?

1. Ringer's solution
2. 5% dextrose in water (D_5W)
3. 0.9% sodium chloride (0.9% NaCl)
4. Lactated Ringer's solution

7 The nurse is caring for a client admitted with heart failure (HF). When assessing the client's risk for fluid imbalances, the nurse should check which laboratory values? Select all that apply.

1. Hemoglobin (Hgb)
2. Hematocrit (Hct)
3. Atrial natriuretic peptide (ANP)
4. Blood glucose
5. Liver enzymes

8 A client with a nursing diagnosis of Excess Fluid Volume has been treated with diuretics and fluid restriction. Which findings would best indicate to the nurse that fluid volume balance has not yet been totally achieved?

1. S_3 heart sounds and moist lung crackles resolving.
2. Return to coherent conversation and appropriate behavior.
3. Oral mucous membranes are no longer sticky and cracked and skin is warm and dry.
4. Skin tenting decreasing and conjunctiva of eyes moist.

9 During intershift report, the nurse is told that a client who has suffered a stroke has also developed diabetes insipidus (DI). The nurse concludes this client is now at risk for which of the following?

1. Severe deficient fluid volume because of excess urine output
2. Severe excess fluid volume because of inadequate urine output
3. Hyperglycemia because of poor insulin production
4. Hypoglycemia because of excess insulin production

10 A father telephones the clinic nurse asking what he should do for his three-year-old son who developed fever, vomiting, and diarrhea today. What would be an appropriate recommendation by the nurse?

1. "Have him drink as much water as you can get him to swallow."
2. "Give small sips of commercial oral rehydration fluids frequently."
3. "Provide frequent sips of fruit juice and commercial sports drinks."
4. "Have him eat only bananas, rice, applesauce, and toast (BRAT diet)."

➤ *See pages 30–32 for Answers and Rationales.*

ANSWERS & RATIONALES

Pretest

1 **Answer: 1** **Rationale:** Infants and older adults cannot compensate as well for fluid losses. Clients with NG suction (loss of fluids and electrolytes in fairly proportional amounts) are at greater risk for fluid volume deficit. The older adult with NG suction has both risk factors, while the child's age is the only risk factor. The client taking glucocorticoids is predisposed to sodium and fluid retention rather than fluid loss. The 30-year-old jogger is a young adult in a moderate climate, which lowers the risk from exertion alone. **Cognitive Level:** Analyzing **Client Need:** Physiological Adaptation **Integrated Process:** Nursing Process: Diagnosis **Content Area:** Adult Health **Strategy:** Recall concepts of fluid balance and factors contributing to losses. Eliminate one option since fluid is gained with steroids and two others because they have fewer risk factors than the correct option. **Reference:** LeMone, P., & Burke, K. (2008). *Medical surgical nursing: Critical thinking in client care* (4th ed.). Upper Saddle River, NJ: Pearson/Prentice Hall, pp. 203–207.

2 **Answer: 3** **Rationale:** Items that are liquid at body temperature are also considered part of the fluid intake, so ice pops, gelatin, and ice cream can be considered as part of overall fluid intake. The color of urine is only one indicator of hydration and many older adults take a diuretic, which would produce more dilute urine, falsely reassuring the client. The client should drink a variety of fluids not just water. With aging, the thirst mechanism becomes less effective. Significant fluid can be lost before thirst is triggered, so the elderly should not rely solely on thirst to indicate when they need to drink fluids. **Cognitive Level:** Applying **Client Need:** Health Promotion and Maintenance **Integrated Process:** Communication and Documentation **Content Area:** Adult Health **Strategy:** Note the critical words *older adult* and *remain hydrated*. Recall knowledge of risk factors for dehydration in older adults and of fluid intake to make a final selection. **Reference:** LeMone, P., & Burke, K. (2008). *Medical surgical nursing: Critical thinking in client care* (4th ed.). Upper Saddle River, NJ: Pearson Education, pp. 195–200.

3 **Answer: 3** **Rationale:** The client has symptoms of fluid volume deficit (FVD) and hypovolemia. The presence of postural hypotension when rising from a lying position indicates the presence of significant hypovolemia. The other vital signs are important for general reasons but do not directly reflect circulating fluid volume. **Cognitive Level:** Analyzing **Client Need:** Physiological Adaptation **Integrated Process:** Nursing Process: Assessment **Content Area:** Adult Health **Strategy:** Recognize that the client has signs and symptoms of an FVD: intravascular and recall clinical manifestations of such. Eliminate two options because they do not reflect intravascular fluid losses.

Choose correctly from the remaining two since it best supports the client symptoms of weakness and dizziness. **Reference:** LeMone, P., & Burke, K. (2008). *Medical surgical nursing: Critical thinking in client care* (4th ed.). Upper Saddle River, NJ: Pearson/Prentice Hall, pp. 203–207.

4 **Answer: 1, 4, 5** **Rationale:** Neck veins are normally flat when the bed is elevated; distended neck veins reflect FVE in the vascular system. An accumulation of fluid in the alveoli and blood vessels will often cause shortness of breath with activity, reflecting FVE. Pitting edema reflects an accumulation of fluid in the interstitial tissues as seen with FVE. Hand veins would remain full or empty slowly if FVE is present. Rapid and weak peripheral pulses reflect a fluid volume deficit, not an excess. **Cognitive Level:** Analyzing **Client Need:** Physiological Adaptation **Integrated Process:** Nursing Process: Evaluation **Content Area:** Adult Health **Strategy:** Note the critical words *hydration status* and *fluid volume excess*. Choose those options that reflect a full vascular bed, which in this case are peripheral edema, venous engorgement, and excessive pulmonary fluid. **Reference:** LeMone, P., & Burke, K. (2008). *Medical surgical nursing: Critical thinking in client care* (4th ed.). Upper Saddle River, NJ: Pearson/Prentice Hall, pp. 208–213.

5 **Answer: 3** **Rationale:** 0.9% sodium chloride is an isotonic solution that does not produce fluid shifts and would be the best choice of solutions. 10% dextrose is a hypertonic solution and would pull water from the GI tract into the vascular space, possibly leading to a fluid volume excess. 5% dextrose is metabolized to a hypotonic solution and could contribute to fluid shifts into the GI tissue. 0.45% sodium chloride is a hypotonic solution and could contribute to fluid shifts into the GI tissue. **Cognitive Level:** Applying **Client Need:** Physiological Adaptation **Integrated Process:** Nursing Process: Planning **Content Area:** Adult Health **Strategy:** Recall principles of osmosis and diffusion, and differences among hypotonic, isotonic, and hypertonic fluids. Eliminate incorrect options since fluid shifts will occur with hypotonic and hypertonic solutions. **Reference:** Kozier, B., Erb, G., Berman, A., & Snyder, S. (2008). *Fundamentals of nursing: Concepts, process, and practice* (8th ed.). Upper Saddle River, NJ: Pearson/Prentice Hall, pp. 1438–1441.

6 **Answer: 4** **Rationale:** A moist cough, dyspnea, and falling pulse oximetry reading in a client with a history of heart disease are signs of developing pulmonary edema secondary to excess fluid volume excess (FVE). The first action should be to reduce IV fluid intake to prevent more fluid from accumulating in the lungs, then further assessment can be done, emergency actions taken, and the physician contacted. **Cognitive Level:** Analyzing **Client Need:** Reduction of Risk Potential

Integrated Process: Nursing Process: Implementation **Content Area:** Adult Health **Strategy:** Note the critical word *first*, indicating one option has a priority action. Use knowledge of cardiovascular disease and EFV to choose correctly. **Reference:** LeMone, P. & Burke, K. (2008). *Medical surgical nursing: Critical thinking in client care* (4th ed.). Upper Saddle River, NJ: Pearson/Prentice Hall, pp. 207–213.

7 Answer: 2 Rationale: Explaining the functioning of the kidneys provides the client with information as to why the fluid restriction is necessary. The client already knows the physician ordered the restriction. There is no evidence that the client drank excessive fluids before becoming ill; this explanation is not accurate. Although explaining effects of excess fluid is accurate information, it is presented in an alarming fashion. **Cognitive Level:** Applying **Client Need:** Physiological Adaptation **Integrated Process:** Communication and Documentation **Content Area:** Adult Health **Strategy:** Note the critical words *best* and *response*. Use knowledge of communication skills and regulation of fluid imbalances to choose the correct option. **Reference:** LeMone, P., & Burke, K. (2008). *Medical surgical nursing: Critical thinking in client care* (4th ed.). Upper Saddle River, NJ: Pearson/Prentice Hall, pp. 207–213.

8 Answer: 1 Rationale: An excess response to diuretic therapy results in an excess loss of water and electrolytes in the urine, leaving the blood hemoconcentrated and causes a high BUN (normal 8–22 mg/dL) and Hct (normal approximately 38–45%). The water loss results in an acute weight loss. Weight gain indicates ineffective response to diuretic therapy. **Cognitive Level:** Analyzing **Client Need:** Physiological Adaptation **Integrated Process:** Nursing Process: Evaluation **Content Area:** Adult Health **Strategy:** Note the critical words *excessive response*, indicating a greater than desired action is achieved. Use knowledge of diuretic action and recall normal values for BUN and Hct to eliminate incorrect options. **Reference:** LeMone, P., & Burke, K. (2008). *Medical surgical nursing: Critical thinking in client care* (4th ed.). Upper Saddle River, NJ: Pearson/Prentice Hall, pp. 207–213.

9 Answer: 4 Rationale: 1/4 NS (0.225% sodium chloride) is a hypotonic solution that provides free water to the cells. Cerebral cells are especially sensitive to fluid gains from hypotonic fluids. If infused too rapidly, the cerebral cells will be the first to gain fluid too quickly, resulting in neurological changes. Monitoring the client for urine output, edema, and oral cavity dryness are important, but this reflects a response to IV therapy rather than detection of a complication. **Cognitive Level:** Analyzing **Client Need:** Physiological Adaptation **Integrated Process:** Nursing Process: Assessment **Content Area:** Adult Health **Strategy:** Note critical words *complications of therapy* and *most important*, indicating one of the options is of higher priority. Recall knowledge of fluid shifts with hypotonic fluids to

choose correctly. **Reference:** LeMone, P., & Burke, K. (2008). *Medical surgical nursing: Critical thinking in client care* (4th ed.). Upper Saddle River, NJ: Pearson/Prentice Hall, pp. 201–213.

10 Answer: 1, 4, 5 Rationale: Priority should be placed on assessment of the neurological system since the 3% NaCl infusion can lead to cellular dehydration and could lead to mental status changes and possibly seizures. 3% NaCl is very hypertonic and, if infused too rapidly, will increase serum sodium and osmolality, causing high volumes of water to be pulled into vessels from cells. This results in cellular dehydration and vascular volume overload. The serum sodium level should be monitored to ensure adequate therapy without too rapid an increase. Urine specific gravity would not provide the most important information to regarding onset of complications as it would be affected later. Serum glucose levels are an indicator of pancreatic function. **Cognitive Level:** Analyzing **Client Need:** Physiological Adaptation **Integrated Process:** Nursing Process: Evaluation **Content Area:** Adult Health **Strategy:** Note critical words *priority* and *detect*. Recall physiology of fluids shifts from hypertonic solutions to choose correctly. Note the wording of the question indicates that more than one option is correct. **Reference:** LeMone, P., & Burke, K. (2008). *Medical surgical nursing: Critical thinking in client care* (4th ed.). Upper Saddle River, NJ: Pearson/Prentice Hall, pp. 195–200.

Posttest

1 Answer: 2 Rationale: Dyspnea and increased respirations are most likely caused by fluid accumulation in the lungs, both signs of fluid volume excess. The jugular vein distention is also a sign of fluid accumulation related to hypervolemia. The client is exhibiting signs of fluid volume excess, not fluid volume deficit. The client is receiving an isotonic solution, not a hypotonic solution. The client does show evidence of fluid accumulation in the abdomen related to ascites, but rather in the lungs and jugular veins. **Cognitive Level:** Analyzing **Client Need:** Physiological Adaptation **Integrated Process:** Nursing Process: Diagnosis **Content Area:** Adult Health **Strategy:** Note the client is elderly and has received too much fluid, indicating a fluid overload. Recall knowledge of fluid volume excess to eliminate options that are incorrect or irrelevant to the client. **Reference:** LeMone, P., & Burke, K. (2008). *Medical surgical nursing: Critical thinking in client care* (4th ed.). Upper Saddle River, NJ: Pearson/Prentice Hall, pp. 220–203.

2 Answer: 1 Rationale: Processed and canned foods (tuna, soup, tomato juice) and sodas are high in sodium. Fresh foods (grilled chicken, fruit, and vegetables) are lower in sodium. **Cognitive Level:** Applying **Client Need:** Health Promotion and Maintenance **Integrated Process:** Nursing Process: Implementation **Content Area:** Adult Health **Strategy:** Note the critical word *best* is used, indicating one of the choices is better than the others. Recall knowledge of the sodium content of various foods to eliminate the incorrect options. **Reference:** LeMone, P., & Burke, K. (2008). *Medical surgical nursing: Critical thinking in client care* (4th ed.). Upper Saddle River, NJ: Pearson/ Prentice Hall, pp. 208–212.

3 **Answer: 1** **Rationale:** Acute bleeding results in isotonic fluid loss and can quickly lead to shock and vascular collapse. The priority is to expand vascular volume and restore circulation using isotonic IV fluid. Hypertonic (3% saline) and hypotonic (D_5W, $D_5\frac{1}{4}NS$) solutions are not indicated. **Cognitive Level:** Applying **Client Need:** Pharmacological and Parenteral Therapies **Integrated Process:** Nursing Process: Planning **Content Area:** Adult Health **Strategy:** The critical words are *most appropriate* and *fluid losses*. Recognize the client needs replacement of isotonic fluids to eliminate incorrect options, since these are either hypertonic or hypotonic. **Reference:** LeMone, P., & Burke, K. (2008). *Medical surgical nursing: Critical thinking in client care* (4th ed.). Upper Saddle River, NJ: Pearson/Prentice Hall, pp. 205–212.

4 **Answer: 1.25** **Rationale:**

$$\frac{\text{Desired dose} \times \text{Quantity}}{\text{Dose on hand}}$$

$$\frac{25 \text{ mg} \times 1 \text{ mL}}{20 \text{ mg}}$$

$$25 \text{ divided by } 20 \times 1 = x$$
$$x = 1.25$$

Cognitive Level: Applying **Client Need:** Pharmacological and Parenteral Therapies **Integrated Process:** Nursing Process: Planning **Content Area:** Adult Health **Strategy:** Specific knowledge of formulas for calculating medication dosage is needed to answer this question Recall the formula and check calculations carefully. **Reference:** Booth, K.A., Whaley, J.E., Sienkiewicz, S., & Palmunen, J. (2012). *Math and dosage calculations for healthcare professionals.* (4th ed.). New York, NY: McGraw Hill, pp. 112–120.

5 **Answer: 3** **Rationale:** The 76-year-old client is most at risk for a fluid volume deficit secondary to increasing age, fluid losses through the NG tube, and having had major surgery. Clients receiving corticosteroids often retain sodium and fluid, placing them at risk for a fluid volume excess, not deficit. An inguinal herniorrhaphy is not considered major surgery and the client is not at risk for large volumes of fluid loss. Although the 68-year-old client has been NPO for the procedure, fluid replacement will be resumed and the risk for deficit is low. **Cognitive Level:** Analyzing **Client Need:** Physiological Adaptation **Integrated Process:** Nursing Process: Assessment **Content Area:** Adult Health **Strategy:** Critical words are *at highest risk* and *deficient fluid volume*. Recall knowledge of risk factors contributing to fluid deficits and determine one option has the greater number of them. **Reference:** LeMone, P., & Burke, K. (2008.). *Medical surgical*

nursing: Critical thinking in client care (4th ed.). Upper Saddle River, NJ: Pearson/Prentice Hall, pp. 199–203.

6 **Answer: 2** **Rationale:** 5% dextrose in water (D_5W) has a hypotonic effect when infused, providing free water to cells, which would worsen this client's cerebral edema. The other fluids listed are isotonic and would primarily remain in the extracellular spaces. **Cognitive Level:** Analyzing **Client Need:** Pharmacological and Parenteral Therapies **Integrated Process:** Nursing Process: Implementation **Content Area:** Adult Health **Strategy:** Note the client has a head injury and recognize the danger of hypotonic fluids that could contribute to cerebral edema. Also note the question requires nurse to question an order, indicating that one option will be incorrect and three are correct. Consider tonicity of IV fluids to make a selection. **Reference:** LeMone, P., & Burke, K. (2008). *Medical surgical nursing: Critical thinking in client care* (4th ed.). Upper Saddle River, NJ: Pearson/Prentice Hall, pp. 205–211.

7 **Answer: 1, 2, 3** **Rationale:** Hemoglobin and hematocrit can decrease or increase secondary to hemoconcentration or hemodilution. ANP is a cardiac hormone released when atria are stretched by increased blood volume, which would occur in HF. Glucose and liver enzymes would not be affected by fluid volume. **Cognitive Level:** Applying **Client Need:** Physiological Adaptation **Integrated Process:** Nursing Process: Assessment **Content Area:** Adult Health **Strategy:** Note that the client has HF. Recall knowledge of fluid imbalances and correlate lab studies associated with them. Eliminate two options since they are not affected by fluid volume. **Reference:** LeMone, P., & Burke, K. (2008). *Medical surgical nursing: Critical thinking in client care* (4th ed.). Upper Saddle River, NJ: Pearson/Prentice Hall, pp. 199–203.

8 **Answer: 1** **Rationale:** S_3 heart sounds are associated with increased workload on the heart and lung crackles are associated with fluid accumulation in the lungs. Since these sounds are resolving, it would support that fluid volume is decreasing, but not yet fully achieved. Although a client with a fluid overload may become confused and incoherent, this would not be the best choice to support resolution of a fluid volume excess. The client may have been inappropriate for reasons unrelated to the fluid excess. Cracked and sticky mucous membranes are associated with a fluid volume deficit, not an excess. A decrease in skin tenting indicates an improvement from a fluid volume deficit, not excess. **Cognitive Level:** Analyzing **Client Need:** Physiological Adaptation **Integrated Process:** Nursing Process: Evaluation **Content Area:** Adult Health **Strategy:** Note the critical phrases *excess fluid volume* and *has not yet been achieved*. Recall signs and symptoms of fluid excess and eliminate one option because it indicates full resolution of these signs. Eliminate two other options because they indicate resolution of deficient fluid volume, which is not the focus of the question. **Reference:** LeMone, P., &

Burke, K. (2008). *Medical surgical nursing: Critical thinking in client care* (4th ed.). Upper Saddle River, NJ: Pearson/Prentice Hall, pp. 200–205.

9 **Answer: 1 Rationale:** DI is associated with insufficient ADH production, which would lead to excessive fluid losses DI would lead to excessive fluid. DI would lead to excessive fluid losses, not fluid volume excesses. Diabetes mellitus, not DI, is associated with poor insulin production. Hypoglycemia can be a complication of diabetes mellitus, not DI. **Cognitive Level:** Analyzing **Client Need:** Physiological Adaptation **Integrated Process:** Nursing Process: Diagnosis **Content Area:** Adult Health **Strategy:** The critical words are *diabetes insipidus* and *at risk for*. Eliminate two options because they relate to diabetes mellitus. Discriminate appropriately between DI and SIADH to choose correctly between the remaining two. **Reference:** LeMone, P., & Burke, K. (2008). *Medical surgical nursing: Critical thinking in client care* (4th ed.). Upper Saddle River, NJ: Pearson/Prentice Hall, pp. 195–200.

10 **Answer: 2 Rationale:** Oral rehydration fluids contain electrolytes that will help to replace what is lost with vomiting and diarrhea. Replacing fluid losses with plain water could lead to electrolyte imbalances since electrolytes are lost with perspiration, vomiting, and diarrhea. Fruit juices and commercial sports drinks are often high in sugar and could worsen the vomiting. Solid foods should not be encouraged when the child is vomiting. **Cognitive Level:** Applying **Client Need:** Physiological Adaptation **Integrated Process:** Nursing Process: Implementation **Content Area:** Child Health **Strategy:** Recall knowledge of age appropriate fluids. Determine symptoms reflect risk for fluid volume deficit to choose correctly. **Reference:** Dudek, S. (2010). *Nutrition essentials for nursing practice* (6th ed.). Philadelphia: Lippincott Williams & Wilkins, pp. 128–130.

References

Ball, J., Bindler, R., & Cowen, K. (2010). *Child health nursing: Partnering with children and families* (2nd ed.). Upper Saddle River, NJ: Pearson Education.

Berman, A., & Snyder, S. (2012). *Kozier & Erb's fundamentals of nursing: Concepts, process, and practice* (9th ed.). Upper Saddle River, NJ: Pearson Education.

Hockenberry-Eaton, M., & Wilson, D. (2010). *Wong's nursing care of infants and children* (9th ed.). St. Louis: Elsevier Mosby.

Hogan, M., & Skrabal, J. (2012). *Pearson comprehensive review for NCLEX-PN®* (2nd ed.). Upper Saddle River, NJ: Pearson Education, p. 441

Ignatavicius, D., & Workman, M. (2010). *Medical-surgical nursing: Patient-centered collaborative care* (6th ed.). Philadelphia: Elsevier Saunders.

Kee, J. L. (2009). *Laboratory and diagnostic tests with nursing implications* (8th ed.). Upper Saddle River, NJ: Pearson/Prentice Hall.

LeMone, P., Burke, K., & Bauldoff, G. (2012). *Medical surgical nursing: Critical thinking in patient care* (5th ed.). Upper Saddle River, NJ: Pearson/Prentice Hall.

London, M., Ladewig, P., Ball, J., Bindler, R., & Cowen, K. (2011). *Maternal & child nursing care* (3rd ed.). Upper Saddle River, NJ: Pearson Education.

Sole, M. L., Klein, O. G., & Moseley, M. J. (2008). *Introduction to critical care nursing* (5th ed.). St. Louis, MO: Elsevier Saunders.

Sodium Balance and Imbalances

2

Chapter Outline

Overview of Sodium Regulation

Hyponatremia

Hypernatremia

Objectives

➤ Review the basic functions of sodium in the body.
➤ Explain the pathophysiology and etiology of sodium imbalances.
➤ Identify specific assessment findings in sodium imbalances.
➤ Identify priority nursing diagnoses for a client experiencing a sodium imbalance.
➤ Describe the therapeutic management of sodium imbalances.
➤ Describe the nursing management of a client who is experiencing a sodium imbalance.

NCLEX-RN® Test Prep

Use the accompanying online resource, NursingReviewsandRationales, to test yourself with hundreds of NCLEX®-style practice questions.

Review at a Glance

anion an ion with a negative charge

cation an ion with a positive charge

cerebral demyelination an adverse outcome of hyponatremia that causes demyelination of the pons in the brain and leads to dysphagia, delirium, coma, and even death

chloride anion found in the ECF that is linked to sodium, bicarbonate, and water in the body and participates in osmotic pressure regulation and acid–base balance

diabetes insipidus (DI) an endocrine disturbance whereby ADH is either not secreted (central DI) or there is

kidney failure (nephrogenic DI) that leads to an increased dilute urine, hypernatremia, and thirst

dilutional hyponatremia a term used to describe hyponatremia where the serum sodium level is diluted by excess fluid

euvolemia normal fluid volume in the body

hypernatremia serum sodium level above 145 mEq/L

hyperosmolar osmotic pressure greater than normal plasma pressure

hypervolemia increase in the circulating volume (intravascular fluid)

hyponatremia serum sodium level below 135 mEq/L; also called dilutional hyponatremia or water intoxication

hypovolemia low-circulating blood volume

syndrome of inappropriate antidiuretic hormone secretion (SIADH) excessive release of ADH hormone that causes fluid and electrolyte imbalances resulting in fluid retention, increased ECF volume, hyponatremia, and concentrated urine

water intoxication another term to describe hyponatremia where the serum sodium level is diluted by excess fluid

PRETEST

1 Which serum electrolyte imbalances would the nurse assess for in a child admitted with a high fever and severe dehydration? Select all that apply.

1. Hypercalcemia
2. Hypokalemia
3. Hypernatremia
4. Hyperchloremia
5. Hypophosphatemia

2 Which of the following clients would the nurse identify as being most at risk to develop a sodium imbalance?

1. An adult client taking corticosteroid therapy
2. An older adult client who drinks eight glasses (eight ounces each) of water each day
3. A school-age client with diabetes mellitus who is under glycemic control
4. A teenager who is drinking Gatorade during exercise workouts

3 When caring for a 79-year-old client who has a sodium level of 149 mEq/L, the nurse identifies the client will be at increased risk to develop dehydration because of which factor?

1. A diminished thirst drive
2. An increased level of aldosterone
3. A decrease in muscle mass
4. ADH (antidiuretic hormone) is no longer produced

4 Which of the following interventions does the nurse complete when caring for a client admitted with a sodium level of 152 mEq/L?

1. Provide extra blankets for warmth
2. Observe client for nausea and malaise
3. Observe and prepare for possible seizures
4. Restrict fluids to 1200 mL per day

5 The nurse is teaching a client who is on a low-sodium diet how to read food labels and check for hidden sodium content. The nurse informs the client that sodium is contained in higher amounts in which of the following products? Select all that apply.

1. Baking goods containing baking powder
2. Seasonings using monosodium glutamate (MSG)
3. Over-the-counter cold and cough preparations
4. Canned vegetables
5. Salad oil

6 The nurse is caring for a client who is experiencing a steady decline in sodium level. The nurse places highest priority on which of the following interventions?

1. Close monitoring of neurological status
2. Preventing weakness and fatigue
3. Spacing activities to conserve energy
4. Providing oral hygiene and skin care

7 When caring for a client with syndrome of inappropriate antidiuretic hormone (SIADH), the nurse plans to carry out which intervention to restore fluid and electrolyte balance?

1. Encourage client to drink plenty of water
2. Restrict dietary salt intake
3. Monitor infusion of hypotonic saline infusions
4. Administer prescribed loop diuretics

8 Lab chemistry results reveal a client's serum sodium is within normal range. Based on this finding, the nurse estimates the client's serum (plasma) osmolality to be no higher than _____ mOsm/kg.

Fill in your answer below:
_____ mOsm/kg

9 A client with abnormal sodium loss is receiving a regular diet. To encourage foods high in sodium, the nurse would recommend which of the following foods for lunch?

1. A cheese and ham sandwich
2. Chicken salad on lettuce
3. Tossed salad with vinegar dressing
4. White fish and plain baked potato

10 Which intervention should the nurse anticipate implementing in a client who is experiencing dilutional hyponatremia?

1. Administration of hypotonic intravenous solutions
2. Restriction of additional oral fluids
3. Increasing sodium intake in the diet
4. Encouraging intake of tap water

➤ *See pages 49–51 for Answers and Rationales.*

PRETEST

I. OVERVIEW OF SODIUM REGULATION

A. **Sodium balance and function**: major extracellular fluid (ECF) **cation** (positively charged ion), making up about 99% of the body's sodium level; the remaining 1% is in the intracellular fluid (ICF) and is responsible for water balance and determination of plasma osmolality; the movement of **chloride** (major **anion**—negatively charged ion—in the ECF) is also closely associated with the movement of sodium

1. Serum levels
   a. Normal ECF range is 135 to 145 mEq/L; normal intracellular level is 10 mEq/L
   b. Sodium works with chloride in the body to affect electrolyte changes; they may occur at the same time or independently
   c. The effect of serum sodium levels has a profound effect on cellular fluid dynamics
   d. Serum sodium levels are used to monitor electrolyte, water, and acid–base balance in the body

2. Determinant of plasma osmolality
   a. Sodium is the major determinant of plasma osmolality
   b. Osmolality determines the movement of water between the ECF and the ICF; water will move from a lower concentration of solute (hypotonic) to a higher concentration of solute (hypertonic)
   c. Osmolality of the ECF and ICF are roughly equal (isotonic) at 270 to 290 mOsm/kg water
   d. Osmotic force helps to move water across the cell membrane to equalize osmotic pressure; water follows sodium, so a sodium imbalance is usually accompanied by an associated imbalance in water
   e. Plasma osmolality can be roughly estimated by doubling the plasma sodium value
   f. Formula used to determine serum osmolality:

$$2 \times \text{serum Na} + \frac{\text{BUN}}{3} + \frac{\text{glucose}}{18} = \text{serum osmolality}$$

   g. Free water (pure water) is available to all body compartments and helps to maintain osmotic balance

3. Functions in the body
   a. Determines plasma osmolality and regulates water balance and distribution
   b. Helps maintain electrolyte balance by exchanging for potassium and attracting chloride
   c. Assists with acid–base balance by combining with bicarbonate and chloride to alter pH
   d. Promotes neuromuscular response and stimulates conduction of nerve impulses and muscle fiber impulse transmission through the sodium potassium pump

Practice to Pass

What methods can the nurse utilize to get an estimate of a client's plasma osmolality?

4. System interactions

    a. The primary regulator of sodium concentration is in the kidneys (renal tubules)

    b. In addition, the posterior pituitary and adrenal glands of the endocrine system help to regulate sodium levels by hormonal control

        1) Aldosterone (a mineralocorticoid) and cortisone increase serum sodium by increasing tubular reabsorption

        2) Antidiuretic hormone (ADH) increases sodium and water renal tubular reabsorption

    c. The movement and regulation of sodium is also affected by the sodium–potassium pump, which is located in the cell membrane; ATP helps to actively move sodium from the cell into the ECF; the process of diffusion offsets the continual movement

    d. The cerebral cells are very sensitive to changes in serum sodium levels and exhibit adaptive changes to sodium imbalances

        1) In acute situations where there is a dramatic change in sodium levels, the brain tries to adapt with a corresponding change in water to maintain fluid balance

        2) It is important to recognize both the acuity and severity of onset in managing the care of clients who exhibit severe sodium disturbances

    e. Since the brain readily responds to sodium imbalances in an attempt to maintain homeostasis, the restoration of normal sodium levels can be especially problematic; too rapid a correction can cause further fluid and cellular shifting, which can further compromise the client's condition; for example, too rapid a correction of hypernatremia leads to fewer particles in serum than in the brain, causing fluid to shift into brain with resultant brain swelling

    f. Sodium imbalances can exist in different volume states: **euvolemia** (normal volume), **hypovolemia** (low volume), and **hypervolemia** (increased volume)

B. Sources of sodium

    1. Cellular level

        a. A greater amount of sodium is found in bones than in the ECF, but it is not involved in electrolyte exchange

        b. Sodium is found in all body fluids, including blood, bile, gastric and intestinal secretions, pancreatic fluid, and saliva

        c. Sodium is found normally in body perspiration

    2. Dietary level

        a. Most people in the United States eat more sodium (average of 4 to 6 grams on a daily basis) than is needed; safe minimum levels have been established for infants and children, adults, and pregnant and lactating women; 500 mg is the minimally safe recommended sodium intake for an adult client (refer to current findings of the National Research Council–National Academy of Sciences for further information)

        b. The primary dietary source of sodium is found in table salt (NaCl); table salt contains approximately 40% sodium

        c. Sodium is found in a variety of foods in the Western diet such as cheese, eggs, fish, milk, poultry, shellfish, canned foods, and processed foods

        d. Hidden sources of sodium in the diet are found in processed foods, preservatives, seasonings, and flavorings; in addition, hidden sources of sodium are found in medications; although this may not be considered a dietary form, it still contributes to the overall dietary intake (see Box 2-1 for hidden sources of sodium)

Practice to Pass

Where does the chief regulation of sodium occur?

Box 2-1	The following items should be evaluated for their hidden sodium content:
Hidden Sources of Sodium	• Processed foods: contain increased amounts of sodium used in the processing and preserving process • Medications: such as OTC cold products, cough syrups, antacids, and Alka-Seltzer • Canned food items: often contain increased amounts of sodium, especially soups • Seasonings: such as MSG (monosodium glutamate), seasoned salts, and soy sauce • Baking products: such as baking powder and baking soda

II. HYPONATREMIA: SERUM SODIUM LEVEL BELOW 135 MEQ/L

A. Etiology and pathophysiology

1. Cellular level transport

a. Sodium deficit is usually associated with hypervolemia (increased volume) states and can also be referred to as **dilutional hyponatremia** or **water intoxication** (excess fluid that dilutes serum sodium)

b. Sodium deficit can also occur in euvolemia (normal volume) and hypovolemia (low volume) states (see Table 2-1 for a summary of this disorder)

c. Water will shift from the ECF (area of lower volume of solutes) to the ICF (area of higher volume of solutes) in an attempt to restore equilibrium, resulting in decreased circulating plasma volume and an increased intracellular fluid volume

d. In response to low-sodium levels, the body responds by using the following compensatory mechanisms:

1) Decreased circulating plasma volume leads to activation of pressure receptors (baroreceptors) in the cardiac atria and thoracic veins in an attempt to increase plasma volume; ADH hormone responds to changes in extracellular volume (ECV) and plasma osmolality

2) Renal sodium excretion is decreased in order to prevent further sodium depletion

3) Hormonal response of aldosterone helps to promote sodium retention and potassium excretion

Practice to Pass

What happens to the fluid balance of the body when the sodium level is decreased?

Table 2-1	Hyponatremia in Various Fluid Volume States		
	Description	**Clinical Presentation**	**Treatment**
Euvolemia	Decrease in fluids in both the intravascular and interstitial space Use of sodium-free solutions that dilute the ECF Serum osmolality remains normal	Medications, hypothyroidism, psychiatric disorders, cerebral salt-wasting syndrome	Water restriction, correction of underlying cause; treat SIADH with demeclocycline (unlabeled use) and increase dietary salt intake
Hypervolemia	High glucose states that pull water from cells leading to cellular dehydration as seen in diabetic ketoacidosis (DKA) Fluid loss from ECF greater than solute loss leading to increased serum osmolality	Congestive heart failure (CHF), cirrhosis, syndrome of inappropriate ADH (SIADH), nephrotic syndrome, and renal failure	Water restriction, treat existing disease states, loop diuretics, and restrict dietary salt intake
Hypovolemia	Glucose in isotonic solutions is oxidized leading to cellular swelling Loss of solute from ECF is greater than excess of water, resulting in a decreased serum osmolality	GI fluid loss, diuretic therapy, osmotic diuresis, adrenal insufficiency, burns, and sweating, hypotonic dehydration	NS to correct ECF deficits, increase dietary salt intake; hypertonic saline to raise sodium level

Figure 2-1

Cellular dynamics in response to sodium levels.
A. Hyponatremia (cells edematous). B. Hypernatremia (cells shrink).

Cell swells as water is pulled in from ECF

Cell shrinks as water is pulled out into ECF

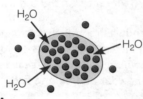

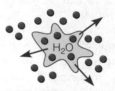

A Hyponatremia: Na less than 135 mEq/L

B Hypernatremia: Na greater than 145 mEq/L

    e. Cellular response results in cellular swelling/edema (see Figure 2-1a)

    f. Cerebral cell response

      1) Osmotic force that causes water to be drawn into brain cells leads to the development of cerebral edema in hyponatremic disorders

      2) If hyponatremia is severe (acuity and severity of onset), **cerebral demyelination** can occur; this is a serious complication whereby the pons is severely affected, leading to mutism, dysphagia, delirium, coma, and possibly death

2. Predisposing clinical conditions

    a. Conditions that cause loss of body fluids

      1) Renal losses through excretion, diuretic administration, and renal disease (salt-wasting nephropathy)

      2) Gastrointestinal (GI) losses through vomiting, diarrhea, suctioning, tap water enemas (TWE), GI surgery, and bulimia

      3) Skin losses through perspiration, environmental conditions, burns, and tissue destruction

      4) Wound drainage; wound suctioning

    b. Conditions that increase extracellular water

      1) Hormone regulation response of ADH and aldosterone, leading to fluid shifting and water gain

      2) Disease states that add to increased volume such as congestive heart failure (CHF), cirrhosis, and nephrotic syndrome

      3) Disease states such as psychiatric disorders that involve compulsive water drinking

      4) Disease states such as tumors, **syndrome of inappropriate antidiuretic hormone secretion** or **SIADH**, and adrenal insufficiency affect hormonal response leading to increased secretion (refer to Box 2-2 for additional information on SIADH)

      5) Hyperglycemic states such as diabetic ketoacidosis (DKA) that cause cellular dehydration

      6) Medications can promote the development of hyponatremia (refer to Table 2-2 for a listing of medications that affect serum sodium levels)

      7) Prolonged or excessive use of hypotonic fluid administration can lead to the development of hyponatremia

    c. Conditions that lead to inadequate dietary intake of sodium

      1) Prolonged use of fluids without sodium replacement by individuals can result in the development of hyponatremia

      2) The presence of anorexia and other eating disorders can lead to inadequate intake of sodium in the diet

3. See Table 2-3 for age-related risk factors for hyponatremia

Box 2-2	
Syndrome of Inappropriate Antidiuretic Hormone Secretion (SIADH)	• Increased ADH secretion occurs due to malignancies, CNS disorders, pulmonary disorders, medications, and in postoperative states. • Plasma osmolality and sodium are decreased, urine sodium is high, and urine osmolality is increased. • Hyponatremia is present. • Clients present with significant fluid retention, GI symptoms, and neurological symptoms related to fluid retention. • Free water restriction is used to treat this clinical condition. • Demeclocycline (blocks ADH secretion) is used if fluid restriction alone does not correct the disturbance. Lithium also blocks ADH secretion, but it is not commonly used as it can reach toxic levels in the body and cause additional complications. • Clients can be placed on a high-salt, high-protein diet to restore normal sodium level and allow the kidneys to excrete more urine (increased solute load). • It is important to identify and correct the underlying cause of the problem. • It is important when restoring normal sodium balance that the correction is done per protocol so as not to cause further complications.

Table 2-2 Medications That Can Affect Sodium Levels

Increase Sodium Levels	Decrease Sodium Levels
Corticosteroids (cortisone, prednisone)	Diuretics
Hypertonic saline solutions	Lithium (Lithobid)
Sodium bicarbonate, sodium phosphate, and sodium salicylate	Antineoplastic agents* (cisplatin, vincristine)
Antibiotics* (Penicillin Na, Ticarcillin)	ACE inhibitors* (captopril, lisinopril)
Amphotericin B	Psychotropic medications* (amitriptyline, thioridazine)
Demeclocycline (Declomycin)	Antidiabetic agents* (chlorpropramide, tolbutamide)
Lactulose cough medicines	CNS depressants* (morphine, barbiturates)
	Ibuprofen (Motrin)
	Nicotine
	Oxytocin (Pitocin)

* For these medications, please refer to a drug textbook for specific names as there are many different types of drugs in each category.

Table 2-3 Lifespan Considerations for Health Maintenance: Hyponatremia

Lifespan Considerations	Fluids	Electrolytes	Acid–Base Balance
Infants	Mature breast milk is present by two weeks postpartum; establish an "on-demand" feeding schedule	Sodium (Na+) is essential for fluid balance, nerve, and muscle function.	Acid–base imbalance in infants is primarily due to respiratory disorders related to respiratory insufficiency
Pediatrics	Give isotonic fluids and avoid hypotonic fluids such as D_5W; possible fluid restriction	Monitor for decreased level of consciousness, anorexia, nausea, vomiting, confusion, headache, respiratory distress, muscle weakness, agitation, and lethargy	Acidosis can occur through the loss of fluid in clients with cystic fibrosis
Adults	Due to a loss of sodium or a gain of water; monitor fluid losses and gains; check urine specific gravity	Hyponatremia leads to swelling of the cells, with resulting confusion, hypotension, edema, muscle cramps, weakness, and dry skin	If the imbalance is due to a loss of sodium, replace the sodium with appropriate fluids; if the imbalance is due to a gain of water (edema), expect to administer diuretics

B. Assessment
1. Clinical manifestations
   a. Common signs are related to the shift of water into cells from vascular space and to sodium's role in nerve impulse transmission and muscle contraction
   b. Cardiovascular: tachycardia, hypotension (with decreased ECV), hypertension with bounding pulse (with increased ECV)
   c. Integument: pale, dry skin and dry mucous membranes (with decreased ECV), edema, "doughy" skin, and weight gain (with increased ECV)
   d. Renal: thirst (decreased ECV), renal failure (increased ECV)
   e. Neuromuscular: lethargy and weakness, headache, confusion, agitation, dizziness, seizures
   f. Gastrointestinal: vomiting, diarrhea, abdominal cramps

Practice to Pass

The pathophysiologic effects of hyponatremia are most evident in which areas of the body?

2. Diagnostic and laboratory findings
   a. Plasma levels and urinary levels
      1) Plasma level less than 135 mEq/L
      2) Change in urine sodium level reflects the cause of the deficit; see Box 2-3 for procedure for collecting 24-hour urine sodium specimen
      3) Urine sodium levels > 20 mEq/L correlate to renal etiology or SIADH
      4) Urine sodium levels < 10 mEq/L correlate with edema etiology (CHF, cirrhosis, and nephrotic syndrome)
   b. Associated electrolyte and other levels
      1) Serum osmolality < 270 mOsm/kg
      2) Serum chloride may be decreased
      3) Urine specific gravity < 1.010 (except in SIADH)
      4) Decreased blood urea nitrogen (BUN), unless the cause is CHF, and hematocrit (Hct)
      5) An increase of 100 mg/dL in blood glucose will decrease serum sodium by 1.7 to 2.4 mEq/L
   c. Trending of results
      1) Identify primary cause of mechanism for sodium deficit
      2) Confirm compensatory response to sodium loss
      3) Determine client fluid balance status and response to treatment measures
3. Identification of risk factors
   a. Aging and gender variables
      1) Very young and older adult clients are more prone to sodium deficit
      2) There is an increased risk for development of acute hyponatremia in female clients and those with human immunodeficiency virus (HIV)
   b. Medications
      1) Obtain pertinent client history of medications that can alter sodium levels (refer again to Table 2-2 for a listing of medications that cause sodium deficit)
      2) Treatment measures that include intravenous solutions (such as D_5W), hypotonic fluids, irrigations, and tap water enema (TWE) as part of the therapeutic plan of care can lead to the development of hyponatremia

Box 2-3	• Obtain large urine collection container labeled with start and stop times.
Measurement of Urine Sodium (24-hour Specimen)	• Explain procedure to client and family to ensure all urine is placed in container.
	• Place container in refrigerator or on ice.
	• Instruct not to mix/contaminate specimen with bathroom tissue or feces.
	• Discard specimen voided at start time but save specimen voided at end time.

3) Clients undergoing operative procedures involving irrigations may develop hyponatremia (such as endometrial ablation and transurethral resection of the prostate [TURP])

   c. Dietary

     1) Prolonged NPO status

     2) Overcorrection with nonelectrolyte solutions, causing free water accumulation

   d. Medical disorders such as heart failure, cancer, or GI disorders

C. Priority nursing diagnoses: Risk for Excess Fluid Volume, Risk for Impaired Sensory/Perception, Risk for Injury, Risk for Impaired Oral Mucous Membranes, Impaired Mental Status, and Risk for Impaired Skin Integrity

D. Therapeutic management: treatment focuses on restoring normal levels, preventing complications, and treating underlying problems

  1. Replacement therapies

   a. Encourage inclusion of high-sodium foods in the diet

   b. Referral to a dietitian for assistance in meal planning and including adequate sources of sodium in the diet (refer to Box 2-4 for sodium food sources)

   c. If a client has hyponatremia with normal fluid volume (euvolemic), then use water restriction and treat the underlying cause to correct the deficit

   d. If a client has hyponatremia with hypovolemic volume, treat with normal saline (NS) or Lactated Ringer's (LR) solution to correct ECF deficit

   e. If a client has hyponatremia with hypertonic dehydration, treat with fluid restriction and treat the underlying cause to correct the deficit

   f. If a client requires irrigation (such as though a nasogastric tube) as a part of therapy, use of appropriate solutions (isotonic saline) should prevent further fluid shifting and sodium deficit

   g. A client with acute hyponatremia can be treated with 3% hypertonic saline (refer to physician order, pharmacy, and hospital protocols for rate of infusion) and loop diuretics to promote water excretion if indicated by the clinical picture

   h. Loop diuretics, sodium and fluid restrictions, and possibly dialysis may be utilized for fluid excess if the clinical picture dictates

  2. Continued monitoring of client

   a. Monitor laboratory results

   b. Keep accurate I&O (intake and output) records

   c. Obtain daily weights

   d. Perform neurological assessment; monitor for central nervous system changes, such as confusion, lethargy, and seizures, and maintain safe environment

   e. Monitor and document routes of fluid loss

  3. Restoration of balance

   a. Depending on acuity and severity of deficit, the client may present as asymptomatic or symptomatic; it is important to look both at the laboratory values and correlate them with the client's overall physical condition in order to maintain sodium and fluid balance

Practice to Pass

You are providing care to a client who is NPO and has intermittent nasogastric suctioning. What will you monitor for and why?

Box 2-4	The following foods are considered ample sources of sodium:
Sodium Food Sources	• Processed food products (highest sources of sodium in the diet; e.g., canned food, especially soups)
	• Ham, bacon, and pork products (high-sodium levels)
	• Dill pickles, corned beef, and products that are "pickled" in brine solutions
	• Potato chips
	• Anchovies, mackerel, and other saltwater fish products

b. If client's sodium deficit is acute and symptomatic, prompt management should be initiated

   1) Follow physician prescription, pharmacy, and hospital protocol for rate of infusion and length of therapy

   2) It is critical to raise sodium levels per established protocols as cerebral cell adaptation can cause further complications

   3) A target goal of 120 to 125 mEq/L should be aimed for, and sodium levels should be raised no more than 25 mEq/L in the first 48 hours with a rate not to exceed 1 to 2 mEq/L/hr

c. It is important to identify and treat the underlying cause in order to prevent reoccurrence of deficit and restore sodium and fluid balance

E. Planning and implementation

1. Monitor pertinent client assessment data for potential effects related to hyponatremia and for response to treatment

   a. Assess for confusion, changes in the level of consciousness, and seizures

   b. As the clinical condition progresses, signs and symptoms may become more acute, ranging from anorexia, nausea, and lethargy in the early phase to disorientation, agitation, focal neurological deficits, coma, and seizures in the advanced phase

2. Protect the client from injury and maintain a safe environment if client experiences neurological changes due to hyponatremia

3. Employ dietary interventions to promote normal sodium levels

   a. Encourage use of high-sodium foods in the diet

   b. Give appropriate amounts of fluids in the diet to prevent dehydration

   c. Avoid caffeinated beverages (such as coffee, tea, sodas)

4. Provide replacement therapy as ordered by physician paying attention to baseline laboratory results, client's response, and therapeutic benefits

   a. Keep accurate fluid I&O records looking at shift and 24-hour totals to determine fluid balance

   b. Depending on acuity and severity, hourly monitoring may be indicated

   c. Weigh client daily, at same time using same scale and in similar clothing

   d. A weight loss of > 0.5 pounds in 24 hours is considered to be due to fluid loss

F. Medication therapy

1. Oral replacement therapy

   a. Salt tablets can be used to correct sodium deficits

   b. There are numerous medications that contain sodium (refer again to Table 2-2 for medications that can affect sodium levels)

   c. Depending on the nature of volume status, diuretic therapy may either be restricted (such as no thiazide diuretics because they promote ADH activity) or used (loop diuretics) to promote fluid loss in order to maintain sodium balance

2. Parenteral replacement therapy

   a. LR or 0.9% sodium chloride (NS) can be used to treat hyponatremia with isotonic dehydration

   b. 3% or 5% hypertonic saline can be used to treat clients with a more severe deficit

3. Dietary therapy

   a. Encourage foods high in sodium, such as bacon, cheese, and table salt

   b. Judiciously use processed foods and foods containing preservatives as one way to add sodium to the diet

G. Client education

1. Awareness of predisposing factors

   a. Older adult and very young clients are at risk for hyponatremia due to potential fluid volume disturbances

   b. Fluid restriction, if applicable

c. Teach clients to recognize environmental conditions (heat and humidity) that may increase sodium and fluid loss and to use appropriate oral replacement therapies to prevent further electrolyte depletion

d. Daily weight!

 2. Dietary education

a. Provide a list of foods that are high in sodium during client education

b. Collaborate with dietitian

3. Teach clients to report early signs and symptoms of hyponatremia such as abdominal cramps, muscle weakness, and nausea

4. Teach clients and family members to report changes in mental status, especially if the client already has contributory medical conditions such as cardiac, renal, and endocrine problems that might exacerbate hyponatremia

H. Evaluation

1. Serum sodium level returns to a normal range (135–145 mEq/L)

2. Client is alert and oriented to time, place, and person

3. Client is free of any signs or symptoms of hyponatremia

4. Client is euvolemic

5. Vital signs are within normal limits

6. Mucous membranes are moist and intact

7. Client remains free from injury

III. HYPERNATREMIA: SERUM SODIUM LEVEL ABOVE 145 MEQ/L

A. Etiology and pathophysiology

1. Cellular-level transport

a. Sodium excess always exists in a **hyperosmolar** (osmotic pressure greater than normal plasma pressure) state

b. Sodium excess can exist in hypovolemic, euvolemic, and hypervolemic states (see Table 2-4 for summary of this disorder)

c. To restore equilibrium between the ECF and the ICF, water will shift from the ICF to the ECF, which results in cellular shrinkage/dehydration (refer back to Figure 2-1b)

 d. Cerebral cells respond to high-sodium levels by shrinking as the osmotic pressure drives fluid out of the cells leading to a decreased brain volume

Table 2-4	**Hypernatremia in Various Fluid Volume States**		
	Description	**Clinical Presentation**	**Treatment**
Euvolemia	Decrease in water that leads to elevation of serum sodium levels Does not present with contracted volume unless there is a severe water loss	Increased fluid loss via skin or lungs (hyperventilation)	Free water replacement either orally or by fluid-hydrating solutions
Hypervolemia	Greater gain of sodium in relation to fluids that leads to elevation of serum sodium levels	Seen with administration of hypertonic saline solutions or $NaHCO_3$, in primary hyperaldosteronism or hypertonic dehydration	Remove sodium source, administer diuretics, and replace water
Hypovolemia	Greater loss of water than sodium, leading to elevation of serum sodium levels	Renal losses with osmotic diuresis, diabetes insipidus (DI), insensible loss with sweating and/or fever, GI losses with diarrhea Young and older adult clients are more prone to develop this	Normal saline to correct intravascular volume deficit, then hypotonic fluids can be used to restore sodium level

Note: All hypernatremic states are hyperosmolar.

        e. High serum sodium levels lead to an increase in neurological activity

        f. In response to high-sodium levels, the thirst mechanism is stimulated

    2. Predisposing clinical conditions

        a. Clients who have disturbances in water regulation such as decreased intake, increased insensible loss, or watery diarrhea are prone to develop hypernatremia

        b. Clients who experience water loss due to fever, hyperventilation, diuretic therapy, hypertonic tube feedings, and burns are prone to develop hypernatremia

        c. Clients who have increased sodium intake either due to dietary intake or infusion of sodium fluids are prone to develop hypernatremia

        d. Clients who have renal losses or disease/hormonal states such as Cushing's syndrome (increased cortisol production) or **diabetes insipidus** or **DI** (a defect in ADH secretion causing sodium retention and increased secretion of a dilute urine) are prone to develop hypernatremia (refer to Box 2-5 for more information on DI)

        e. Clients who experience near drowning in salt water are at risk for developing hypernatremia

B. Assessment

    1. Clinical manifestations

        a. Common signs are related to the water shift from the cells (cellular dehydration) into the vascular space and sodium's role in nerve impulse transmission and muscle contraction

        b. Cardiovascular: tachycardia, hypertension, decreased cardiac contractility

        c. Integument: dry and sticky mucous membranes, rough, dry tongue, flushed skin that has poor turgor and tenting

        d. Renal: thirst, increased urine output

        e. Neuromuscular: twitching, tremor and hyperreflexia, agitation, hallucinations, central nervous system irritability, seizures, coma; worsening hypernatremia can result in hyporeflexia, paralysis, and coma

        f. Gastrointestinal: watery diarrhea, nausea, thirst

        g. Clients whose levels rise slowly may be asymptomatic for some time

Box 2-5 **Diabetes Insipidus (DI)**	• DI is characterized by decreased secretion of ADH or failure to respond to ADH secretion due to malignancies, excessive water intake, medications (demeclocycline and lithium), and genetic defects. • DI can be further classified as central (insufficient production) or nephrogenic (related to decreased renal sensitivity). • Plasma osmolality is increased, urine osmolality and specific gravity are decreased; water deprivation test reveals inability to concentrate urine. • Hypernatremia is present. • Clients present with polyuria (increased dilute urine) and polydipsia (increased thirst). • Treatment for central DI consists of desmopressin acetate (DDAVP) nasal spray administration or, if critically ill, vasopressin IV. • Treatment for nephrogenic DI consists of a low-salt diet and thiazide diuretics to increase sodium excretion, as well as fluid replacement. • Assessing I&O is critical to clients with this disorder. • Complications of treatment: therapy can lead to water intoxication so client must be closely monitored by looking at labs/diagnostics and performing frequent physical assessment. • Continued monitoring of fluid status upon discharge is necessary for clients who experience this type of disorder so as to prevent further recurrences. • Correction of underlying disorder and recognition of clients at risk in the clinical setting will lead to better client outcomes.

2. Diagnostic and laboratory findings
   a. Plasma levels and urinary levels
      1) Plasma levels greater than 145 mEq/L
      2) May see increased urine output
   b. Associated electrolyte and other levels
      1) Chloride may be elevated
      2) Serum osmolality greater than 290 mOsm/kg
      3) Urinary specific gravity (SG) greater than 1.015 unless diabetes insipidus is present, leading to dilute urine with SG of less than 1.005
      4) Increased BUN and Hct
   c. Trending of results
      1) Identify primary cause of sodium excess
      2) Confirm compensatory response to sodium excess
      3) Determine client fluid balance status and response to treatment measures
3. Identification of risk factors
   a. Age-related risk factors (see also Table 2-5)
      1) Very young clients can be at risk for fluid deprivation due to poor nutritional care or having an activity level that overlooks hydration (so busy playing that they don't eat or drink enough)
      2) Older adult clients are at risk due to decreased thirst mechanism and renal functioning
      3) Infant clients can be placed at risk due to improper reconstitution, usage, and storage of prepared formula
   b. Medications
      1) Obtain pertinent client history of medications because some medications have hidden sodium, and the client may not be aware of this (refer again to Table 2-2 for a listing of medications that can affect sodium levels)
      2) OTC medications with high-sodium content such as Alka-Seltzer, cough syrups, and aspirin may contribute to increased sodium levels
      3) Treatment measures that include the use of sodium, such as sodium bicarbonate administration during a code, use of hypertonic saline solutions, and saline-induced abortions, can contribute to increased sodium levels
      4) Clients who receive medical treatment with cortisone therapy, loop diuretics, or who experience saltwater ingestion can have increased sodium levels

Table 2-5 Lifespan Considerations for Health Maintenance: Hypernatremia

Lifespan Considerations	Fluids	Electrolytes	Acid–Base Balance
Infants	Breastfeeding (colostrum); formula (Similac Advance, Enfamil Lipil); whole milk	Sodium (Na^+) is essential for fluid balance, nerve and muscle function	Acid–base imbalance in infants is primarily due to respiratory disorders related to respiratory insufficiency
Pediatrics	Increase water intake; do not give undiluted formula concentrate or evaporated milk due to high-sodium content; popsicles, both hypotonic and isotonic fluids	Monitor for diarrhea, vomiting, and excessive sweating without fluid replacement	Isotonic fluids may be ordered first to replenish the volume, followed by hypotonic fluid to correct the osmolality
Adults	Hypotonic and isotonic fluids; increase water intake	Sodium is the most abundant electrolyte in the ECF; increased risk: heart failure, tuberculosis, cirrhosis, head injury, surgical clients	Central nervous system is especially affected, resulting in signs of neurological impairment (e.g., restlessness, weakness, disorientation, delusion, and hallucinations)

   c. Dietary
      1) Diet that contains large amount of salt
      2) Use of salt as a flavoring agent in the diet can contribute to increased sodium levels as the diet normally contains adequate salt
C. Priority nursing diagnoses: Risk for Injury, Risk for Deficient Fluid Volume, Impaired Physical Mobility, Risk for Impaired Sensory/Perception, Risk for Impaired Oral Mucous Membranes
D. Therapeutic management: treatment focuses on restoring normal levels, preventing complications, and treating underlying problems
   1. Decrease sodium intake
      a. Restrict sodium use in the diet; restrictions vary depending on severity of clinical condition and may be set at 3 grams, 2 grams, 1 gram, or 500 mg/day
      b. Adhere to sodium restrictions in treatment plan
      c. Refer client to a dietitian to evaluate dietary intake for hidden sodium sources
   2. Promote sodium excretion
      a. If a client has hypernatremia with normal fluid volume (euvolemic), then use water replacement and treat the underlying cause to promote sodium loss
      b. If a client has hypernatremia with hypovolemia, treat with NS initially to correct the intravascular deficit
      c. If a client has hypernatremia with hypervolemia, remove source of sodium excess, administer diuretics, and replace water as needed
   3. Continued monitoring of client
      a. Monitor laboratory results
      b. Keep accurate I&O records, assessing for trends
      c. Obtain daily weights at the same time using same equipment and similar clothing in order to accurately trend results
      d. Assess central nervous system for neurological changes such as agitation, hallucinations, and seizures, and maintain a safe environment
   4. Restoration of balance
      a. With hypernatremia, it is important to use a gradual reduction to restore serum sodium levels to normal, as cerebral cells are both adaptive and sensitive to changes in sodium levels
      b. The usual protocol with chronic hypernatremia is to correct 50% of calculated water deficit in the first 12 to 24 hours with the remainder corrected in one to two days; follow physician order and pharmacy and hospital protocols as directed when correcting hypernatremia in the clinical setting
      c. It is important to look at the volume status of the client before and during attempts to restore sodium balance in order to prevent further complications
      d. If the client has hypernatremia as a result of solute excess, then the use of diuretics with water replacement may be warranted
      e. It is important to identify and treat the underlying cause in order to prevent recurrence of excess and to restore sodium and fluid balance
E. Planning and implementation
   1. Monitor pertinent client assessment data for potential effects related to hypernatremia and for response to treatment
      a. Serum sodium levels and plasma osmolality
      b. Urine sodium levels and urine osmolality
      c. Monitor neurological status closely as client is likely to have CNS irritability, possibly leading to seizures
   2. Maintain safe environment as a result of CNS irritability and risk of seizure activity; initiate seizure precautions
   3. Dietary interventions to decrease sodium levels
      a. Place client on a salt-restricted diet (refer to Box 2-6)
      b. Refer client to a dietitian as needed to assist with dietary measures

Box 2-6	The following interventions should be employed when following a sodium-restricted diet:
Sodium-Restricted Diet Instructions	• Do not routinely add salt to foods prior to tasting. • The physician should order the amount of sodium restriction as there can be confusion between following a low-sodium diet and a sodium-restricted diet. A restricted diet can range from a severe restriction (500 mg) to a mild restriction (3000–4000 mg). • Limit or avoid use of bottled or canned sauce products, as they are usually higher in sodium than homemade preparations. • Use pure herbs, seasonings, and wine in cooking preparation, as many "seasoned" products and cooking wine contain sodium. • When eating outside the home at restaurants, have food items prepared without salt. • Eat freshly prepared bakery products; commercially prepared and frozen products contain more sodium due to processing and use of preservative agents. • Be aware that artificial sweeteners used in soft drinks and other products can contain additional sodium. Limit your intake of such products. • There are a wide range of "low-sodium" and "sodium-free" products available. Learn to read and interpret nutrition labels so as to make wise food selections.

4. Provide therapy as ordered by physician, paying attention to baseline labs, client's response, and therapeutic benefits
5. Assess I&O
   a. Keep accurate fluid I&O records looking at shift and 24-hour totals to determine fluid balance
   b. Depending on acuity and severity, hourly monitoring may be indicated
   c. Weigh client on daily basis using the same equipment and similar clothing
   d. Weight gain can be a consequence of fluid retention from hypernatremia, which could lead to further clinical compromise

Practice to Pass

In caring for a client with hypernatremia, what should the nurse do to help ensure client safety?

F. **Medication therapy**
1. Diuretic therapy
   a. Loop diuretics can be used to treat sodium excess
   b. Thiazide diuretics can be used in the treatment of diabetes insipidus
2. Parenteral administration of fluids
   a. NS to correct intravascular volume deficit
   b. D_5W solution can be used once volume deficit has been restored
3. Dietary restrictions
   a. Limit sodium intake
   b. Use low-sodium foods and fluids
G. **Client education**
1. Awareness of predisposing factors
   a. Older adult clients are also at risk for hypernatremia due to limited mobility, multiple medication profile, and restricted access to fluids
   b. Teach clients potential signs and symptoms of hypernatremia and have them report problems to their health care provider
2. Dietary education (refer again to Box 2-6)
   a. Teach clients about the daily sodium requirement needed in the diet along with proper fluid management; the majority of individuals ingest a daily intake above the needed RDA
   b. Teach clients about the sodium content of foods and the sources of hidden sodium in the diet
   c. Teach client to follow a low-sodium diet after discharge
   d. Teach client to read all labels for sodium content prior to ingestion

e. Teach client to use herbs, lemon juice, spices, and vinegar instead of salt to season foods; salt substitutes are useful but should be avoided by clients with impaired renal function because they contain potassium
  f. Teach clients not to routinely salt their food prior to tasting

H. Evaluation
1. Serum sodium level returns to normal range (between 135 and 145 mEq/L)
2. Client is free of any signs or symptoms of hypernatremia
3. Client is alert and oriented to time, place, and person
4. Client is euvolemic
5. Vital signs are within normal limits
6. Client remains free from injury

Case Study

A 45-year-old construction company owner was brought from work to the emergency department reporting dizziness, nausea, weakness, abdominal cramps, and headache. During the admission assessment, the following information was obtained:

- *Onset of symptoms occurred three days ago but were mild until today when client stated that he "almost fell off a building at work."*
- *Previously diagnosed with hypertension (HTN) six weeks ago.*
- *Has been following a low-sodium diet and has been taking hydrochlorothiazide (Hydrodiuril) as directed since being diagnosed six weeks ago.*

1. What does the initial data provided by the client suggest?
2. What questions will you ask of the client prior to performing your physical examination?
3. What data do you expect your physical assessment to reveal?
4. What do you expect the laboratory tests to reveal?
5. What discharge teaching would be important to perform?

For suggested responses, see pages 202–203.

POSTTEST

1 When assessing a client with diabetes insipidus (DI), the nurse expects to find which of the following?

1. Nausea and vomiting
2. Polyuria and polydipsia
3. Dysuria
4. Confusion

2 A client receiving treatment for hypernatremia is being monitored for signs and symptoms of complications of therapy. The nurse would assess this client for which of the following?

1. Cellular dehydration
2. Cerebral edema
3. Red blood cell (RBC) destruction
4. Renal shutdown

3 A client is semiconscious and restless, and exhibits tremors and muscle weakness. Physical examination reveals a dry, swollen tongue and a body temperature of 99.8°F. The nurse anticipates that the serum sodium value for this client is most likely to be which of the following?

1. 120 mEq/L
2. 132 mEq/L
3. 142 mEq/L
4. 155 mEq/L

4 A client was brought to the hospital following a near-drowning experience in the Atlantic Ocean. In providing care to this client, the nurse plans to carefully monitor for which of the following?

1. Hypernatremia
2. Hyponatremia
3. Hypocalcemia
4. Hypercalcemia

5 When caring for an adult client diagnosed with hyponatremia, the nurse plans to restrict which of the following?

1. Water
2. Sodium
3. Potassium
4. Chloride

6 Which of the following manifestations should the nurse assess for when developing a plan of care for a client with hypernatremia?

1. Muscle weakness
2. Moist mucous membranes
3. Subnormal temperature
4. Complaints of thirst

7 The nurse is providing care to a client with syndrome of inappropriate antidiuretic hormone (SIADH). What should the nurse explain to the unlicensed assistant about water intake?

1. It should be encouraged
2. It should be restricted
3. It is given according to the client's preference
4. It is given via intravenous fluids only

8 A client with a diagnosis of bipolar disorder has been drinking copious amounts of water and voiding frequently. The client is experiencing a bounding pulse and confusion and is reporting a headache. The nurse checks laboratory test results for which of the following?

1. Low platelet count
2. Low-sodium level
3. High serum osmolality
4. High urine specific gravity

9 A client with a feeding tube has been experiencing severe watery diarrhea. The client is lethargic with decreased skin turgor, a pulse rate of 110, and hyperactive reflexes. The nurse would include which of the following interventions on the client's plan of care? Select all that apply.

1. Monitor and record intake, output, and daily weights
2. Administer salt tablets
3. Withhold tube feedings until diarrhea subsides
4. Avoid adding additional water before and after tube feedings
5. Initiate seizure precautions

10 The nurse assigned to a client with hyponatremia would conclude that which of the following client factors probably contributed to this electrolyte imbalance? Select all that apply.

1. Osmotic diuretic therapy
2. Fever
3. Fluid retention
4. Excessive hypertonic intravenous infusion
5. Heart failure

➤ *See pages 51–53 for Answers and Rationales.*

ANSWERS & RATIONALES

Pretest

1 **Answer: 3, 4 Rationale:** The combination of high fever and severe dehydration leads to insensible water loss. This indicates a loss of pure water and does not contain electrolytes. Therefore, excessive amounts of insensible water loss result in a hypertonic dehydration that leads to a state of hypernatremia and hyperchloremia. Calcium levels usually decrease in the presence of dehydration and fever. Phosphate levels usually increase in the presence of dehydration and fever. Potassium levels can usually remain normal in the serum and are increased in the urine. **Cognitive Level:** Applying **Client Need:** Physiological Adaptation **Integrated Process:** Nursing Process: Assessment **Content Area:** Child Health **Strategy:** The critical words in this question are *imbalance, high fever,* and *severe dehydration.* Systematically eliminate options containing an imbalance not associated with water losses and dehydration. **Reference:** LeMone, P., & Burke, K. (2008). *Medical surgical nursing: Critical thinking in client care* (4th ed.). Upper Saddle River, NJ: Pearson Education, pp. 213–217.

2 Answer: 1 Rationale: The use of corticosteroids can lead to the development of hypernatremia because they cause sodium to be retained and potassium to be excreted. The elderly client drinking eight glasses of water each day is within a normal range of fluid intake and is not at risk for developing sodium imbalances. The diabetic client whose blood glucose is within normal range is not at risk for developing sodium imbalances. The teenager who is using Gatorade as an oral replacement therapy to compensate for fluid and electrolyte loss during exercise is not at risk for developing sodium imbalances. **Cognitive Level:** Analyzing **Client Need:** Physiological Adaptation **Integrated Process:** Nursing Process: Assessment **Content Area:** Adult Health **Strategy:** The critical word *most* indicates all or some of the options are correct, but one will have a greater influence on creating the imbalance. Eliminate one option because it is not an abnormal amount of water to consume. Eliminate another as it is not associated with sodium, and a third because the client is young and better able to accommodate an imbalance. **Reference:** LeMone, P., & Burke, K. (2008). *Medical surgical nursing: Critical thinking in client care* (4th ed.). Upper Saddle River, NJ: Pearson/Prentice Hall, pp. 213–217.

3 Answer: 1 Rationale: The thirst mechanism is decreased in older adults and would normally serve as a compensatory mechanism to provide water intake. Aldosterone production would be decreased in the presence of hypernatremia. Muscle mass may be reduced in older adults but the decreased thirst poses a greater risk. ADH is still produced. **Cognitive Level:** Analyzing **Client Need:** Reduction of Risk Potential **Integrated Process:** Nursing Process: Assessment **Content Area:** Adult Health **Strategy:** Critical items to note include an older adult client, hypernatremia, and risk for dehydration. Knowledge of compensatory mechanisms of fluid balance is required to answer this question. **Reference:** LeMone, P., & Burke, K. (2008). *Medical surgical nursing: Critical thinking in client care* (4th ed.). Upper Saddle River, NJ: Pearson/Prentice Hall, pp. 213–217.

4 Answer: 3 Rationale: Clients with hypernatremia (normal 135–145 mEq/L) should be assessed for potential development of neurological complications such as seizures. Blankets are not needed because temperature is often elevated with hypernatremia. Malaise and nausea are symptoms of hyponatremia. Clients with hypernatremia have an increased need for fluids, not a

decreased need. **Cognitive Level:** Analyzing **Client Need:** Reduction of Risk Potential **Integrated Process:** Nursing Process: Implementation **Content Area:** Adult Health **Strategy:** The core concept of the question is knowledge of interventions that are necessary when a client has hypernatremia. Recall high-sodium levels cause temperature elevations to eliminate one option, and eliminate another because fluids need to be encouraged. Remember that seizures are a risk with high-sodium levels in order to choose correctly between the remaining two options. **Reference:** LeMone, P., & Burke, K. (2008). *Medical surgical nursing: Critical thinking in client care* (4th ed.). Upper Saddle River, NJ: Pearson/Prentice Hall, pp. 213–217.

5 Answer: 1, 2, 3, 4 Rationale: Processed foods and some baking products contain sodium. Clients need to be taught to look for products containing sodium as part of the ingredient. Monosodium glutamate has the word *sodium* as part of its name. Many over-the-counter cough, cold, and flu remedies contain sodium. Canned goods often contain sodium and these food labels should be read carefully. Salad oil is typically low in sodium and is a good diet option. **Cognitive Level:** Applying **Client Need:** Health Promotion and Maintenance **Integrated Process:** Teaching and Learning **Content Area:** Adult Health **Strategy:** Recall knowledge of foods or products containing sodium. The wording of the question indicates that more than one option is correct. **Reference:** Dudek, S. (2010). *Nutrition essentials for nursing practice* (6th ed.). Philadelphia: Lippincott Williams & Wilkins, p. 124.

6 Answer: 1 Rationale: As sodium levels decrease, fluid shifts in the brain can lead to cerebral edema and seizures. Clients should be assessed for headaches, lethargy, decreased responsiveness, and seizure activity. Hyponatremia will also cause weakness and fatigue, and the client needs to conserve energy, but neurological status is of highest priority. Energy conservation is important with fatigue, but is not the greatest concern at this time. Oral and skin care are routine aspects of care. **Cognitive Level:** Analyzing **Client Need:** Physiological Adaptation **Integrated Process:** Nursing Process: Planning **Content Area:** Adult Health **Strategy:** Critical words are *highest priority,* indicating all options will be appropriate, but one is more important. Note similarity in two options to eliminate them. Choose correctly, recalling neurological status is higher priority than skin care. **Reference:** LeMone, P., & Burke, K. (2008). *Medical surgical nursing: Critical thinking in client care* (4th ed.). Upper Saddle River, NJ: Pearson/Prentice Hall, pp. 213–217.

7 Answer: 4 Rationale: SIADH is caused by excessive production of ADH or an ADH-like substance, resulting in decreased serum sodium and hypervolemia. Loop diuretics are given to promote diuresis. Oral fluids are restricted due to hypervolemia. Dietary sodium is encouraged. Hypertonic or isotonic intravenous solutions are administered to provide needed sodium.

Cognitive Level: Analyzing Client Need: Physiological Adaptation Integrated Process: Nursing Process: Planning Content Area: Adult Health Strategy: The concept being tested is knowledge of SIADH. Recall the client experiences fluid retention and sodium losses to eliminate incorrect options. Reference: LeMone, P., & Burke, K. (2008). *Medical surgical nursing: Critical thinking in client care* (4th ed.). Upper Saddle River, NJ: Pearson/Prentice Hall, pp. 213–217.

8 Answer: 290 Rationale: An estimate of serum osmolality is obtained by multiplying the sodium level by two. The normal range of sodium is 135 to 145. If the highest normal sodium value is 145, then the highest normal serum osmolality should be no higher than 290. Cognitive Level: Applying Client Need: Reduction of Risk Potential Integrated Process: Nursing Process: Assessment Content Area: Adult Health Strategy: Recall normal serum sodium level and multiply by two. Reference: LeMone, P., & Burke, K. (2008). *Medical surgical nursing: Critical thinking in client care* (4th ed.). Upper Saddle River, NJ: Pearson/Prentice Hall, p. 213.

9 Answer: 1 Rationale: Cheese can be high in sodium and ham is high in sodium because it is cured as a preservative process. The addition of these types of foods will supply extra sodium in the diet. Chicken salad on lettuce is lower in sodium content. Tossed salad with vinegar dressing is not high in sodium. White fish and plain baked potato do not provide excessive sodium. Cognitive Level: Applying Client Need: Health Promotion and Maintenance Integrated Process: Nursing Process: Implementation Content Area: Adult Health Strategy: The question requires knowledge of sodium content of foods. Note foods high in sodium is the correct answer. Choose the first option because processed and preserved foods contain a lot of sodium. Reference: Dudek, S. (2010). *Nutrition essentials for nursing practice* (6th ed.). Philadelphia: Lippincott, Williams & Wilkins, pp. 126–127.

10 Answer: 2 Rationale: Hyponatremia is caused by an excess of water, which dilutes the amount of sodium present in the plasma, leading to a fluid volume excess (FVE). It is important to restrict additional fluids as they can further increase the sodium deficit. In addition, the client already is an FVE state, which can lead to development of further disturbances of fluid balance. Hypotonic fluids would further complicate the hyponatremia. Sodium usually does not need to be replaced in dilutional states. When the excess fluid is removed, the sodium is often within normal range. Tap water is a hypotonic fluid and hypotonic fluids would further complicate the hyponatremia. Cognitive Level: Applying Client Need: Physiological Adaptation Integrated Process: Nursing Process: Planning Content Area: Adult Health Strategy: The critical word is *dilutional*. Eliminate two options because additional water is not needed. Eliminate a third option because additional sodium is not needed. Reference: LeMone, P., & Burke, K. (2008). *Medical

surgical nursing: Critical thinking in client care* (4th ed.). Upper Saddle River, NJ: Pearson/Prentice Hall, pp. 213–217.

Posttest

1 Answer: 2 Rationale: DI is characterized by a decrease in ADH secretion, resulting in loss of fluids through polyuria. Polyuria in turn leads to increased thirst. Nausea and vomiting are not characteristic of DI. Dysuria would occur with a disorder or infection of the bladder. Confusion has many causes, but DI is not among them. Cognitive Level: Applying Client Need: Physiological Adaptation Integrated Process: Nursing Process: Assessment Content Area: Adult Health Strategy: Recall physiology of DI. If you have trouble recalling information, a clue might be the common word *diabetes*—although diabetes mellitus is different from diabetes insipidus, they share the common symptoms of polyuria and polydipsia. Reference: LeMone, P., & Burke, K. (2008). *Medical surgical nursing: Critical thinking in client care* (4th ed.). Upper Saddle River, NJ: Pearson/Prentice Hall, pp. 213–217.

2 Answer: 2 Rationale: Too rapid a correction of hypernatremia can lead to changes in vascular tone, which can affect blood vessels and cause increased fluid entry into the brain, thereby causing cerebral edema. Cellular dehydration is caused by hypernatremia. RBC destruction is not viewed as a risk when treating hypernatremia. Renal shutdown could be of concern because of the original state of hypernatremia but not because of treatment. Cognitive Level: Analyzing Client Need: Physiological Adaptation Integrated Process: Nursing Process: Assessment Content Area: Adult Health Strategy: Critical words are *hypernatremia* and *complications*. Note the question addresses the complications of treatment. Recall treatment involves fluid replacement and increasing risks of fluid shifts to choose option correctly. Reference: LeMone, P., & Burke, K. (2008). *Medical surgical nursing: Critical thinking in client care* (4th ed.). Upper Saddle River, NJ: Pearson/Prentice Hall, pp. 215–217.

3 Answer: 4 Rationale: This client has signs and symptoms of hypernatremia, and the serum sodium level of 155 mEq/L matches the expected value, which would be greater than 145 mEq/L. A value of 120 mEq/L indicates a significant state of hyponatremia, which does not match the client's symptoms. This reflects a mild decrease in serum sodium levels and is not consistent with the client's symptoms. A value of 142 mEq/L reflects a normal serum sodium level. Cognitive Level: Applying Client Need: Reduction of Risk Potential Integrated Process: Nursing Process: Assessment Content Area: Adult Health Strategy: Recognize that symptoms in the question reflect hypernatremia. Systematically eliminate options less than 145 mEq/L. Reference: LeMone, P.,

& Burke, K. (2008). *Medical surgical nursing: Critical thinking in client care* (4th ed.). Upper Saddle River, NJ: Pearson/Prentice Hall, p. 215.

4 **Answer: 1** **Rationale:** Near drowning in saltwater often results in hypernatremia due to the high-sodium level in sea/saltwater. Hyponatremia and disturbances in calcium levels are not seen in this clinical situation. Hyponatremia may be seen in fresh water near drowning. Hypocalcemia is not the concern in this clinical situation. Hyerpcalcemia is not seen in this clinical situation. **Cognitive Level:** Applying **Client Need:** Physiological Adaptation **Integrated Process:** Nursing Process: Assessment **Content Area:** Adult Health **Strategy:** Critical words are *near drowning* and *ocean*, indicating ingestion of salt water. Recognize this constitutes a sodium load to choose correctly. **Reference:** LeMone, P., & Burke, K. (2008). *Medical surgical nursing: Critical thinking in client care* (4th ed.). Upper Saddle River, NJ: Pearson/ Prentice Hall, pp. 215–217.

5 **Answer: 1** **Rationale:** In hyponatremia, water is already present in an excessive amount compared to the amount of sodium present. This can result in water intoxication or dilutional hyponatremia; therefore, water restriction is a primary cornerstone of therapy. Sodium should not be restricted but rather should be included in the treatment plan to prevent further electrolyte imbalances from occurring. Potassium should not be restricted but rather should be included in the treatment plan so as to prevent further electrolyte imbalances from occurring. Chloride intake usually accompanies sodium intake. **Cognitive Level:** Applying **Client Need:** Physiological Adaptation **Integrated Process:** Nursing Process: Planning **Content Area:** Adult Health **Strategy:** The critical word is *restrict*. Recall dangers related to further dilution of sodium to choose correctly. **Reference:** LeMone, P., & Burke, K. (2008). *Medical surgical nursing: Critical thinking in client care* (4th ed.). Upper Saddle River, NJ: Pearson/ Prentice Hall, pp. 214–215.

6 **Answer: 4** **Rationale:** Thirst is a primary indicator of sodium excess (hypernatremia) and should be assessed for in a plan of care for a client with hypernatremia. Muscle weakness is not reflective of hypernatremia but is more likely to be found with a sodium deficit. The presence of moist mucous membranes is a normal parameter. An elevated temperature would be expected with hypernatremia. **Cognitive Level:** Applying **Client Need:** Physiological Adaptation **Integrated Process:** Nursing Process: Assessment **Content Area:** Adult Health **Strategy:** Critical words are *manifestations* and *hypernatremia*. Recall the primary compensatory mechanism for fluid balance to choose correctly. **Reference:** LeMone, P., & Burke, K. (2008). *Medical surgical nursing: Critical thinking in client care* (4th ed.). Upper Saddle River, NJ: Pearson/Prentice Hall, p. 95.

7 **Answer: 2** **Rationale:** In SIADH, the antidiuretic hormone is present in excess amounts. This causes excessive water reabsorption. Water must be restricted to avoid water

intoxication. Giving additional fluids would only further serve to increase fluid levels and increase sodium deficit. While it is important to consider a client's preference in fluid selection, fluid restriction is the major priority. While fluid therapy can be given via IV, it is important to allow the client to take PO fluids even if they are on a restricted basis. **Cognitive Level:** Applying **Client Need:** Management of Care **Integrated Process:** Nursing Process: Implementation **Content Area:** Adult Health **Strategy:** The question addresses the relationship between water and SIADH. Note the incorrect options are similar in that all provide fluids in some form; therefore, these should be eliminated. **Reference:** LeMone, P., & Burke, K. (2008). *Medical surgical nursing: Critical thinking in client care* (4th ed.). Upper Saddle River, NJ: Pearson/Prentice Hall, pp. 213–215.

8 **Answer: 2** **Rationale:** The client has consumed excessive amounts of water, which is hypotonic and contributes to fluid intoxication, and is actually exhibiting signs of hyponatremia. The nurse would check the electrolyte levels, expecting to find a low-sodium level. Monitoring the CBC for a platelet level is not indicated, as there is no correlation between sodium levels and platelet activity. The client's serum osmolality would be low due to water intoxication. The client's urine specific gravity is expected to be low because of water intoxication. **Cognitive Level:** Applying **Client Need:** Physiological Adaptation **Integrated Process:** Nursing Process: Assessment **Content Area:** Adult Health **Strategy:** Recognize that symptoms are reflective of a fluid volume excess and hyponatremia to choose correctly. **Reference:** LeMone, P., & Burke, K. (2008). *Medical surgical nursing: Critical thinking in client care* (4th ed.). Upper Saddle River, NJ: Pearson/Prentice Hall, pp. 213–215.

9 **Answer: 1, 5** **Rationale:** The client is exhibiting signs of hypernatremia and dehydration. Appropriate nursing interventions are to measure and record I&O (intake and output) and daily weight. The client is at risk to develop seizures secondary to an elevated sodium level. Administering salt tablets would further contribute to the client's hypernatremic state. Restricting fluid intake and holding feedings could worsen the hypernatremia and fluid volume deficit (hypertonic dehydration) as the client already has extensive fluid loss due to diarrhea, elevated pulse rate, and decreased skin turgor. Avoiding adding additional water would worsen the hypertonic dehydration. **Cognitive Level:** Analyzing **Client Need:** Reduction of Risk Potential **Integrated Process:** Nursing Process: Implementation **Content Area:** Adult Health **Strategy:** Recognize that symptoms reflect dehydration and hypernatremia. Eliminate two options because fluids need to be replaced. Eliminate a third option because additional salt is not needed. **Reference:** LeMone, P., & Burke, K. (2008). *Medical surgical nursing: Critical thinking in client care* (4th ed.). Upper Saddle River, NJ: Pearson/Prentice Hall, pp. 213–217.

ANSWERS & RATIONALES

10 **Answer: 3, 5** **Rationale:** Fluid retention can result in hyponatremia through a dilutional effect. Fluid is retained in heart failure leading to dilutional hyponatremia. Osmotic diuretic therapy could lead to hypernatremia. Fever could result in hypernatremia secondary to increased metabolism and loss of free water. Excessive hypertonic intravenous infusion would lead to hypernatremia. **Cognitive Level:** Applying **Client Need:** Physiological Adaptation **Integrated Process:** Nursing Process: Assessment **Content Area:** Adult Health **Strategy:** Analyze options to identify potential for sodium losses or dilution. Eliminate two options since more water than sodium is lost. Eliminate a third option since sodium would be gained. **Reference:** LeMone, P., & Burke, K. (2008). *Medical surgical nursing: Critical thinking in client care* (4th ed.). Upper Saddle River, NJ: Pearson/Prentice Hall, pp. 213–217.

References

Ball, J., Bindler, R., & Cowen, K. (2010). *Child health nursing: Partnering with children and families* (2nd ed.). Upper Saddle River, NJ: Pearson Education.

Berman, A., & Snyder, S. (2012). *Kozier & Erb's fundamentals of nursing: Concepts, process, and practice* (9th ed.). Upper Saddle River, NJ: Pearson Education.

Black, J., & Hawks, J. (2009). *Medical surgical nursing: Clinical management for positive outcomes* (8th ed.). Philadelphia.

Ignatavicius, D., & Workman, M. (2010). *Medical-surgical nursing: Patient-centered collaborative care* (6th ed.). Philadelphia: Elsevier Saunders.

Kee, J. L. (2009). *Laboratory and diagnostic tests with nursing implications* (8th ed.). Upper Saddle River, NJ: Pearson Education.

Kee, J. L., Paulanka B. L., & Polek, C. (2009). *Handbook of fluid, electrolyte, and acid-base imbalances* (3rd ed.). Albany, NY: Thomson Delmar Learning.

LeMone, P., Burke, K., & Bauldoff, G. (2011). *Medical surgical nursing: Critical thinking in patent care* (5th ed.). Upper Saddle River, NJ: Pearson Education.

Lewis, S., Dirksen, S., Heitkemper, M., & Bucher, L. (2011). *Medical surgical nursing: Assessment and management of clinical problem* (8th ed.). St. Louis, MO: Elsevier.

London, M., Ladewig, P., Ball, J., Bindler, R., & Cowen, K. (2011). *Maternal & child nursing care* (3rd ed.). Upper Saddle River, NJ: Pearson Education.

Smeltzer, S., Bare, B., Hinkle, J., & Cheever, K. (2010). *Textbook of medical-surgical nursing* (12th ed.). Philadelphia: Lippincott Williams & Wilkins.

Taylor, C., Lillis, C., LeMone, P., & Lynn, P. (2011). *Fundamentals of nursing: The art and science of nursing care* (7th ed.). Philadelphia, PA: Lippincott Williams & Wilkins.

Wagner, K., Johnson, K., & Hardin-Pierce, M. (2009). *High acuity nursing* (5th ed.). Upper Saddle River, NJ: Pearson Education.

ANSWERS & RATIONALES

3 Potassium Balance and Imbalances

Chapter Outline

Overview of Potassium
    Regulation

Hypokalemia

Hyperkalemia

Objectives

➤ Review the basic functions of potassium in the body.
➤ Explain the pathophysiology and etiology of potassium imbalances.
➤ Identify specific assessment findings in potassium imbalances.
➤ Identify priority nursing diagnoses for a client experiencing a
potassium imbalance.
➤ Describe the therapeutic management of potassium imbalances.
➤ Describe the nursing management of a client who is experiencing a
potassium imbalance.

Review at a Glance

hyperkalemia serum potassium
level above the laboratory normal value
(usually 5.1 mEq/L)

hypokalemia serum level of potassium falls below 3.5 mEq/L

relative hyperkalemia movement
of potassium from the intracellular fluid to
the extracellular fluid, leading to elevated
serum potassium levels without a true

body increase of potassium, such as
occurs with acidosis

relative hypokalemia movement
of potassium from the extracellular
fluid to the intracellular fluid, leading to
lowered serum potassium levels without
a true decrease of potassium in the
body, such as occurs with insulin
therapy

sodium-potassium pump controls the concentration of potassium by
removing three sodium ions from the cell
for every two potassium ions that return
to the cell; fueled by the breakdown of
ATP and responsible for causing muscle
cells to generate action potentials and
transmit impulses

PRETEST

1 Which of the following potassium levels would be of greatest concern to the nurse when seen in a client who is taking furosemide (Lasix)?

1. 5.4 mEq/L
2. 4.3 mEq/L
3. 3.4 mEq/L
4. 3.1 mEq/L

2 Which statement should the nurse include when teaching a client about oral potassium supplementation?

1. "When you take your potassium pill, if you cannot swallow it, you can crush it up and put it in orange juice."
2. "Potassium should only be taken in the morning on an empty stomach."
3. "Take your potassium tablet after you have eaten breakfast."
4. "You can continue to use a salt substitute while you are taking your potassium supplement."

3 The nurse anticipates the client with which condition would be most at risk to develop hyperkalemia?

1. Chronic renal failure
2. Newly diagnosed cirrhosis
3. Partial bowel obstruction requiring nasogastric suctioning
4. Diarrhea for the last four days

4 The nurse should place highest priority on which nursing intervention for a client with renal failure who has a potassium level of 6.8 mEq/L?

1. Obtain an electrocardiogram (ECG)
2. Evaluate level of consciousness
3. Measure urinary output
4. Draw arterial blood gases

5 The nurse should include dietary teaching regarding addition of potassium-rich foods if the client is receiving which diuretic? Select all that apply.

1. Hydrochlorothiazide (HCTZ)
2. Spironolactone (Aldactone)
3. Triamterene with hydrochlorothiazide (Maxide)
4. Amiloride (Midamor)
5. Furosemide (Lasix)

6 A client has a potassium level of 6.2 mEq/L. The nurse identifies which ECG tracing to correlate with this electrolyte level?

1. 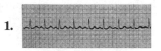   2.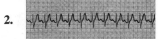

3. 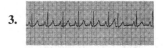   4.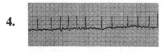

Source: LeMone, P., Burke, K., & Bauldoff, G. (2011). Medical-surgical nursing: Critical thinking in patient care (5th ed.). Upper Saddle River, NJ: Pearson Education.

7 When caring for a client who has a potassium level of 2.8 mEq/L, the nurse should assess for which of the following?

1. Perforated bowel
2. Paralytic ileus
3. Renal failure
4. Diabetes mellitus

8 The nurse determines that the intravenous (IV) administration of calcium gluconate to a client with hyperkalemia has been effective when which finding is seen on assessment?

1. Urine output increases
2. Bowel movements are loose
3. Cardiac dysrhythmia is corrected
4. Muscles are relaxed and weak

9 Which of the following statements by a client indicates a need for further instruction regarding treatment for hypokalemia?

1. "I will eat more bananas and cantaloupes for breakfast."
2. "I will eat more bran flakes to increase my potassium level."
3. "I will take my potassium in the morning after breakfast so it does not upset my stomach."
4. "I will tell my primary care provider if I start having muscle cramps or weakness."

10 What is the best response by the nurse to the 22-year-old daughter of a 56-year-old client admitted with hypokalemia and who reports being dizzy upon standing?

1. "Your mother has been lying in bed too long and when she stands up she will get dizzy."
2. "Once we correct your mother's potassium level, the dizziness should improve."
3. "Your mother is probably dizzy because her heart is not pumping as effectively, making her blood pressure low."
4. "Your mother is dizzy because her nervous system is not functioning correctly; once her potassium level goes up, she will improve."

➤ *See pages 71–72 for Answers and Rationales.*

I. OVERVIEW OF POTASSIUM REGULATION

A. **Potassium balance and function:** major cation of the intracellular fluid (ICF); 98% of the body's potassium store is located in ICF; the remaining 2% is in the extracellular fluid (ECF) (i.e., the intravascular and interstitial spaces outside the cells; responsible for neuromuscular function)
   1. Serum levels
      a. Normal serum concentration ranges:
         1) Newborn: 3.7–5.9 mEq/L
         2) Infant: 4.1–5.3 mEq/L
         3) Child: 3.4–4.7 mEq/L
         4) Adult: 3.5–5.1 mEq/L
      b. Even small changes in potassium level have a profound effect on the body and are poorly tolerated
   2. Role in acid–base balance
      a. Hydrogen and potassium ions shift back and forth between the ICF and ECF to maintain the pH
      b. Hydrogen ions move out of cells in alkalotic states to help correct the high pH, and potassium ions move in to maintain an electrically stable state; the reverse happens in acidosis
   3. Functions in the body
      a. ECF potassium (K^+) is responsible for maintaining action potentials in excitable cells of muscles, neurons, and other tissues
      b. ECF K^+ assists in controlling cardiac rate and rhythm, conduction of nerve impulses, skeletal muscle contraction, and function of smooth muscles and endocrine tissues
      c. Intracellular K^+ has a role in cellular metabolism and functions in the regulation of protein and glycogen synthesis
      d. Due to the fact that K^+ is the primary intracellular cation, it has some control over intracellular osmolarity and volume via the sodium-potassium ion exchange mechanism

Table 3-1	Lifespan Considerations for Health Maintenance: Potassium Balance
Lifespan Considerations	**Risk Factors for Imbalances**
Infants	Diarrhea, vomiting, pyloric stenosis
Pediatrics	Diarrhea, poor dietary intake
Adults	Increased use of diuretics Heart failure Poor nutrition

4. System interactions
  a. The primary control of ECF K^+ concentration is the **sodium-potassium pump**, contained within the cell membrane of all cells in the body
  b. The sodium-potassium pump controls the concentration of potassium by removing three sodium ions from the cell for every two potassium ions that return to the cell
  c. The pump is fueled by the breakdown of ATP and is responsible for causing muscle cells to generate action potentials and transmit impulses
5. See Table 3-1 for lifespan factors affecting potassium balance

B. Sources of potassium
  1. Cellular level: Factors that affect the movement of potassium in and out of the cells contribute to the level of potassium in the ICF and the ECF
    a. The kidneys eliminate approximately 90% of potassium lost
    b. The remaining amount is excreted through stool and perspiration
    c. Cellular release can lead to additional potassium circulating in the body and may be due to disease processes and/or medications
  2. Dietary levels
    a. Adequate intake is approximately 40–60 mEq daily
    b. Western diets consist of adequate intake of potassium daily in the form of fruits, dried fruits, and vegetables
    c. Many salt substitutes contain potassium
    d. Intake can also occur when parenteral fluid with potassium is infused
    e. Excessive intake of black licorice can lead to decreased K^+ levels due to the effect of glyceric acid (aldosterone effect)

Practice to Pass

A client asks the nurse why potassium levels are so important in the body. How will the nurse respond?

II. HYPOKALEMIA: SERUM POTASSIUM LEVEL BELOW 3.5 MEQ/L

A. Etiology and pathophysiology (see Table 3-2)
  1. Cellular level transport
    a. The amount of potassium in the ECF is so small that small changes in the K^+ level can lead to major alterations in membrane excitability in muscle and neural cells, making them less responsive to stimuli (such as in paralytic ileus) or can cause cardiac irritability (such as premature ventricular contractions or PVCs)
    b. Rapid changes in ECF potassium cannot be compensated for quickly and can result in profound changes in body function
    c. If this decrease is not corrected very quickly, death can occur from cardiac and respiratory arrest
    d. **Relative hypokalemia** occurs when potassium moves from the ECF to the ICF (the total body level of potassium remains unchanged), leading to abnormal distribution of potassium
      1) Alkalosis causes K^+ to migrate into the cell as hydrogen ions move out to correct the high pH

Practice to Pass

How are you going to ensure client safety when that client has hypokalemia?

Table 3-2	Overview of Hypokalemia	
Etiology	**Manifestations**	**Nursing Interventions**
Inadequate intake Use of potassium-wasting diuretics Excessive loss of GI fluid Heat-induced diaphoresis Starvation High glucose levels leading to diuresis Increased secretion of aldosterone as seen in adrenal adenomas, cirrhosis, nephrosis, heart failure, and hypertensive crisis Diabetes insipidus	Weak, thready pulse Pedal pulses difficult to palpate ECG changes—ST segment depression, flattened T wave, appearance of U wave, ventricular dysrhythmias (especially PVCs), heart block Enhanced effect of digoxin leading to toxicity at therapeutic levels Decreased breath sounds Shallow respiratory pattern Dyspnea Polyuria; difficulty in concentrating urine Decreased deep tendon reflexes Muscle weakness Anxiety Lethargy Depression Confusion Paresthesias Weakness Leg cramps Abdominal distention Hypoactive bowel sounds Vomiting Nausea Constipation Paralytic ileus	Monitor vital signs, especially blood pressure; orthostatic hypotension common Monitor serum potassium levels Assess heart rate and rhythm Assess ECG changes Assess respiratory rate, depth, and pattern Assess for signs of hypokalemia if client taking diuretics Protect from injury Monitor serum magnesium and calcium levels Monitor I&O (intake and output) Check for signs of metabolic alkalosis Give potassium supplements as ordered with food to prevent gastric irritation Use an infusion pump when administering parenteral potassium and assess IV site frequently for infiltration, phlebitis, and tissue necrosis Assess mental status and cognition Client education about food sources of potassium (Box 3-1, p. 62) and other measures (Box 3-2, p. 63)

      2) Increased secretion of insulin causes K^+ to move into skeletal muscles and hepatic cells when there is increased secretion of insulin

      3) Tissue repair causes shifting of K^+ concentration

      4) Water intoxication causes dilution of serum potassium

  2. Predisposing clinical conditions: actual hypokalemia is the actual loss of potassium or lack of adequate intake of potassium

    a. Increased secretion of aldosterone leads to the excretion of K^+ from the renal tubules and is seen in clients with the following:

      1) Adrenal adenomas

      2) Cirrhosis

      3) Nephrosis

      4) Heart failure and hypertensive crisis

      5) Cushing's syndrome

      6) Diabetes insipidus

      7) Hyperaldosteronism

    b. Excessive loss of potassium by use of certain medications, such as loop diuretics (such as furosemide [Lasix]), thiazide diuretics (such as hydrochlorothiazide [Hydrodiuril]), corticosteroids, cardiac glycosides (digoxin [Lanoxin]), penicillin derivatives (such as ampicillin, sodium penicillin, carbenicillin), amphotericin B, gentamicin (Garamycin), theophylline (Theo-Dur), cisplatin (Platinol), and terbutaline (Brethine), a tocolytic and respiratory agent; refer to Table 3-3 for a summary of medication classes that affect potassium levels

Table 3-3 Common Medications That Affect Potassium Levels

Increase Potassium Levels	Decrease Potassium Levels
Potassium chloride and salts	Laxatives, enemas, and sodium polystyrene sulfonate (Kayexalate)
Angiotensin converting enzyme (ACE) inhibitors*	Corticosteroids (Cortisone, Prednisone)
Heparin	Antibiotics*
Barbiturates, sedatives, heroin, and amphetamines	Insulin and glucose
Nonsteroidal anti-inflammatory drugs (NSAIDs)*	Beta$_2$ agonists (terbutaline, estrogen, albuterol)
Beta blockers and alpha agonists*	Potassium-wasting diuretics*
Cyclophosphamide	Amphotericin
Potassium-sparing diuretics*	

For these medications, please refer to a drug textbook for specific names because there are many different types of drugs in each category.

    c. Gastrointestinal (GI) loss by vomiting, diarrhea, prolonged nasogastric (NG) suctioning, newly created ileostomy, villous adenoma on the intestinal tract, laxative abuse, or enema administration

    d. Heat-induced diaphoresis

    e. Renal disease affecting the reabsorption of potassium seen in the diuretic phase of renal failure

    f. Hemodialysis and peritoneal dialysis

    g. Altered intake

        1) Potassium-restricted diets

        2) NPO status without sufficient IV replacement therapy

        3) Starvation, malnutrition, alcoholism, and anorexia

        4) High glucose levels, which increase osmotic pressure and lead to diuresis

        5) Large ingestion of black licorice (causes aldosterone effects)

    h. Intravenous insulin therapy to treat diabetic ketoacidosis, which drives potassium into cells temporarily

B. Clinical manifestations

    1. Rarely develop before potassium level falls below 3.0 mEq/L unless the rate of fall is rapid

    2. See Table 3-4 for manifestations of hypokalemia in specific body systems

    3. See Figure 3-1 (p. 61) for electrocardiogram changes with hypokalemia

C. Assessment

    1. Monitoring expectations

        a. Serum potassium levels

        b. ECG changes

        c. Electrolyte levels

        d. I&O

            1) Diuresis can lead to excessive loss of potassium

            2) One liter of urine contains about 40 mEq of potassium

    2. Identification of risk factors

        a. Assess for factors that increase the risk of hypokalemia such as the following:

            1) Age: aging decreases the kidneys' ability to concentrate urine, leading to diuresis; older adults are also more likely to be taking medications that can alter potassium levels

            2) Alcoholism

Practice to Pass

Why is an understanding of actual versus relative hypokalemia important to client safety?

Table 3-4	Clinical Manifestations of Hypokalemia
Body System	**Manifestations**
Cardiovascular	Variable pulse rate Weak, thready pulse Decreased blood pressure Pedal pulses difficult to palpate ECG changes: ST segment depression, flattened T wave, appearance of U wave, ventricular dysrhythmias (especially premature ventricular contractions [PVCs]), and heart block Hypokalemia prolongs repolarization, leading to flattened, prolonged T waves and production of possible U waves. U waves are small, low-amplitude waveforms occurring after the T wave Digitalis toxicity is potentiated
Respiratory	Decreased breath sounds Shallow respiratory pattern Dyspnea
Renal	Polyuria and nocturia Decreased specific gravity
Neuromuscular	Deep tendon hyporeflexia Muscle weakness, paresthesias, leg cramps, and soft flabby muscles Fatigue and lethargy, which can proceed to depression and coma in clients with severe hypokalemia Coma Anxiety
Gastrointestinal	Hypermotility with hyperactive bowel sounds Abdominal cramping Nausea, vomiting, and diarrhea Weight loss

      b. Medications
         1) Obtain pertinent client history of medications that can alter potassium levels (refer back to Table 3-3)
         2) Examine both prescription and over-the-counter medications and supplements that the client is taking for possible interactions
      c. Dietary
         1) Obtain pertinent client history regarding food intake
         2) Determine whether the client is taking nutritional supplements and check for potential interactions
   D. Diagnostic and laboratory findings
      1. Plasma levels
         a. Hypokalemia is confirmed by a serum level less than 3.5 mEq/L (or the normal value indicated by a particular laboratory)
         b. Trending of serum K^+ levels is necessary in order to establish a baseline and monitor response to therapy
      2. Associated electrolyte levels
         a. Elevated pH and bicarbonate levels (alkalosis)
         b. Elevated serum glucose levels (increased insulin secretion and increased osmotic pressure)
         c. Decreased serum chloride levels

Figure 3-1

Electrocardiogram (ECG) changes caused by altered potassium levels. A. Normal ECG, B. Changes resulting from hyperkalemia, C. Changes resulting from hypokalemia.

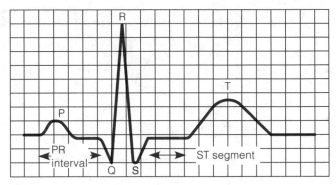

A

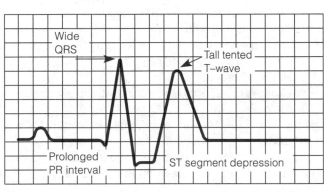

B

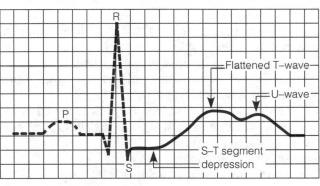

C

    d. Decreased magnesium levels (because hypomagnesemia can potentiate hypokalemia)

    e. Decreased calcium levels can also be seen in conjunction with decreased potassium and magnesium levels

  3. Trending of results

    a. ECG tracings demonstrate characteristic changes with hypokalemia (described earlier in this chapter and as shown in Figure 3-1c above)

    b. Trending ECG changes can help to monitor a client's status and response to therapeutic treatment

E. Priority nursing diagnoses

  1. Risk for Injury related to muscle weakness and hyporeflexia

  2. Risk for Ineffective Breathing Pattern related to neuromuscular impairment

Box 3-1	The following foods are considered adequate sources of potassium:
Good Food Sources of Potassium	• Vegetables such as spinach, broccoli, carrots, green beans, tomatoes and tomato juice, acorn squash, and potatoes • Fruits such as bananas, cantaloupe, oranges, apricots, and strawberries • Milk, milk products, yogurt, and meat • Legumes, nuts, and seeds • Whole grains

    3. Decreased Cardiac Output related to dysrhythmias
    4. Constipation related to smooth muscle atony
    5. Imbalanced Nutrition related to poor dietary levels
    6. Fatigue related to neuromuscular weakness
    7. Impaired Physical Mobility related to muscle weakness

F. Therapeutic management: treatment focuses on restoring normal levels, preventing complications, and treating underlying problems
    1. Replacement therapies
        a. For clients at risk, provide a diet containing adequate potassium, about 50–100 mEq daily
        b. If the diet is insufficient to meet needs, administer potassium supplements as ordered
        c. Initiate a referral to a dietitian for assistance with meal planning to ensure adequate sources of potassium in the diet (refer to Box 3-1 for dietary sources of potassium)
    2. Continued monitoring of client (lab values and physical manifestations) to assess efficacy of treatment
    3. Restoration of balance (normal serum K^+ level) to maintain homeostasis and prevent development of further complications
        a. It is important to monitor serum calcium and magnesium levels in clients who are hypokalemic, because sometimes, even with appropriate potassium replacement, serum levels do not rise
        b. If client is also found to have hypocalcemia and/or hypomagnesemia, then correction must be aimed at restoring all three electrolyte levels in order to correct serum potassium

G. Planning and implementation
    1. Monitor pertinent client assessment data for potential effects related to hypokalemia, and for response to therapeutic treatment
        a. Vital signs, especially blood pressure (hypokalemia can cause the client to develop orthostatic hypotension) and respiratory rate, depth, and pattern
        b. Serum electrolyte levels
        c. ECG changes and heart rate and rhythm
        d. I&O and possibly daily weight
    2. Monitor therapeutic serum drug levels for clients taking cardiac glycosides (Digoxin) and serum potassium levels for clients taking loop and thiazide diuretics
    3. Protect the client from injury and maintain a safe environment as client may experience weakness due to hypokalemia
    4. Dietary interventions to promote normal potassium levels
        a. Encourage use of high-fiber diets and increased fluid intake, if not on fluid restriction, to prevent constipation that can occur because of ileus secondary to hypokalemia
        b. Provide adequate dietary sources of potassium in the diet
        c. Maintain accurate I&O

5. Check for signs of metabolic alkalosis (including irritability and paresthesias) because hypokalemia is present in alkalotic states

6. Provide replacement therapy as ordered by health care provider paying attention to baseline labs, client's response, and therapeutic benefit

7. Always use an infusion pump when administering parenteral potassium
   a. Observe IV site frequently for signs of infiltration, phlebitis, and tissue necrosis as potassium-containing solutions are irritating to veins
   b. Verify additive K^+ in solution prior to hanging infusion
   c. Do not exceed maximum safe infusion rate (see section that follows)

8. Observe client's mental status and cognition during course of therapy

H. **Medication therapy (note: potassium supplements should not be given unless the client has a urine output of at least 0.5 mL/kg/hour)**

1. Oral replacement therapy
   a. Clients should be started on oral supplements if they take potassium-wasting diuretics, have poor nutritional intake, and/or have disease processes that cause further potassium losses
   b. The usual oral preparation is potassium chloride or KCl, which is available in many preparations (K-Dur, K-Lyte, K-Lyte/Cl, K-Tab, Klotrix, Micro-K, and Slow-K)
   c. The daily prophylactic dose is 20 mEq
   d. Therapeutic treatment can be given at higher doses (up to 100 mEq in divided doses), depending on the client's baseline
   e. The medication can be given in either liquid or pill form
   f. Refer to Box 3-2 for client teaching points regarding oral potassium therapy

2. Parenteral replacement therapy
   a. Dilute potassium in a solution that provides no more than 1 mEq/10 mL
   b. Most potassium infusions are run at a rate not exceeding 5–10 mEq/hr unless there is moderate hypokalemia; peripheral IV potassium should not be infused more quickly than 20 mEq/hr or in concentrations greater than 40 mEq/L unless severe hypokalemia exists; higher concentration potassium solutions should be administered through a central line, and the client should have hemodynamic monitoring throughout the course of therapy
   c. The solution should be dextrose free, if possible, to prevent the release of insulin
   d. If more than 20 mEq/hour is given, the client should have continuous ECG monitoring, and the serum levels should be checked every 4–6 hours until a normal level is achieved

Practice to Pass

What nursing interventions should be used with clients receiving intravenous solutions containing KCl?

Box 3-2	Prior to discharge, teach client and family to do the following:
Client Education Regarding Hypokalemia	• Take potassium supplements with at least four ounces fluid or with food. • Never crush or break potassium tablets or capsules. • Dissolve powder form of potassium in at least four ounces of water or juice (no carbonated beverages). • Take potassium after meals to prevent GI upset. • Do not use salt substitutes when taking potassium supplements. • Know the signs and symptoms of hyperkalemia and report any of these to the health care provider. • Get regular serum potassium levels drawn as per health care provider recommendations. • Teach client about side effects of potassium supplements and to report them to health care provider if they occur.

e. Monitor IV site closely as KCl is irritating to vessels and can lead to infiltration, phlebitis, and tissue necrosis

       f. Use an infusion pump to control the infusion, paying attention to rate, intake, and output

       g. Potassium should never be administered by the IV push or intramuscular routes because this can lead to development of fatal arrhythmias

    3. Diet therapy

       a. Foods high in potassium include raisins, bananas, apricots, oranges, avocados, beans, beef, potatoes, tomatoes, cantaloupe, and spinach

       b. Avoid foods such as black licorice that, when eaten in large quantities, can cause hypokalemia

I. Client education

    1. Teach awareness of predisposing factors

       a. Older adult clients are at risk for hypokalemia due to multiple medication profile

       b. Clients taking diuretics (loop and thiazide) and/or digoxin (Lanoxin) are at risk to develop K^+ depletion

    2. Teach clients signs and symptoms of hypokalemia and have them report potential problems to their health care provider

    3. Teach clients about potassium supplement medication

       a. Take with at least four ounces of fluid or food to prevent GI upset

       b. Do not crush slow-release tablets, as this can trigger a quick release of potassium

    4. Dietary education

       a. If client takes a potassium-sparing diuretic, do not encourage the use of foods high in potassium

       b. Provide list of foods that are high in potassium during client education (refer to Box 3-1 for a listing of adequate food sources of potassium)

       c. Collaborate with dietitian as needed

J. Evaluation

Practice to Pass

What foods would you suggest to a client who is hypokalemic?

    1. Client returns to and maintains a normal serum potassium level

    2. Client complies with drug and diet therapies as ordered

    3. Client states the early signs and symptoms of hypokalemia

    4. Client has normal bowel pattern

    5. Client maintains adequate gas exchange

    6. Client maintains regular cardiac rate and rhythm

III. HYPERKALEMIA: SERUM POTASSIUM LEVEL ABOVE 5.1 MEQ/L

A. Etiology and pathophysiology (see Table 3-5)

    1. Cellular level transport

       a. Potassium moves from the ECF to the ICF and increases cell excitability, so that cells respond to stimuli of less intensity and may actually discharge independently without a stimulus

       b. The myocardium is most sensitive to increases in potassium levels

       c. Manifestations seen with hyperkalemia depend on how rapidly the increase occurs

          1) Sudden increases show profound functional changes at 6–7 mEq/L

          2) Slower increases may not lead to changes until levels of 8 mEq/L are reached

    2. Predisposing clinical conditions

       a. Actual hyperkalemia (potassium level in the ECF is elevated)

          1) Excessive potassium intake due to overingestion of potassium-rich food or medications, use of salt substitutes, or rapid infusion of K^+-containing IV solutions

Table 3-5 Overview of Hyperkalemia

Etiology	Manifestations	Nursing Interventions
Excessive potassium intake from foods, medications, salt substitutes, IV infusions of KCl	Irregular, slow heart rate	Restrict potassium intake
Decreased excretion due to adrenal insufficiency, renal failure, potassium-sparing diuretics; decreased secretion of aldosterone	Decreased blood pressure	Monitor serum potassium levels
Massive tissue trauma	ECG changes—tall, peaked T waves, widened QRS, frequent ectopy, ventricular tachycardia or fibrillation, standstill	Assess for signs and symptoms
Metabolic acidosis	If levels are extremely high, can lead to muscle weakness, paralysis, and respiratory failure	Monitor cardiac status
Gastrointestinal bleeds	Muscle twitching, paralysis	Monitor for metabolic acidosis and implement treatment for same
Digoxin use	GI hypermotility	Monitor ECG changes
Overdose	Hyperactive bowel sounds	If blood transfusions necessary, give fresh packed red blood cells
Insulin deficiency	Abdominal cramping	Encourage compliance with therapeutic regimen
Hyperuricemia	Diarrhea	Discontinue use of IV KCl
Burns	Muscle cramps	Implement safety precautions
	Irritability	Administer diuretics or other medications that lower serum potassium levels
	Anxiety	
	Flaccid paralysis	
	Oliguria	

2) Decreased excretion of potassium due to adrenal insufficiency (Addison's disease), renal insufficiency or failure, K$^+$-sparing diuretics, or use of ACE inhibitors

  b. **Relative hyperkalemia** (movement of potassium from the ICF to the ECF leading to elevated serum potassium levels without a true body increase of potassium)

  1) Conditions that affect cellular release

   a) Massive cell damage, crush injuries

   b) Burns

   c) Tumor lysis syndrome, in which potassium is released from cells along with phosphates and uric acid

   d) Gastrointestinal bleeds

   e) Major surgeries and hypercatabolism

  2) Conditions that are considered to cause pseudohyperkalemia

   a) Hemolysis of blood sample due to prolonged tourniquet use

   b) Clenched fist during blood draws may cause RBC hemolysis

  3) Conditions that affect transcellular shifting

   a) Metabolic acidosis, which causes K$^+$ to move out of the cell as hydrogen ions move into it to correct the pH.

   b) Insulin deficiency leads to a decrease in K$^+$ utilization.

   c) Rapid increase in blood osmolality causes an increased blood concentration of K$^+$

  4) Conditions that result from medication therapy

   a) Overdose of replacement therapy

   b) Administration of stored blood, which causes hemolysis of RBCs in solution and increases serum levels

   c) Use of potassium-sparing diuretics

> **Practice to Pass**
>
> Why does a client who has massive tissue destruction get hyperkalemia?

Table 3-6	Clinical Manifestations of Hyperkalemia
Body System	**Manifestations**
Cardiovascular	Irregular, slow heart rate Decreased blood pressure ECG changes (refer again to Figure 3-1b): narrow, peaked T waves, widened QRS complexes, prolonged PR intervals, flattened P waves, frequent ectopy, ventricular fibrillation, and ventricular standstill
Respiratory	Unaffected until levels are very high, leading to muscle weakness and paralysis and causing respiratory failure
Renal	Oliguria (seen when renal failure is the cause of hyperkalemia)
Neuromuscular	Early: paresthesias, muscle twitching Muscle cramps Irritability Anxiety Difficulty with phonation Late: ascending flaccid paralysis involving arms and legs
Gastrointestinal	Hypermotility with hyperactive bowel sounds Abdominal cramping Nausea, vomiting, and diarrhea Weight loss

     5) Addison's disease due to decreased aldosterone that leads to sodium depletion and potassium retention

  c. Hyperkalemia occurs rather rarely in clients who have normally functioning kidneys

B. Clinical manifestations (see Table 3-6)

C. Assessment

  1. Monitoring expectations

    a. Serum potassium levels

    b. ECG changes (see Figure 3-1 again)

    c. I&O (adequate renal function is needed for potassium excretion; measure I&O accurately and frequently)

  2. Identification of risk factors

    a. Assess for factors that increase the risk of hyperkalemia, such as the following:

      1) Age: aging leads to a decrease in renal functioning

      2) Medications that can increase serum potassium levels, such as K^+-sparing diuretics or K^+ supplements, blood products, ACE inhibitors, beta adrenergic blockers, nonsteroidal anti-inflammatory drugs (NSAIDs), heparin, and sulfamethoxazole/trimethoprim (Bactrim)

    b. Dietary

      1) High intake of potassium-rich foods

      2) Salt substitutes

      3) Potassium supplements

    c. Clients with disease states, both acute and chronic

      1) Diabetes mellitus and renal failure can lead to hyperkalemia

      2) Acute disease such as massive trauma or burns can lead to hyperkalemia

    d. Clients undergoing therapeutic treatment

      1) Recent medical or surgical intervention

      2) Blood transfusions

D. Diagnostic and laboratory findings
1. Plasma levels: a value greater than 5.1 mEq/L confirms the diagnosis of hyperkalemia
2. Associated electrolyte levels
   a. If dehydration is causing hyperkalemia, then hematocrit, hemoglobin, sodium, and chloride levels should be drawn
   b. If associated with renal failure, creatinine and BUN levels should also be drawn
   c. An arterial blood gas (ABG) is needed to monitor for metabolic acidosis
3. Trending of results
   a. ECG monitoring to determine cardiac changes
   b. ABGs to determine acid–base balance

E. Priority nursing diagnoses
1. Risk for Injury related to muscle weakness and seizures
2. Risk for Decreased Cardiac Output related to dysrhythmias
3. Imbalanced Nutrition related to decreased renal function or increased intake
4. Diarrhea related to neuromuscular changes and irritability

F. Therapeutic interventions
1. Decrease potassium intake
   a. Stress importance of adherence to prescribed potassium restrictions
   b. Do not administer potassium supplements either orally or in parenteral fluids
   c. Refer client to a dietitian to evaluate dietary intake for hidden potassium sources
2. Promote potassium excretion
   a. Increase urinary output
   b. Ensure adequate renal function
3. Continued monitoring of client
   a. Serum potassium levels; report abnormals
   b. Signs and symptoms of hyperkalemia
   c. Cardiac status
   d. Metabolic acidosis

4. Restoration of balance
   a. Because small elevations can lead to profound myocardial changes, a normal potassium level should be restored as soon as possible to prevent lethal dysrhythmias
   b. Treatment is based on serum levels and client presentation; aggressive therapeutic management may be required to return serum levels to baseline in a timely manner
   c. Whenever possible, determine and treat the underlying cause of hyperkalemia to restore balance
5. Dialysis may be performed for intractable conditions if hyperkalemia cannot be controlled in a timely manner to prevent development of potentially lethal problems or if the client's clinical condition warrants immediate intervention

G. Planning and implementation
1. Monitor pertinent client assessment data for potential effects related to hyperkalemia and for response to therapeutic treatment
   a. Notify health care provider of levels exceeding 5.1 mEq/L as elevations can cause serious cardiac consequences
   b. Serum electrolyte levels
   c. ECG changes and heart rate and rhythm pattern
2. Monitor client for potential serum elevations due to concomitant drug therapy (as noted in Table 3-2)

3. Check for signs of metabolic acidosis because relative hyperkalemia frequently accompanies acidotic states (and often self-corrects when the pH is corrected)
4. Do not provide any additional potassium in the form of medications (IV, supplements, and/or stored blood)
5. Dietary interventions to promote normal potassium levels
    a. Decrease catabolism by encouraging the client to consume prescribed amounts of dietary protein and carbohydrates
    b. Limit or stop additional potassium sources in the diet (such as use of salt substitutes)
    c. Refer client to a dietitian for individualized instruction as needed
6. Encourage compliance with therapeutic regimen, treat infections promptly, and decrease hypermetabolic responses

H. **Medication therapy**
1. Exchange resins
    a. Sodium polystyrene sulfonate (Kayexalate) can be given either as an enema or orally with an osmotic agent to decrease possible constipation
    b. Medication works to exchange sodium with potassium in the GI tract and excrete the resin formed with potassium in the stool
    c. Sorbitol 70% can also be used as a cation exchange resin and is available in both oral and rectal forms
2. Intravenous medications
    a. Calcium gluconate
        1) Antagonizes the effect of potassium on the myocardium and decreases myocardial irritability
        2) Calcium administration does not promote K^+ loss, thus it only temporarily manages symptoms
        3) Carefully monitor clients who are taking digoxin (Lanoxin) because calcium administration can promote digitalis toxicity
    b. Regular insulin and dextrose (usually 50%) solution
        1) Combination therapy is used to shift the potassium from ECF to ICF
        2) This is not a long-term treatment method but rather an emergency treatment to reduce potassium levels
    c. Sodium bicarbonate
        1) This is used to make the cells more alkaline (elevating pH); should only be used with documented acidosis unresponsive to other treatment such as proper ventilation
        2) This shifts the potassium back into the cells (causes transcellular shifting), and therefore is used to temporarily manage symptoms
3. Diuretic therapy with potassium-wasting diuretics (loop diuretics and thiazide and thiazide-like diuretics) will promote potassium excretion from renal tubules
4. Aerosolized beta$_2$ agonist will drive potassium into cells
5. In the presence of Addison's disease, hydrocortisone succinate can be given via IV initially, then hydrocortisone by mouth plus fludrocortisone acetate

I. **Client education**
1. Awareness of predisposing factors
    a. Older adult clients are at risk for hyperkalemia due to multiple medication profile as are clients with multiple disease profiles (such as diabetes and renal failure)
    b. Clients taking medications that promote potassium retention should have periodic lab testing to determine serum levels
    c. Teach clients potential signs and symptoms of hyperkalemia and have them report problems to their health care provider

2. Dietary education
 a. Diet education includes knowledge of foods to avoid and permissible foods that contain very little potassium
 b. Teach clients to examine food labels and medication packages to determine potassium content
 c. Teach clients to avoid salt substitutes
J. **Evaluation**
 1. The client returns to and maintains normal serum potassium level
 2. The client complies with drug and diet therapies as ordered
 3. The client states the early signs and symptoms of hyperkalemia
 4. The client maintains adequate gas exchange
 5. The client maintains regular cardiac rate and rhythm

Case Study

A 68-year-old male client is admitted to the hospital with complaints of diarrhea for three days. The client reports being weak and feels like his heart is racing.

1. What questions will the nurse ask when assessing the client's medical history?

2. What other manifestations might be present?

3. What laboratory and diagnostic tests might be ordered for this client?

For suggested responses, see page 203.

4. What type of medical interventions would the nurse expect this client to receive?

5. What information will be provided for this client by the nurse before being discharged and what are the most effective teaching methods for this client?

POSTTEST

POSTTEST

1 Which serum potassium level would the nurse anticipate seeing in a child with a three-day history of diarrhea?

1. 3.0 mEq/L
2. 3.6 mEq/L
3. 4.1 mEq/L
4. 5.8 mEq/L

2 The nurse is instructing a client diagnosed with hyperkalemia about foods to avoid. Which of the following statements by the client indicates to the nurse a need for further instruction?

1. "I should avoid eating a lot of bananas."
2. "It will be nice to be able to eat a lot of fresh tomatoes this summer."
3. "I will avoid using salt substitutes instead of real salt."
4. "No more avocado salads for me."

3 A client is admitted to the hospital with a serum potassium level of 2.8 mEq/L. The nurse anticipates that assessment findings will include which of the following?

1. Elastic skin turgor and vomiting a small amount of bile-stained emesis
2. Pink nail beds, and ECG showing a normal sinus rhythm with a rate of 76
3. Respiratory rate of 16 with equal bilateral breath sounds, and two loose stools this morning
4. Irregular pulse rate and shallow respirations

4 The nurse instructs a client receiving hydro-chlorothiazide (HCTZ) to report which of the following symptoms to the health care provider?

1. Leg cramps and muscle weakness
2. Muscle weakness and diarrhea
3. Fatigue and irritability
4. Nausea and irritability

5 Which of the following foods should the nurse instruct the client with end stage renal disease (ESRD) to avoid?

1. Bread
2. Cantaloupe
3. Green beans
4. Apple juice

6 A postoperative client with a serum potassium level of 3.6 mEq/L is ordered to receive an IV with a potassium supplement (KCl) via a peripheral line. The nurse checks to determine that the amount of KCl ordered does not exceed the standard hourly replacement rate of _____ mEq/hr. Record your answer rounding to the nearest whole number.

Fill in your answer below:
_____ mEq/hr

7 The nurse concludes that a client understands the side effects of furosemide (Lasix) and its relationship to potassium levels when the client makes which statement?

1. "I do not need to take my pulse anymore when I take my Digoxin."
2. "I should call the doctor if I develop diarrhea."
3. "I should call my doctor if I feel myself becoming dizzy when I stand up."
4. "I do not need to eat bananas for breakfast any more because I am taking this medication."

8 The nurse provides which instruction to a client going home with a prescription for spironolactone (Aldactone)?

1. "Be sure to take this medication on an empty stomach."
2. "Take this pill just before you go to bed."
3. "Cut back on your intake of those foods on your list that are high in potassium."
4. "You do not have to watch your intake of fluid while you are taking this medicine."

9 The nurse identifies which of the following clients admitted to the hospital to be at risk for developing hypokalemia? Select all that apply.

1. A client whose arterial blood gases indicate metabolic acidosis
2. A client who had developed metabolic alkalosis
3. A client with acute renal failure
4. A client with adult respiratory distress syndrome (ARDS)
5. The client with a nasogastric tube to low intermittent suction

10 The nurse plans to administer which intravenous (IV) treatment to a client for treatment of hyperkalemia associated with severe acidosis?

1. Calcium gluconate to make the potassium shift from the intracellular fluid (ICF) to the extracellular fluid (ECF)
2. Insulin and dextrose to make the client hypoglycemic
3. Sodium bicarbonate to make the client alkalotic so the potassium will shift into the ICF
4. Normal saline (NS) to provide extra sodium so the potassium will move out of the ICF into the ECF

➤ *See pages 72–74 for Answers and Rationales.*

ANSWERS & RATIONALES

Pretest

1 **Answer: 4** **Rationale:** Potassium is lost when taking a loop diuretic such as furosemide (Lasix); a level of 3.1 mEq/L is below the normal range of potassium and would be of greatest concern to the nurse. A potassium level of 5.4 mEq/L is elevated, reflecting retention of potassium. A potassium level of 4.3 mEq/L is within the normal range of potassium levels. A potassium level of 3.4 mEq/L is at the low end of the normal range of potassium levels and may be of concern to the nurse, but it does not reflect the level that is of most concern. **Cognitive Level:** Analyzing **Client Need:** Reduction of Risk Potential **Integrated Process:** Nursing Process: Assessment **Content Area:** Adult Health **Strategy:** The critical word is *greatest*. Recall normal potassium levels and eliminate two options since one is elevated and one is normal. Eliminate a third option as less abnormal than the most abnormal option. **Reference:** LeMone, P., & Burke, K. (2008). *Medical surgical nursing: Critical thinking in client care* (4th ed.). Upper Saddle River, NJ: Pearson/ Prentice Hall, pp. 218–223.

2 **Answer: 3** **Rationale:** Potassium can irritate the stomach and should be taken just after eating. Many potassium supplements are time released and should not be crushed. To prevent gastric irritation, oral potassium supplements should be taken with at least four ounces of fluid or with food. Salt substitutes may contain potassium and, if taken with a potassium supplement, could cause hyperkalemia. **Cognitive Level:** Applying **Client Need:** Pharmacological and Parenteral Therapies **Integrated Process:** Teaching and Learning **Content Area:** Adult Health **Strategy:** Recall that potassium should not be crushed and is irritating to the stomach to eliminate two options. Recall that salt substitutes contain potassium to eliminate a third option. Note that two options are opposites, indicating that one could be true. **Reference:** LeMone, P., & Burke, K. (2008). *Medical surgical nursing: Critical thinking in client care* (4th ed.). Upper Saddle River, NJ: Pearson/Prentice Hall, pp. 219–220.

3 **Answer: 1** **Rationale:** Clients in renal failure have difficulty excreting potassium, leading to its accumulation in the bloodstream. Clients with cirrhosis tend to retain sodium and lose potassium, which would contribute to hypokalemia. Intestinal and nasogastric suctioning lead to the loss of potassium and hypokalemia. Potassium is lost with diarrhea, leading to hypokalemia. **Cognitive Level:** Analyzing **Client Need:** Physiological Adaptation **Integrated Process:** Nursing Process: Evaluation **Content Area:** Adult Health **Strategy:** The critical word is *hyperkalemia*. Review ways in which potassium is lost from the body to eliminate two options and choose the correct one. **Reference:** LeMone, P., & Burke, K. (2008).

Medical surgical nursing: Critical thinking in client care (4th ed.). Upper Saddle River, NJ: Pearson/Prentice Hall, pp. 224–226.

4 **Answer: 1** **Rationale:** A potassium level of 6.8 mEq/L is a critically high potassium level and could cause life-threatening cardiac arrhythmias; an ECG should be obtained. Although the client's level of consciousness may be affected by the hyperkalemia and decreased cardiac output, this is not of highest priority. The client with renal failure has a decreased urinary output that needs to be measured, but this is not the most critical nursing intervention with this critically high potassium level. Arterial blood gases may be indicated to determine state of acidosis and respiratory status, but is not a greater priority than obtaining an ECG. **Cognitive Level:** Analyzing **Client Need:** Reduction of Risk Potential **Integrated Process:** Nursing Process: Implementation **Content Area:** Adult Health **Strategy:** The critical words are *highest priority*. Eliminate one option since the client is in renal failure. Remember ABCs—airway, breathing, and circulation—to choose the correct option. **Reference:** LeMone, P., & Burke, K. (2008). *Medical surgical nursing: Critical thinking in client care* (4th ed.). Upper Saddle River, NJ: Pearson/Prentice Hall, pp. 224–226.

5 **Answer: 1, 5** **Rationale:** HCTZ and Lasix are diuretics that increase the excretion of potassium, so clients should be taught to increase the intake of potassium in their diet. All of the other medications are considered potassium-sparing or combination diuretics and, as such, dietary supplementation would not be indicated. **Cognitive Level:** Analyzing **Client Need:** Pharmacological and Parenteral Therapies **Integrated Process:** Teaching and Learning **Content Area:** Pharmacology **Strategy:** The question is testing knowledge of potassium-wasting diuretics. Recall that thiazide and loop diuretics decrease potassium to choose correctly. **Reference:** Adams, M., Josephson, D., & Holland, L. (2011). *Pharmacology for nurses: A pathophysiologic approach* (3rd ed.). Upper Saddle River, NJ: Pearson/ Prentice Hall, pp. 641–646.

6 **Answer: 2** **Rationale:** A potassium level of 6.2 mEq/L reflects hyperkalemia. An ECG tracing associated with this electrolyte imbalance shows tall, tented T waves, which occur during repolarization of the cardiac conduction system. Normal sinus rhythm, premature atrial contractions, and atrial fibrillation are not associated with hyperkalemia. **Cognitive Level:** Analyzing **Client Need:** Physiological Adaptation **Integrated Process:** Nursing Process: Diagnosis **Content Area:** Adult Health **Strategy:** First identify that a potassium level of 6.2 mEq/L is elevated. Recall the ECG changes associated with hyperkalemia to choose the correct option. **Reference:** LeMone, P., Burke, K., & Bauldoff, G. (2011). *Medical surgical* *nursing: Critical thinking in patient care* (5th ed.). Upper Saddle River, NJ: Pearson Education, pp. 947–948.

7 **Answer: 2** **Rationale:** Hypokalemia can lead to alterations in smooth muscle functioning. Smooth muscle alterations in the gastrointestinal tract can lead to development of a paralytic ileus. Complications of hypokalemia are usually not associated with renal failure, diabetes, or a perforated bowel because these conditions are more likely to lead to increased potassium levels. **Cognitive Level:** Analyzing **Client Need:** Physiological Adaptation **Integrated Process:** Nursing Process: Assessment **Content Area:** Adult Health **Strategy:** Recall action of potassium on body systems and its action on the neuromuscular system to choose the correct option. **Reference:** LeMone, P., & Burke, K. (2008). *Medical surgical nursing: Critical thinking in client care* (4th ed.). Upper Saddle River, NJ: Pearson/Prentice Hall, pp. 218–223.

8 **Answer: 3** **Rationale:** Calcium gluconate is given to antagonize the effects of potassium on the conduction system of the heart. It is not given to promote potassium excretion (either in urine or stool). The medication acts to blunt the effects of elevated potassium on the myocardium. **Cognitive Level:** Analyzing **Client Need:** Pharmacological and Parenteral Therapies **Integrated Process:** Nursing Process: Evaluation **Content Area:** Adult Health **Strategy:** The question requires recall of the use in calcium in treating hyperkalemia. Eliminate three options since it is not given to eliminate potassium from the body. **Reference:** LeMone, P., & Burke, K. (2008). *Medical surgical nursing: Critical thinking in client care* (4th ed.). Upper Saddle River, NJ: Pearson/Prentice Hall, pp. 224–227.

9 **Answer: 2** **Rationale:** Bran flakes are not a source of potassium in the diet. It is important for the client to communicate to the physician if symptoms of hypokalemia develop during the course of therapy. Bananas and cantaloupe are excellent sources of dietary potassium. Taking potassium supplements on a full stomach will help to minimize gastric irritation, which is commonly associated with this medication. **Cognitive Level:** Analyzing **Client Need:** Reduction of Risk Potential **Integrated Process:** Teaching and Learning **Content Area:** Adult Health **Strategy:** The question requires reverse thinking; three options are correct statements and one is wrong. Note similarities between two options, noting that bran is not a good source of potassium to choose that as the incorrect response. **Reference:** LeMone, P., & Burke, K. (2008). *Medical surgical nursing: Critical thinking in client care* (4th ed.). Upper Saddle River, NJ: Pearson/Prentice Hall, pp. 218–223.

10 **Answer: 3** **Rationale:** Potassium works to maintain cardiac contractility and normal heart rate. Hypokalemia leads to the development of potential arrhythmias that can result in ischemia and death. While the length of bedrest and actual potassium level could be associated with a complaint of dizziness, it is more likely that the dizziness

is associated with orthostatic hypotension and inefficient heart pumping action due to hypokalemia. It is important for the client (and family) to understand that electrolyte imbalances may have significant complications that can affect the entire body. **Cognitive Level:** Analyzing **Client Need:** Physiological Adaptation **Integrated Process:** Communication and Documentation **Content Area:** Adult Health **Strategy:** The question asks for the best answer, indicating that all options may be completely or partially correct, but one is better. Eliminate one option since it does not relate to potassium. Eliminate two other options since they do not address the source or correct reason for the client's dizziness. **Reference:** LeMone, P., & Burke, K. (2008). *Medical surgical nursing: Critical thinking in client care* (4th ed.). Upper Saddle River, NJ: Pearson/Prentice Hall, pp. 218–223.

Posttest

1 **Answer: 1** **Rationale:** A client who has diarrhea will be more likely to develop hypokalemia. A serum potassium of 3.0 mEq/L is considered to be hypokalemic. A level of 3.6 mEq/L is just within the normal range but one would expect a greater K+ loss given the client's history of three days of diarrhea. A level of 4.1 mEq/L is within the normal range and does not reflect potassium loss. A level of 5.8 mEq/L reflects hyperkalemia. **Cognitive Level:** Applying **Client Need:** Reduction of Risk Potential **Integrated Process:** Nursing Process: Assessment **Content Area:** Child Health **Strategy:** Critical words are *three-day history of diarrhea*. Review normal potassium levels and recall that potassium is lost with diarrhea to choose the lowest level. **Reference:** LeMone, P., & Burke, K. (2008). *Medical surgical nursing: Critical thinking in client care* (4th ed.). Upper Saddle River, NJ: Pearson/Prentice Hall, pp. 218–222.

2 **Answer: 2** **Rationale:** Bananas, tomatoes, avocados, and salt substitutes are all high in potassium and should be limited in a client with hyperkalemia. Clients should be aware of foods to avoid that are high in potassium if teaching has been successful. **Cognitive Level:** Applying **Client Need:** Reduction of Risk Potential **Integrated Process:** Teaching and Learning **Content Area:** Adult Health **Strategy:** Review foods high in potassium. Note the question asks for need for further instruction and look for the one incorrect response. Recall content of salt substitutes to choose correctly. **Reference:** LeMone, P., & Burke, K. (2008). *Medical surgical nursing: Critical thinking in client care* (4th ed.). Upper Saddle River, NJ: Pearson/Prentice Hall, pp. 217–218; 224–226.

3 **Answer: 4** **Rationale:** A serum level of 2.8 mEq/L reflects hypokalemia, which often manifests as cardiac and respiratory problems related to the ineffective smooth muscle contractions. One option reflects normal findings. The symptoms listed in two other options do not indicate severe hypokalemia. A serum potassium of

2.8 mEq/L in conjunction with irregular pulse and shallow respirations is a symptomatic presentation in this client and suggests severe hypokalemia. It is important to look at the whole clinical picture and not just the serum level to determine the severity of an electrolyte imbalance. **Cognitive Level:** Analyzing **Client Need:** Reduction of Risk Potential **Integrated Process:** Nursing Process: Assessment **Content Area:** Adult Health **Strategy:** Recognize the value is indicative of severe hypokalemia. Eliminate one option since findings are normal and two other options since they are not as severe as those in the correct option. **Reference:** LeMone, P., & Burke, K. (2008). *Medical surgical nursing: Critical thinking in client care* (4th ed.). Upper Saddle River, NJ: Pearson/Prentice Hall, pp. 219–223.

4 **Answer: 1** **Rationale:** HCTZ is a potassium-wasting diuretic, and its use can lead to hypokalemia. Leg cramps and muscle weakness are two of the symptoms seen in a client with hypokalemia. Diarrhea, fatigue, nausea, and irritability are not usually seen with the use of this class of diuretics. **Cognitive Level:** Analyzing **Client Need:** Pharmacological and Parenteral Therapies **Integrated Process:** Teaching and Learning **Content Area:** Pharmacology **Strategy:** Recall that this diuretic is potassium wasting to direct you to the correct option. **Reference:** LeMone, P., & Burke, K. (2008). *Medical surgical nursing: Critical thinking in client care* (4th ed.). Upper Saddle River, NJ: Pearson/Prentice Hall, pp. 221–224.

5 **Answer: 2** **Rationale:** Clients with ESRD are unable to excrete potassium and need to restrict intake of foods high in potassium. Cantaloupes are very high in potassium and should be avoided. Bread, green beans, and apple juice are not considered to be good sources of potassium. These foods do not need to be restricted in the diet. **Cognitive Level:** Analyzing **Client Need:** Reduction of Risk Potential **Integrated Process:** Teaching and Learning **Content Area:** Adult Health **Strategy:** This a reverse response question where three options are correct. Recall aldactone is potassium sparing to choose the food item highest in potassium. **Reference:** LeMone, P., & Burke, K. (2008). *Medical surgical nursing: Critical thinking in client care* (4th ed.). Upper Saddle River, NJ: Pearson/Prentice Hall, pp. 224–226.

6 **Answer: 10** **Rationale:** The maximum routine rate of infusion for KCl is 10 mEq/hour (may range from 5–10) via infusion pump. Clients who are moderately hypokalemic may have potassium administered at a rate between 10 to 20 mEq/hour, but this client is not moderately hypokalemic. Higher concentrations of potassium can be administered via a central line in critically ill clients who are hemodynamically monitored. **Cognitive Level:** Applying **Client Need:** Pharmacological and Parenteral Therapies **Integrated Process:** Nursing Process: Implementation **Content Area:** Adult Health **Strategy:** The critical words are *exceed* and *hourly replacement rate*. Note the question indicates a peripheral line to help

you identify an amount that is not high. **Reference:** LeMone, P., & Burke, K. (2008). *Medical surgical nursing: Critical thinking in client care* (4th ed.). Upper Saddle River, NJ: Pearson/Prentice Hall, p. 223.

7 **Answer: 3** **Rationale:** Lasix is a potassium-wasting diuretic that can cause the client to become hypokalemic. This can manifest as a weak, thready pulse and onset of orthostatic hypotension. Diarrhea is not usually seen as a side effect of this medication. Monitoring of one's pulse is not required for clients taking diuretic therapy but is necessary for clients taking digoxin or who have a pacemaker. Bananas are a good source of dietary potassium and may be warranted for this client in order to maintain normal serum potassium levels. **Cognitive Level:** Analyzing **Client Need:** Physiological Adaptation **Integrated Process:** Nursing Process: Evaluation **Content Area:** Adult Health **Strategy:** The core concept of the question is the relationship of low potassium to the diuretic. Eliminate two options as these are still important actions to take but do not necessarily indicate the client's understanding. Eliminate a third option that is not a usual effect of Lasix. **Reference:** LeMone, P., & Burke, K. (2008). *Medical surgical nursing: Critical thinking in client care* (4th ed.). Upper Saddle River, NJ: Pearson/Prentice Hall, pp. 221–224.

8 **Answer: 3** **Rationale:** Aldactone is a potassium-sparing diuretic and the intake of potassium-rich foods should be discouraged. Diuretics should be taken with food to decrease GI upset. Diuretics should not be taken before going to bed because their primary effect is diuresis. This time frame could cause the client to experience altered sleep patterns due to nocturia. Clients taking diuretics should be aware of their fluid intake and monitor accordingly. **Cognitive Level:** Analyzing **Client Need:** Pharmacological and Parenteral Therapies **Integrated Process:** Teaching and Learning **Content Area:** Pharmacology **Strategy:** Recall knowledge of diuretics to eliminate three options. **Reference:** Adams, M., Josephson, D., & Holland, L. (2011). *Pharmacology for nurses: A pathophysiologic approach.* (3rd ed.). Upper Saddle River, NJ: Pearson/Prentice Hall, pp. 645–646.

9 **Answer: 2, 5** **Rationale:** A client with metabolic alkalosis is at risk for developing hypokalemia due to the shift of potassium to the ICF from the ECF. Clients with NG tubes lose potassium from the stomach and the NPO status limits their intake. Clients with acute renal failure are usually hyperkalemic due to a decreased ability to excrete potassium. Clients with ARDS are usually hyperkalemic due to compromised ventilation, resulting in metabolic acidosis. Metabolic acidosis is associated with hyperkalemia because potassium shifts from the ECF to the ICF as a result of increase in hydrogen ion concentration. **Cognitive Level:** Analyzing **Client Need:** Physiological Adaptation **Integrated Process:** Nursing Process: Assessment **Content Area:** Adult Health **Strategy:** Recall knowledge of conditions in which potassium is lost or shifts into the cell to choose the correct options. **Reference:** LeMone, P., & Burke, K. (2008). *Medical surgical nursing: Critical thinking in client care* (4th ed.). Upper Saddle River, NJ: Pearson/Prentice Hall, pp. 221–224.

10 **Answer: 3 Rationale:** Sodium bicarbonate will temporarily alkalinize the plasma, causing the potassium to move into the cells. NS is an isotonic solution and therefore will not cause fluid or electrolyte shifting. Calcium gluconate is given to blunt the effects on the myocardium; it does not decrease the serum K^+ level. Insulin and dextrose are given to decrease K^+ levels by increasing K^+ uptake at the cellular level. **Cognitive Level:** Applying **Client Need:** Reduction of Risk Potential **Integrated Process:** Nursing Process: Planning **Content Area:** Adult Health **Strategy:** A critical word is *acidosis*. Recall that potassium is increased in acidosis to direct you to the option in which alkalosis is the goal of treatment. **Reference:** LeMone, P., & Burke, K. (2008). *Medical surgical nursing: Critical thinking in client care* (4th ed.). Upper Saddle River, NJ: Pearson/Prentice Hall, pp. 223–227.

References

Adams, M. P., Josephson, D. C., & Holland, C. N. (2011). *Pharmacology for nurses: A pathophysiologic approach* (3rd ed.). Upper Saddle River, NJ: Pearson Education.

Berman, A., & Snyder, S. (2012). *Kozier & Erb's Fundamentals of nursing: Concepts, process, and practice* (9th ed.). Upper Saddle River, NJ: Pearson Education.

Hockenberry, M. J., & Wilson, D. (2009). *Wong's essentials of pediatric nursing,* (8th ed.). St. Louis, MO: Mosby, Elsevier.

Ignatavicius, D., & Workman, M. (2010). *Medical surgical nursing: Patient-centered collaborative care* (6th ed.). St. Louis, MO: Elsevier.

Kee, J. L. (2009). *Laboratory and diagnostic tests with nursing implications* (8th ed.). Upper Saddle River, NJ: Pearson Education.

LeMone, P., Burke, K., & Bauldoff, G. (2011). *Medical-surgical nursing: Critical thinking in client care* (5th ed.). Upper Saddle River, NJ: Pearson Education.

London, M., Ladewig, P., Ball, J., Bindler, R., & Cowen, K. (2011). *Maternal & child nursing care* (3rd ed.). Upper Saddle River, NJ: Pearson Education.

Smeltzer, S., Bare, B., Hinkle, J., & Cheever, K. (2010). *Textbook of medical-surgical nursing* (12th ed.). Philadelphia, PA: Lippincott Williams & Wilkins.

Calcium Balance and Imbalances

4

Chapter Outline

Overview of Calcium
   Regulation

Hypocalcemia

Hypercalcemia

Objectives

➤ Review the basic functions of calcium in the body.
➤ Explain the pathophysiology and etiology of calcium imbalances.
➤ Identify specific assessment findings in calcium imbalances.
➤ Identify priority nursing diagnoses for a client experiencing a calcium imbalance.
➤ Describe the therapeutic management of calcium imbalances.
➤ Describe the nursing management of a client who is experiencing a calcium imbalance.

NCLEX-RN® Test Prep

Use the accompanying online resource, NursingReviewsandRationales, to test yourself with hundreds of NCLEX®-style practice questions.

Review at a Glance

calcitonin also called thyrocalcitonin; a calcium-lowering hormone, produced by the thyroid gland, which lowers calcium by inhibiting bone-resorbing osteoclasts and promoting osteoblasts that lead to bone formation

calcitriol active hormone form of vitamin D; promotes absorption of calcium in intestines, decreases calcium excretion via kidneys, and acts with PTH to maintain homeostasis

calcium pump a "pump" driven by ATP that takes calcium into and out of cells; initiated by mechanical or electrical stimulus during relaxation and contraction of skeletal muscles (involves a change in membrane potential) and smooth muscle (intracellular calcium causes contraction)

Chvostek sign tapping over facial nerve just anterior to ear that causes ipsilateral facial muscle contraction or twitching; indicates a positive response and is a sign of hypocalcemia; a form of latent tetany

hypercalcemia increased total serum calcium concentration to > 10.5 mg/dL

hyperparathyroidism a condition caused by excess levels of parathyroid

hormone, demonstrated by a PTH > 55 pg/dL

hypocalcemia decreased total serum calcium concentration to < 8.5 mg/dL; any condition that causes a decrease in PTH production may lead to hypocalcemia

hypoparathyroidism a condition caused by insufficient or absent secretion of parathyroid glands, demonstrated by a PTH level < 11 pg/dL

ionized calcium represents approximately 40 to 50% of calcium that is free or not bound to albumin; calcium level that is physiologically useful and elicits the signs and symptoms of hypocalcemia

osteoblasts bone-forming cells that lay down new bone; responsive to PTH and are stimulated by activated vitamin D; adapt to stress on bone by strengthening bone mass; a form of osteocyte

osteoclasts cells that resorb (remove) calcium from the bone during processes of bone growth and repair; derived from monocytes produced in bone marrow; monocytes travel through bloodstream and collect at sites of bone resorption, where they fuse together to

become osteocytes (cells that erode old bone)

osteoporosis reduction of bone mass (or density) or presence of a fragility fracture

parathyroid hormone (PTH) hormone produced by the parathyroid glands; regulates serum calcium via a negative feedback system; main role is to increase serum calcium by stimulating bone resorption, increasing renal calcium absorption, and promoting renal conversion of vitamin D to its active metabolite, calcitriol; under normal conditions, when calcium is low, PTH increases; conversely, when calcium is high, PTH decreases; normal PTH level is 11 to 55 pg/dL

tetany neurologic disorder marked by intermittent spasms that are usually paroxysmal and involve extremities; calls for immediate intervention

Trousseau sign inflation of a blood pressure cuff on upper arm to 20 mm Hg above the client's systolic pressure for about three minutes leads to carpal spasm; a form of latent tetany

vitamin D a fat-soluble vitamin absorbed from food and synthesized in skin exposed to sunlight

1 The nurse is preparing to administer alendronate (Fosamax) to a client with osteoporosis, secondary to hypercalcemia. Place the interventions in the correct order in which the nurse should perform them.

1. Ensure that the client did not eat or drink any fluids except water.
2. Place client in an upright position.
3. Determine if client has a history of GERD or any condition predisposing the client to esophageal reflux.
4. Prepare the correct dose of the medication.
5. Instruct the client to drink a full glass of water with the medication.

2 Keeping in mind the potential electrolyte imbalances possible with DiGeorge syndrome, the nurse plans to implement which nursing intervention when caring for an infant with this diagnosis? Select all that apply.

1. Place the infant on seizure precautions.
2. Position the infant on the right side.
3. Provide additional padding in the bassinette.
4. Place the infant in a prone position.
5. Provide additional oral stimulation to the infant.

3 A client develops hypocalcemia as a result of prolonged nasogastric (NG) tube suctioning. The nurse concludes that which of the following is the primary cause for hypocalcemia at this time?

1. Metabolic alkalosis
2. Fluid shifts from hypoalbuminemia
3. Hypermagnesemia
4. Metabolic acidosis

4 A client has a diagnosis of ovarian cancer and is undergoing chemotherapy. After noting that the client's serum calcium level is 11.8 mg/dL, the nurse suspects which of the following?

1. Antineoplastic medications are the cause for this elevation in calcium.
2. The ovarian cancer has metastasized, causing the increase in calcium.
3. The client is not eating enough dairy products as a result of decreased appetite.
4. The client is developing pancreatitis.

5 A client with hypocalcemia has been started on intravenous (IV) corticosteroids. Which of the following findings would indicate to the nurse a further decrease in calcium level in the client?

1. Absence of Trousseau sign
2. Positive Chvostek sign
3. Muscle weakness
4. Frequent urination

6 When assessing a client with hypercalcemia, the nurse concludes that which finding in the neuromuscular examination is consistent with that electrolyte imbalance?

1. Tetany
2. A positive Trousseau sign
3. Muscle weakness
4. Hyperactive deep tendon reflexes

7 When caring for a client with hypercalcemia who is on a cardiac monitor, the nurse checks the cardiac rhythm strip for which typical change?

1. Development of atrial fibrillation
2. Shortening of the QT interval
3. Shortening of the PR interval
4. Peaked T wave

8 A nurse prepares to administer calcium gluconate to a client post-thyroidectomy. The nurse explains to the licensed practical/vocational nurse (LPN/LVN) that this medication is being given for which reason?

1. Because of accidental removal of the parathyroid gland
2. Because it is related to increased parathyroid hormone (PTH) release during surgery
3. To prevent complications from immobility postoperatively
4. Due to hypophosphatemia after this type of surgery

9 A client presents with reports of fatigue, headache, and increasing muscle weakness, and has blood work drawn to evaluate the serum calcium level. The nurse anticipates medical management for an abnormal value to include which of the following?

1. Thiazide diuretics
2. Vitamin D supplements
3. Fluid restriction
4. Increased hydration

10 The nurse evaluates that discharge teaching has been effective when the client with hypocalcemia makes which statement?

1. "I shouldn't take antacids such as Tums."
2. "I should notify my health care provider if I start to feel tingling or numbness around my mouth."
3. "I will need to cut down on the amount of protein I include in my diet each day."
4. "I will watch my urine for signs of kidney stones."

➤ *See pages 96–97 for Answers and Rationales.*

I. OVERVIEW OF CALCIUM REGULATION

   A. Calcium balance and function: major extracellular cation; mainly found in the hard part of the bones where it is stored; concentration of calcium is kept constant by a **calcium pump** that constantly moves calcium in and out of cells

   1. Serum levels
      a. Normal total serum concentration is approximately 8.5 to 10.5 mg/dL
      b. Ionized calcium level is 4.0 to 5.0 mg/dL
      c. Slightly different laboratory reference ranges may appear due to differences in laboratory calibration; always check reference ranges with regard to established laboratory criteria
      d. Three forms of calcium exist in the body

   1) 45% is bound to protein, mostly albumin; part of the total serum calcium concentration

   2) 40% is **ionized calcium** (calcium that is free or unbound from proteins, specifically albumin), which is physiologically active and clinically important for neuromuscular transmission; many symptoms of low calcium are often not apparent until ionized calcium is < 4.0 mg/dL; though many laboratories perform total serum calcium levels most often, ionized calcium levels are recommended for the critically ill client
   3) 15% is bound to other substances such as phosphate, citrate, or carbonate

   e. The concentration of serum proteins, specifically albumin, is an important determinant of calcium concentration; remember to evaluate the calcium in relation to the serum albumin because changes in the serum protein level can cause changes in the serum calcium level
      f. Certain formulas can be used to obtain a calcium level corrected for an albumin level; for example, the total serum calcium will decrease or increase 0.8 mg/dL for every 1 gram/dL decrease or increase in albumin above or below 4 grams/dL
   2. Functions in the body

   a. Important in enzyme activation to stimulate many essential chemical reactions required for hormone secretion and the function of cell receptors

b. Significant role in skeletal and heart muscle relaxation, activation, excitation, and contraction

c. Exerts a sedating, or calming, effect on nerve cells

d. Plays a major role in nerve impulse transmission as it determines the speed of ionic influxes through nerve membranes

e. Plays a role in blood clotting by activating specific steps as an enzymatic cofactor in blood coagulation, the most important being the conversion of prothrombin to thrombin

f. Assists in regulation of acid–base balance

g. Gives firmness and rigidity to bones and teeth

h. Maintains membrane permeability by holding body cells together

i. Is essential for lactation

3. System interactions

a. **Parathyroid hormone (PTH)** raises the plasma calcium level by promoting the transfer of calcium from the bone to plasma

1) PTH responds to the ionized calcium level, regulates the concentration of calcium in the ECF, and has bone-resorbing (removal of calcium from the bone) effects

2) PTH helps with intestinal absorption of calcium by activating **vitamin D** (a fat-soluble vitamin)

3) PTH also aids in calcium reabsorption (where calcium is taken up) in the kidneys

4) The overall effect of PTH is to increase calcium and decrease phosphorus

5) Under normal conditions, PTH responds to changes in the ionized calcium via a negative feedback system; if the ionized calcium level is low, the PTH will be elevated; conversely, if the ionized calcium level is high, the PTH will be low

6) Normal PTH level is 11–54 pg/mL

b. Calcium is dependent upon **calcitriol**, the most active form of vitamin D

1) Calcitriol makes calcium and phosphate available for new bone formation

2) It plays a major role in the prevention of symptomatic **hypocalcemia** (abnormally low serum calcium level) and hypomagnesemia (decreased serum magnesium, clinically noted by increased neuromuscular irritability)

3) Calcitriol also promotes calcium absorption from the intestine (duodenum), helps PTH mobilize calcium from the bone, and limits calcium excretion if the client has hypocalcemia

c. **Calcitonin**, a calcium-lowering hormone produced by the thyroid gland, acts against PTH by transferring calcium from the plasma to the skeletal system

1) Calcitonin is directly secreted when serum calcium level is high (**hypercalcemia**), thus lowering the plasma calcium level when it is elevated

2) Calcitonin inhibits osteoclastic activity and promotes osteoblasts that result in bone formation; **osteoclasts** resorb (remove) bone during the process of growth and repair, while **osteoblasts** are bone-forming cells that respond to PTH, which in turn is stimulated by the activated form of vitamin D

d. Calcium interferes with the absorption of iron, so those with high levels of calcium may be prone to iron deficiency and may need iron supplements

e. Calcium has inverse or reciprocal relationship with phosphorus; when calcium goes up, phosphorus levels go down; conversely, when calcium levels decrease, phosphorus levels increase

4. See Table 4-1 for lifespan factors affecting calcium balance

Practice to Pass

Can you identify the system interactions that control calcium concentrations in the body?

Table 4-1	Lifespan Considerations for Health Maintenance: Calcium Balance	
Lifespan Considerations	**Common Risk Factors for Imbalances**	**Nursing Implications**
Infants	*Hypocalcemia* Di George Syndrome: immaturity of parathyroid glands in first few days of life *Hypercalcemia* Excessive use of cow's milk	Assess infants with DiGeorge syndrome for signs of hypocalcemia. A deficit of calcium in the bones; may not be able to make up later in life. Newborns may exhibit flaccid muscles or failure to thrive.
Pediatrics	*Hypocalcemia* DiGeorge Syndrome *Hypercalcemia* Prolonged immobilization following surgery, trauma, casting Excessive intake of calcium rich foods	Assess for signs of increased neuromuscular excitability and muscle cramps. Institute seizure precautions. Assess child for signs of decreased cardiac output, decreased level of consciousness, constipation, and neuromuscular impairment. Child may exhibit activity intolerance and/or developmental delay. Child is at increased risk for injury and spontaneous fractures. Teach parents to avoid giving excessive amounts of calcium-rich foods.
Adults	*Hypocalcemia* Excessive use of magnesium-based antacids Renal failure *Hypercalcemia* Thiazide diuretics	Instruct clients to avoid use of magnesium-based antacids. Review common OTC names containing magnesium. Instruct on foods high in calcium. Encourage liberal intake of fluids. Assess client for signs of renal calculi. Instruct client to avoid excessive use of calcium-based antacids.

B. Sources of calcium
   1. Cellular level
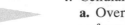
      a. Over 99% of the body's calcium is deposited in the bones, but can be mobilized from bones to keep blood level constant when dietary intake is inadequate
      b. The < 1% outside the bone is located in the extracellular fluid and soft tissues
      c. A total of 1 to 2 kg of calcium is present in the average adult
      d. Calcium pump in the body helps to regulate the flow of calcium at the cellular level
      e. Thirty percent is absorbed in GI tract
      f. In the kidneys, 98% of the filtered calcium is reabsorbed in the proximal renal tubules, and the rest is excreted by the kidneys; rates of reabsorption of filtered calcium are high
   2. Dietary level
      a. Calcium is obtained from ingested foods; about 40% of calcium consumed is absorbed
      b. Adults should consume at least 1000–1200 mg (1–1.2 grams) of calcium daily
      c. Infants require 270 mg, children ages 1 to 3 need 500 mg, children ages 4 to 8 should have 800 mg, and the requirement of children ages 9 to 18 is 1300 mg daily
      d. Pregnant, lactating, and postmenopausal women should consume 1.2 to 1.5 grams of calcium daily
      e. Upper limit for calcium intake is 2.5 grams daily
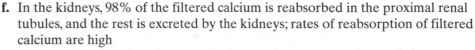
      f. Foods high in dietary calcium include milk, yogurt, cheese, calcium-fortified orange juice, ice cream, canned salmon, sardines, broccoli, tofu, rhubarb, spinach, almonds, figs, and turnip greens

Box 4-1	The following factors promote calcium absorption:

Factors that Affect Calcium Absorption in the Body

- Vitamin D
- Milk products
- Adequate stomach acid
- Growth hormones

The following factors decrease calcium absorption:

- Vitamin D deficiency
- High intake of phosphorus, protein, and/or fiber in the diet
- Phytates, oxalates, and polyphenols (tannins)
- Decreased absorption with aging

   g. Dietary factors that decrease calcium absorption include oxalic acids found in beets, spinach, and peanuts, phytic acids found in grains, excess phosphorus consumption, and polyphenols (tannins) found in teas (see Box 4-1 for a listing of factors affecting calcium absorption)

II. HYPOCALCEMIA: SERUM CALCIUM LEVEL BELOW 8.5 MG/DL) OR IONIZED CALCIUM BELOW 4 MG/DL

A. Etiology and pathophysiology

   1. Cellular level transport
      a. Moves in and out of cells via a calcium pump
      b. Adds to bone by osteoblasts—bone-forming cells that lay down new bone
      c. Calcium is responsive to PTH and is stimulated by activated vitamin D
   2. Predisposing clinical conditions result from decreased physiologic availability of calcium, decreased calcium intake or absorption, or increased calcium excretion (see Box 4-2 for a listing of clinical conditions that can lead to hypocalcemia)

   a. Hypoparathyroidism: a condition caused by insufficient or lack of secretion of PTH by the parathyroid glands
      1) Primary (or idiopathic) hypoparathyroidism (rare) is due to tumor, depressed function, or a hereditary disorder; secondary hypoparathyroidism is related to surgical removal of parathyroid glands

Box 4-2	• Hypoparathyroidism

Clinical Conditions that Lead to the Development of Hypocalcemia

- Hypoparathyroidism
- Hypomagnesemia or hyperphosphatemia
- Alkalotic states
- Multiple blood transfusions (citrate-buffered blood products)
- Medications (loop diuretics, antiepileptics, phosphates, antineoplastic agents, radiographic contrast media, corticosteroids, bisphosphonates, antacids, and heparin)
- Hypoalbuminemia
- Acute pancreatitis
- Vitamin D deficiency
- Malabsorptive states
- Renal disease
- Alcoholism
- Gram-negative sepsis
- Medullary thyroid carcinoma
- Burns
- Chronic diarrhea
- DiGeorge syndrome
- Cardiac surgery using cardiopulmonary bypass

    2) Postsurgical symptoms of hypocalcemia may be due to impaired blood supply to the remaining parathyroid tissue or possibly the release of calcitonin from the thyroid gland

  b. Hypomagnesemia: abnormally low magnesium levels (< 1 mg/dL)

    1) Magnesium helps regulate the mechanisms that keep serum calcium within normal; magnesium is needed for synthesis and release of parathormone, or PTH

    2) If magnesium is low, PTH release is impaired, lowering the serum calcium

    3) Hypomagnesemia lowers the threshold for **tetany**, the neurologic disorder marked by intermittent spasms that are usually paroxysmal and involve the extremities

    4) Hypomagnesemia is also seen with hypokalemia and hypocalcemia

    5) Many medications that decrease magnesium also cause hypocalcemia

  c. Alkalosis: an actual or relative increase in the alkalinity of the blood due to accumulation of bases or reduction in acid (pH > 7.45)

    1) In alkalosis, more ionized calcium binds to albumin

    2) Though serum calcium may be normal, symptoms such as tetany occur due to the decrease in physiologically active ionized calcium

    3) Tetany may result if the pH rises above 7.6; prolonged nasogastric tube (NGT) suctioning or diarrhea lead to metabolic alkalosis

  d. Massive blood transfusion: citrate is a preservative added to units of red blood cells that acts as an anticoagulant; in massive rapid transfusions, citrate can combine with ionized calcium and render this inactive, leading to a transient hypocalcemia (due to citrate toxicity)

  e. Medications that can lead to development of hypocalcemia are listed in Table 4-2

    1) Loop diuretics such as furosemide (Lasix) and bumetanide (Bumex) promote renal excretion of calcium

    2) Phenytoin (Dilantin) and phenobarbital: may alter hepatic metabolism of vitamin D

    3) Citrate-buffered blood and blood products: citrate prevents calcium from becoming ionized and causes transient hypocalcemia

    4) Phosphates: oral, IV, or enema; increase phosphorus levels, thus decreasing calcium level

Table 4-2   Medications That Can Lead to Hypocalcemia

Medication	Action
Loop diuretics	Promote renal excretion of calcium.
Phenytoin (Dilantin) and phenobarbital	Alter hepatic metabolism of vitamin D.
Citrated blood products	Citrate prevents calcium from becoming ionized, causing transient hypocalcemia.
Phosphates	Have inverse relationship; increased phosphate levels lead to low calcium levels.
Plicamycin, calcitonin, and etidronate disodium (Didrone)	Inhibit bone resorption of calcium.
Antineoplastic drugs (cisplatin), and antibiotics (gentamycin and tetracyclines)	These drugs lower magnesium levels, thus lowering calcium levels.
Some radiographic contrast media, such as gallium nitrate	Inhibit bone resorption.
Corticosteroids in large doses	Intestinal calcium absorption is reduced; renal calcium excretion increased.
Bisphosphonates in excessive doses	Inhibit bone resorption.
Magnesium containing antacids	Compete with calcium for absorption in the intestines.

5) Plicamycin (Mithracin), calcitonin, and etidronate disodium (Didrone): inhibit bone resorption of calcium
6) Antineoplastic drugs such as cisplatin (Platinol) and antibiotics such as gentamicin (Garamycin) and tetracycline (Achromycin): lower the magnesium level, thus lowering calcium
7) Some radiographic contrast media such as gallium nitrate: inhibit bone resorption
8) Corticosteroids: large doses can reduce calcium absorption in intestine and increase calcium excretion
9) Biphosphonate drugs, such as pamidronate (Aredia): inhibit bone resorption in excess doses
10) Antacids containing magnesium: compete with calcium in the intestines
11) Heparin, protamine, and glucagon: promote bone resorption and lead to **osteoporosis**, a condition resulting from a reduction in bone mass or density or the presence of a fragility fracture
f. Hypoalbuminemia (low serum albumin levels < 3.5 grams/dL): can result in low total serum calcium concentration although the ionized calcium may be normal; signs of hypocalcemia occur when the ionized calcium level falls below normal; among the causes are malnutrition, malabsorption syndromes, burns, and chronic renal failure
g. Acute pancreatitis
1) PTH secretion is inadequate with this disorder, thereby preventing uptake of calcium from bones to correct the hypocalcemia
2) There is also a lack of pancreatic lipase from impaired fat digestion
3) Dietary calcium and calcium secreted into the intestine from the ECF bind to undigested fat in the intestine and are excreted, which results in decreased calcium absorption and increased calcium excretion
4) May also result from secretion of calcitonin when the inflamed pancreas secretes excessive glucagon
h. Hyperphosphatemia—excessive phosphorus levels (> 4.5 mg/dL): phosphorus has a reciprocal relationship with calcium; is commonly seen in clients with renal failure; may also occur with excess treatment of hypercalcemia resulting in the lowering of calcium; excessive phosphorus in total parenteral nutrition (TPN) may also contribute to hypocalcemia
i. Inadequate vitamin D: due to inadequate dietary consumption, insufficient exposure to sunlight, or malabsorption states; recall that calcium absorption occurs in the duodenum only in the presence of activated vitamin D
j. Malabsorption syndromes: may occur in conditions when effective intestinal surfaces are lost, making fewer available sites for calcium absorption
1) It is important to remember that calcium absorption occurs primarily in the small intestine
2) Conditions such as Crohn's disease, small bowel resection, partial gastrectomy with gastrojejunostomy, and jejunoileal bypass or excessive laxative use may interfere with calcium absorption
k. Renal disease: kidneys cannot produce activated form of vitamin D (calcitriol), which leads to reduced absorption of calcium, thus hypocalcemia; this also associated with renal disease, which decreases calcium levels
l. Alcoholism: may lead to intestinal malabsorption, dietary deficiencies, hypoalbuminemia, pancreatitis, and hypomagnesemia, all of which contribute to deceased calcium levels
m. Neonatal hypocalcemia: due to functional immaturity of the parathyroid glands during the first three days of life; after the first three days, hypocalcemia may be

caused by milk with high phosphate content; those at high risk are those with asphyxia at birth and infants born to Type 1 diabetic mothers

n. Gram-negative sepsis: leads to a decrease in ionized calcium and as such is a true hypocalcemia; possible causes are parathyroid gland insufficiency, inadequate dietary vitamin D, or renal hydroxylase insufficiency

o. Medullary thyroid carcinoma: may produce hypocalcemia if excess calcitonin is secreted by the tumor

p. Burns: fluid shifts outside the cell with burn or wound injuries cause hypoalbuminemia

B. Assessment

   1. Clinical manifestations: due to increased neuromuscular irritability (see Table 4-3)

      a. Cardiovascular: decreased blood pressure and myocardial contractility leading to pulse rate and rhythm changes; ECG changes include prolonged QT interval and lengthened ST segment; cardiac arrest can occur

      b. Respiratory: laryngospasm can occur leading to respiratory compromise and airway failure; respiratory arrest can occur

      c. Renal: low serum calcium levels are associated with renal failure; other electrolyte disturbances are seen in conjunction with clinical manifestations of renal failure

Practice to Pass

What are the predisposing conditions that lead to calcium imbalance in the body?

Table 4-3	Comparison of Clinical Manifestations of Hypocalcemia and Hypercalcemia	
System	**Manifestations of Hypocalcemia**	**Manifestations of Hypercalcemia**
Neuromuscular	Parasthesias, muscle spasms, tetany Positive Chvostek and Trousseau signs Hyperactive deep tendon reflexes (DTRs) Laryngospasm	Muscle weakness Increased fatigue Depressed DTRs
Gastrointestinal	Hyperactive bowel sounds Abdominal cramps Diarrhea	Hypotonic bowel sounds Nausea/vomiting Constipation Anorexia
Central nervous system	Irritability Depression Apprehension or anxiety Confusion Delusions Hallucinations Memory impairment Seizures	Headache Personality changes Acute psychosis Bizarre behavior Confusion Lethargy to coma Memory impairment
Cardiac	Hypotension Decreased myocardial contractility Prolonged QT interval Lengthened ST segment Cardiac arrest	Hypertension Heart block Shortened QT interval Shortened ST segment Cardiac arrest
Respiratory	Respiratory arrest	No major manifestations
Renal	Oliguria Anuria	Polyuria Polydipsia Renal colic and kidney stones
Hematologic	Increased bleeding and bruising	No major manifestations
Integumentary	Dry, brittle nails and hair Pathological fractures	Bone pain Osteomalacia Pathological fractures

   d. Neuromuscular
   1) Positive **Trousseau sign**: inflation of blood pressure cuff on upper arm to
      20 mm above the systolic BP for about three minutes results in carpal spasm
      (see Figure 4-1)
   2) Positive **Chvostek sign**: tapping over the facial nerve just anterior to the ear
      results in ipsilateral facial muscle contracting or twitching (see Figure 4-2)
   3) Above signs are clinical indicators of tetany; characterized by hyperactive
      deep tendon reflexes; seizures can occur
   4) Other: paresthesias and tingling in the hands and feet; muscle spasms of the
      extremities and face; hyperactive reflexes and increased irritability and appre-
      hension; mental status changes ranging from depression, memory impairment,
      delusion, and hallucinations to convulsions

Figure 4-1

Positive Trousseau sign

Source: Kozier, B., Erb, G., Berman, A., & Burke, K. (2008). *Fundamentals of nursing: Concepts, process, and practice* (8th ed.). Upper Saddle River, NJ: Pearson Education, p. 1441, Fig. 52-13 B.

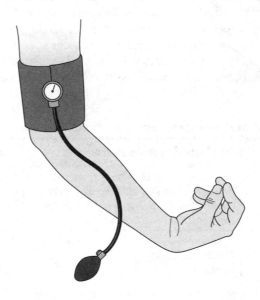

Figure 4-2

Positive Chvostek sign

Source: Kozier, B., Erb, G., Berman, A., & Burke, K. (2008). *Fundamentals of nursing: Concepts, process, and practice* (8th ed.). Upper Saddle River, NJ: Pearson Education, p. 1441, Fig. 52-13 A.

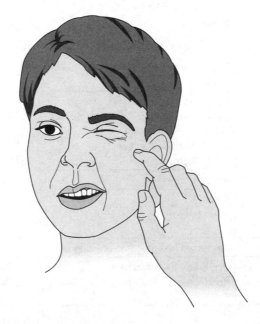

     e. Gastrointestinal: possible hyperactive bowel sounds and diarrhea

     f. Musculoskeletal: possible bone fractures due to demineralization; in children, chronic hypocalcemia may retard growth and cause rickets; can lead to osteomalacia and osteoporosis in adults

     g. Other systems: increased bleeding or bruising from abnormal clotting mechanisms; development of cataracts and calcification of basal ganglia; intestinal cramps; dry, brittle nails and dry hair; complaints of bone pain; increased bleeding or bruising may occur

2. Diagnostic and laboratory findings

     a. Plasma levels, urinary levels, and radiology measurements

        1) Total serum calcium < 8.5 mg/dL

        2) Ionized calcium level < 4.0 mg/dL or < 40%

        3) Twenty-four-hour urinary calcium level (reference levels): low calcium diet < 150 mg/24 hours; average calcium diet 100–250 mg/24 hours; high calcium diet 250–300 mg/24 hours; useful for determining parathyroid gland disorders

        4) X-rays to detect bone fractures and thinning

        5) Bone mass density tests for signs of osteoporosis

        6) CT scan to detect tumors of the parathyroid gland

     b. Associated electrolyte levels

        1) Hypomagnesemia (< 1 mg/dL)

        2) Hypokalemia (< 3.5 mg/dL)

        3) Hyperphosphatemia (> 2.6 mg/dL)

        4) Albumin < 3.5 grams/dL

        5) PTH < 11 mg/dL if caused by hypoparathyroidism

        6) Elevated creatinine from renal insufficiency

        7) Elevated alkaline phosphatase

     c. Trending of results

        1) ECG tracings demonstrate characteristic changes with hypocalcemia; trending ECG changes can help to monitor client's status and response to therapeutic treatment

        2) Monitor appropriate electrolyte levels (calcium, phosphorus, magnesium, potassium) and serum chemistry findings (albumin, BUN, and creatinine levels)

        3) Monitor albumin and PTH levels

        4) Review results of x-rays and bone density tests

3. Identification of risk factors

     a. Assess for factors that increase the risk of hypocalcemia

        1) Postmenopausal women not taking estrogen

        2) Post-thyroidectomy or parathyroidectomy

        3) Family history of hereditary hypoparathyroidism

        4) Clients with history of Crohn's or small bowel dysfunction

        5) Clients with an increased incidence of fractures

        6) Clients who are immobile (or bedfast), due to inadequate calcium stores present in the body as a consequence of immobility

        7) Clients who have osteoporosis and/or osteopenia

     b. Medications

        1) Obtain pertinent client history of medications that can alter calcium levels

        2) Examine both prescription and over-the-counter (OTC) medications and supplements that the client is taking for possible interactions

     c. Dietary

        1) Dietary patterns that lack adequate calcium and vitamin D sources

        2) Excessive use of dietary phosphorus supplements

        3) Clients with eating disorders who use laxatives as part of their dietary pattern

       4) Lactose-intolerant clients who may be at risk for not meeting adequate calcium intake needs unless alternative form products are used

       5) Dietary factors that limit absorption of calcium (oxalates, phytates, and tannins)

C. Priority nursing diagnoses: Potential complication: Hypocalcemia; Decreased Cardiac Output; Risk for Injury related to tetany and seizures; Risk for Impaired Gas Exchange; Potential complication: Fracture; Potential complication: Respiratory Arrest; Potential complication: Osteoporosis; Imbalanced Nutrition: Less Than Body Requirements for calcium; Deficient Knowledge; Risk for Noncompliance

D. Therapeutic management: treatment focuses on restoring normal levels, preventing complications, and treating underlying problems

  1. Replacement therapies

    a. Calcium gluconate 10% solution, 500 mg to 2 grams at a rate of < 0.5 mL/min (10–20 mL) by slow IV push or calcium chloride 10% solution, 500 mg to 1 gram (5–10 mL) at a rate of < 1 mL/min by slow IV push in an emergency

    b. All calcium preparations can cause venous irritation, but calcium chloride causes more venous irritation and may cause sloughing of tissue, so calcium gluconate is the most commonly used preparation

    c. Administer with D_5W or normal saline (NS) and do not add to solutions containing bicarbonate because rapid precipitation may occur

    d. May give slow IV infusion of calcium gluconate until tetany has been controlled or until calcium reaches 8–9 mg/dL

    e. Daily oral doses of elemental calcium, usually 1.0–3.0 grams/day

    f. Postoperative clients may require an additional supplement with calcitriol 0.5–1.0 mcg/dL; dosage range based upon cause or complication of hypocalcemia

    g. Vitamin D supplements may be ordered: 1–3 mg/dL with supplemental calcitriol 0.25–1.0 mcg/dL if hypocalcemia from vitamin D dietary deficiency

    h. Phosphorus-binding antacids may be ordered to increase calcium

    i. Because magnesium is needed for proper calcium function, if hypomagnesemia is present, it must be corrected with 50% magnesium sulfate 2–4 mL over 15 minutes, followed by infusion of 48 mEq in one liter or more over 24 hours; see Chapter 5 for detailed information on hypomagnesemia

    j. Thiazide diuretics may be used to decrease urinary excretion of calcium

  2. Continued monitoring of client (laboratory values and physical manifestations) to watch for efficacy of treatment

    a. Continuous ECG monitoring, especially during calcium gluconate or calcium chloride administration

    b. Continually reassess neurologic, respiratory, and cardiac status

    c. Monitor clients receiving calcium replacement who are also on digoxin for enhanced digitalis effect—check pulse

    d. Monitor clients who may experience hypocalcemia as a result of surgical intervention and/or possible endocrine dysfunction

  3. Restoration of balance (normal serum Ca^{++} level) to maintain homeostasis and prevent development of further complications

    a. Monitor serum magnesium and potassium levels in clients who are hypocalcemic because sometimes there can be concurrent electrolyte abnormalities that may require correction

    b. Monitor endocrine function and evaluate PTH status

E. Planning and implementation

  1. Obtain thorough nursing history and physical examination

    a. Subjective: such as symptoms, family history, previous thyroid or parathyroid surgeries

Practice to Pass

Explain how the neurologic system is affected by hypocalcemia.

    b. Objective: such as signs of hypocalcemia, predisposing clinical conditions, risk factors

    c. Medication history: medications that may cause hypocalcemia, hypomagnesemia, or hyperphosphatemia; OTC and herbal therapies that may interfere with calcium function

2. Monitor pertinent client assessment data for potential effects related to hypocalcemia and for response to therapeutic treatment

    a. Monitor serum calcium, phosphate, magnesium, albumin, creatinine, PTH, and potassium levels and report abnormal findings to health care provider

    b. ECG changes and heart rate and rhythm pattern

    c. Observe for signs of tetany and document findings relative to Chvostek and Trousseau signs; check reflexes

3. Monitor therapeutic serum drug levels for clients taking cardiac glycosides because calcium replacement therapy can enhance effects of digoxin

4. Assess for signs of dehydration that may result from diarrhea or renal insufficiency

5. Assess I&O (intake and output): maintain intake of 2000–3000 mL/day and an output of 1000–1500 mL/day; monitor daily weight

6. Protect the client from injury and maintain a safe environment, as the client is likely to present with neuromuscular changes

    a. Be knowledgeable and prepared for emergencies as a result of hypocalcemia, such as tetany, seizures, laryngospasm, and respiratory and cardiac arrest

    b. Initiate seizure precautions and maintain a quiet environment

    c. Closely observe respiratory and airway status; have emergency tracheostomy kit available and IV calcium gluconate at bedside for postoperative thyroidectomy clients (may have inadvertent removal of parathyroid gland)

    d. Observe for signs of tetany for clients receiving multiple blood transfusions

    e. Observe for signs of bleeding or increased bruising

7. Monitor for the possibility of hypercalcemia as a result of replacement therapy

F. Medication therapy

1. Oral replacement therapy

    a. Approximately 1.5–3.0 grams/day of oral calcium gluconate is needed to raise total calcium by 1 mg/dL

    b. Calcium citrate and calcium lactates are other oral calcium salts that are more soluble and may be better absorbed in the elderly; calcium is best absorbed when taken in divided doses vs. all at once

    c. Calcitonin may by be prescribed instead of calcium salts for postmenopausal women who cannot take estrogen; subcutaneous or IM salmon calcitonin doses are 100 IU/day or intranasally: 1 spray (200 IU) daily, alternating nostrils

    d. Vitamin D supplements may be ordered, initially 400–1000 IU/day if dietary deficiency is present or calcitriol (Rocatrol) 0.25–0.5 mg/capsule, then maintenance

2. Parenteral replacement therapy

    a. For severe hypocalcemia, 10% calcium gluconate solution, 500 mg–2 grams at a rate of < 0.5 mL/min (10–20 mL) by slow IV push or 10% calcium chloride solution, 500 mg–1 gram (5–10 mL) at a rate of < 1 mL/min by slow IV push in emergency; too rapid administration can cause bradycardia and cardiac arrest; may give slow IV infusion of calcium gluconate in D_5W or NS until signs of tetany are controlled or calcium is 8–9 mg/dL; may cause precipitation with bicarbonate

    b. Calcium chloride produces a higher ionized calcium level and is more irritating to the vein, so it is used less frequently than calcium gluconate

        c. For postoperative hypocalcemia from thyroidectomy, radical neck dissection, or parathyroidectomy, an infusion of calcium gluconate may be needed in the first 24 to 48 hours; titrate to clinical signs and calcium levels; this hypocalcemia is usually transient

  3. Dietary therapy

        a. Recommendation for older clients is 1000–1500 mg daily

        b. Encourage adequate calcium intake from the various food groups daily; encourage foods high in calcium, such as dairy products

        c. Be aware of foods that decrease the absorption of calcium and possibly limit them in the diet pattern

G. Client education

  1. Awareness of predisposing factors associated with developing hypocalcemia and how to reduce them

        a. Paresthesias and tingling and numbness in extremities are early warning signs of tetany

        b. Report the onset of signs of tetany or seizures immediately to health care provider

        c. Take oral replacements as prescribed

        d. Avoid overuse of antacids or laxatives containing phosphorus

        e. Use with caution bisphosphonates for prevention of osteoporosis

        f. Importance of regular exercise

  2. Dietary education

        a. Foods rich in calcium and protein

        b. Sources of vitamin D and protein are important to keep calcium level normal

        c. Use appropriate substitutes for milk and dairy products if client is lactose intolerant

        d. Avoid foods or antacids high in phosphorus

        e. Limit foods that decrease absorption of calcium in the diet

        f. Collaborate with dietitian to meet dietary goals

H. Evaluation

  1. Total serum calcium is between 8.5–10.5 mg/dL; ionized calcium level is between 4.0 and 5.0 mg/dL; urine calcium within normal reference range

  2. Resolution of signs and symptoms of hypocalcemia

  3. Levels of magnesium, potassium, and phosphorus are within normal limits

  4. PTH levels are within normal limits if caused by hypoparathyroidism

  5. I&O are within normal limits; daily weight is stabilized

  6. Priority nursing diagnosis goals are met

  7. Client demonstrates compliance with interventions

Practice to Pass

A client has received a calcium gluconate IV push for severe hypocalcemia. How will you evaluate the therapeutic response to calcium gluconate and what nursing interventions are appropriate for this therapy?

III. HYPERCALCEMIA: SERUM CALCIUM LEVEL ABOVE 10.5 MG/DL

A. Etiology and pathophysiology

  1. Cellular level transport

        a. Movement occurs via a calcium pump

        b. Removed from bone by osteoclasts that are derived from monocytes that are produced in the bone marrow

        c. Monocytes travel through the bloodstream and collect at sites of bone resorption, where they fuse together to become osteocytes (cells that erode old bone)

  2. Predisposing clinical conditions

        a. Can result from increased calcium intake or absorption, a shift from calcium from the bone to the ECF, or decreased calcium excretion (see Box 4-3 for a listing of clinical conditions that can lead to hypercalcemia); symptoms may not appear until serum calcium level is greater than 12 mg/dL

Box 4-3	• Hyperparathyroidism

Clinical Conditions that Lead to the Development of Hypercalcemia

- Hyperparathyroidism
- Metastatic cancer
- Use of thiazide diuretics
- Sarcoidosis
- Immobility
- Hypophosphatemia
- Hyperthyroidism (thyrotoxicosis)
- Renal tubular acidosis
- Milk-alkali syndrome
- Familial hypocalciuric hypercalcemia
- Lithium therapy
- Vitamin D intoxication
- Steroid therapy

b. Hyperparathyroidism: increased PTH causes calcium release from bone, adds to absorption of calcium in the intestines, and increases renal absorption of calcium; adenoma of the parathyroid gland is most common cause

c. Metastatic cancer: most common cause of hypercalcemia, especially with myeloma, pulmonary, breast, and ovarian cancers; related to increased release of calcium from bone that is destroyed; occurs locally when tumor cell products stimulate osteoclastic bone resorption or systemically stimulate bone resorption and increased calcium excretion

d. Thiazide-diuretic use: potentiates action of PTH on kidneys and decreases calcium excretion; results in small to moderate increases in calcium

e. Sarcoidosis: from increased active metabolite of vitamin D made in the cells with this and other granulomatous diseases

f. Immobility: related to an imbalance between the rates of bone formation and bone resorption

g. Paget's disease

h. Hypophosphatemia (< 3.0 mg/dL): phosphorus is inversely related to calcium

i. Thyrotoxicosis (hyperthyroidism): associated with high bone turnover; excessive bone resorption

j. Renal tubular acidosis: increases ionized portion of the calcium

k. Milk-alkali syndrome: can occur in clients with peptic ulcer disease who use milk or antacids, especially calcium carbonate (TUMS or Oscal), for prolonged periods of time

l. Familial hypocalciuric hypercalcemia: a rare autosomal dominant disorder

m. Lithium therapy: competes with calcium and other important cations affecting neurotransmitters, cell membranes, and body water

n. Vitamin D intoxication: increases absorption of calcium

o. Steroids increase calcium resorption from bone

B. Assessment
1. Clinical manifestations: occur because of decreased neuromuscular irritability (refer again to Table 4-3)

a. Cardiovascular: hypertension, decreased ST segments, and shortened QT interval on ECG; cardiac dysrhythmias such as heart block and cardiac arrest

b. Neuromuscular: depressed neuromuscular excitability as evidenced by decreased deep tendon reflexes; impairment of memory, personality changes or bizarre behavior or acute psychosis, lethargy, headache, confusion, fatigue, or coma (seizures are rare)

        c. Gastrointestinal: hypotonic bowel sounds, constipation, history of peptic ulcer disease; anorexia, nausea and vomiting; abdominal pain

        d. Renal: polyuria and polydipsia due to altered renal function; decreased ability of the kidneys to concentrate urine; renal colic can occur from development of kidney stones due to excess calcium levels; renal failure may occur; altered voiding patterns due to polyuria and polydipsia

        e. Musculoskeletal: pathologic bone fractures; bone thinning; bone pain, impaired mobility with transfer

   2. Diagnostic and laboratory findings

        a. Plasma, urinary levels, and radiology measurements

           1) Plasma level of > 11 mg/dL; in malignancies, total serum calcium may be >14 mg/dL

           2) Ionized plasma level of > 5.0 mg/dL or > 40%

           3) Twenty-four-hour urinary level of > 400 mg/24 hours

           4) PTH level > 55 pg/dL if due to hyperparathyroidism

           5) Radiology findings that confirm the presence of pathologic fractures, presence of kidney stones, and bone mineral density evaluations

        b. Associated electrolyte levels: hypophosphatemia (< 3.0 mg/dL)

        c. Trending of results

           1) Monitor calcium and phosphorus levels

           2) Assess for signs and symptoms of resolving hypercalcemia

           3) Monitor creatinine and BUN

           4) Monitor daily weight in response to therapeutic regimens

           5) Monitor strict I&O

           6) Monitor ECG for shortening of the ST segment and QT interval

           7) Results of x-rays for bone changes and fractures; results of bone density tests

           8) Monitor for renal calculi and calcium deposits in renal parenchyma on x-ray

           9) If parathyroid tumor, surgical removal should bring PTH to normal; control of tumor from malignancy should aid in restoration of balance

   3. Identification of risk factors: assess for factors that increase the risk of hypercalcemia

        a. Cancer or known metastasis

        b. Overactive parathyroid glands (hyperparathyroidism)

        c. Renal impairment

        d. Immobility due to clinical conditions or sedentary lifestyle

        e. Excessive dietary intake of calcium-rich foods

        f. Excessive intake of antacids for gastric distress

C. Priority nursing diagnoses: Potential complication: Hypercalcemia; Potential complication: Renal Insufficiency; Decreased Cardiac Output; Risk for Constipation; Risk for Injury related to neuromuscular and sensorium changes; Excess Fluid Volume; Deficient Fluid Volume; Potential complication: Dysrrhythmias; Imbalanced Nutrition: More Than Body Requirements for calcium; Deficient Knowledge; Risk for Noncompliance

D. Therapeutic management

   1. Decrease calcium intake

        a. Limit milk and dairy products

        b. Eliminate use of calcium carbonate antacids until calcium levels return to within normal limits

   2. Promote calcium excretion

        a. Use loop diuretics, such as furosemide (Lasix) or bumetanide (Bumex), to promote increased urine output, thus more calcium will be excreted

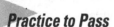

Practice to Pass

How would you compare the differences and similarities that occur in the central nervous system between hypocalcemia and hypercalcemia?

> **b.** Maintain hydration of 3000–4000 mL (3–4 L) of fluid/day; oral fluids should be high in acid ash, such as cranberry or prune juice

> **c.** Give 0.9% saline (NaCl) infusion of 300–500 mL/hour up to 6 liters as ordered until volume status restored, then 0.45% NaCl may be used; watch for fluid overload as a consequence of therapy, especially if the client has preexisting cardiac or respiratory disease

> **d.** Corticosteroids to decrease GI absorption of calcium: prednisone 20–50 mg orally BID is usual dose or 40–100 mg daily in four divided doses; may take 5–10 days for calcium levels to fall

> **e.** Chronic management of hypercalcemia is effective only with parathroidectomy for primary hyperparathyroidism

3. Continued monitoring of client

   a. Monitor serum calcium and phosphorus levels

   > **b.** Continuous ECG monitoring to detect cardiac arrhythmias

   c. Strict I&O

   d. Daily weight

   > **e.** If plicamycin (Mithracin) is used, monitor client for tissue sloughing at IV site as plicamycin (Mithracin) has vesicant properties; it is also nephrotoxic, therefore closely monitor renal function

   > **f.** Monitor client for side effects of corticosteroids such as hyperglycemia, weight gain and mood changes, bearing in mind the long-term side effects

4. Restoration of balance

   a. Monitor calcium and phosphorus levels

   b. Monitor neurologic and cardiac status

   c. Monitor for therapeutic effect of medications to reduce calcium

   d. Monitor parathyroid function

   e. Monitor for balanced I&O

   f. Monitor for stable daily weight

   g. Monitor for absence of signs of heart failure from treatment

   h. Monitor for absence of signs of hypocalcemia from treatment

> **5.** Treatment of hypercalcemic crisis

   a. Isotonic saline (0.9% NaCl) at 300–500 mL/hr initially and up to 6 liters until intravascular volume restored or calcium 8–9 mg/dL; promotes calcium excretion; loop diuretics should be used if heart failure develops

   b. Biphosphonates such as pamidronate (Aredia) intravenously to inhibit bone resorption—90 mg in 1 liter NS or D_5W over 4 hours for severe hypercalcemia (> 13.5 mg/dL), returns calcium to normal within 24–48 hours with effects lasting for weeks in most clients

   c. Plicamycin (Mithracin) intravenously to inhibit bone resorption specifically if hypercalcemia induced by metastasis; doses of 24 mcg/kg in 500 mL D_5W over 4–6 hours gradually reduce calcium

   d. Salmon calcitonin may temporarily lower level by 1–3 mg/dL in clients with severe hypercalcemia; starting dose is 2–8 units/kg intramuscularly, subcutaneously every 6–12 hours; effective within 2 hours after initial dose, peaks in 24–48 hours, and duration is 4–7 days

   e. Intravenous phosphorus to decrease calcium by increasing phosphorus: dose greater than or equal to 1500 mg over 6–8 hours in emergency situations only

6. Dialysis: during oliguric/anuric stage, severe renal dysfunction can lead to life-threatening fluid and electrolyte imbalances

E. Planning and implementation
1. Monitor pertinent client assessment data for potential effects of hypercalcemia and for response to therapeutic treatment
   a. Obtain a thorough nursing history
      1) Subjective (family history, history of previous cancer, history of kidney stones, postoperative parathyroidectomy)
      2) Objective (signs of hypercalcemia, predisposing conditions, risk factors)
      3) Medication history (medications that may cause hypercalcemia or excess of medications to treat hypocalcemia)
      4) OTC or herbal therapies that may lead to hypercalcemia
   b. Assess particular systems for specific findings
      1) Neurologic system for changes in level of consciousness or subtle personality changes
      2) Cardiovascular system to determine if client is on digitalis preparations (because hypercalcemia can enhance digitalis effects) and to detect presence of arrhythmias
      3) Genitourinary system for flank and thigh pain from renal calculi and for polyuria
      4) Gastrointestinal system for nausea, vomiting, constipation, and decreased bowel sounds
      5) Musculoskeletal system for weakness of muscles, diminished deep tendon reflexes, and observable fractures
   c. Hypercalcemic crisis is considered a medical emergency; report laboratory results immediately to health care provider for therapeutic treatment
   d. Monitor PTH if hypercalcemia is from primary hyperparathyroidism
   e. Frequently assess for heart failure in clients receiving hydration therapy
   f. Identify symptoms of digitalis toxicity when client has hypercalcemia and is also receiving digitalis
   g. Monitor client for signs of hypocalcemia as a result of treatment
2. Prevent injuries and maintain safe environment
   a. Monitor for pathologic fractures in clients with long-term hypercalcemia
   b. Assist client with mobility and transfer attempts in order to prevent injury and maintain safety
3. Administer medications as ordered, checking for therapeutic response and evaluating client condition during the course of drug therapy
4. Assess I&O
   a. Encourage clients to drink 3–4 liters of fluid per day, especially fluids such as cranberry juice or prune juice so that calcium salts will not deposit in the urine
   b. Monitor color and characteristics of urine
   c. Observe urine for presence of kidney stones
   d. Obtain daily weight
5. Assess for signs of fluid volume excess from treatment or dehydration from polyuria
6. Dietary interventions to decrease calcium levels
   a. Limit calcium sources in the diet
   b. Limit medications that provide hidden sources of calcium in the diet
   c. Refer to a dietitian
7. If client's hypercalcemic state is due to malignancy, long-term treatment may be indicated to correct this problem
8. Encourage compliance with therapeutic regimen

F. Medication therapy

1. Hydration therapy
   a. Isotonic saline (0.9% sodium chloride or NaCl) at a rate of 300–500 mL/hr, up to 6 liters, in emergency or 0.45% NaCl until serum calcium level is diluted
   b. Titrate to prevent signs of heart failure

2. Specific drug therapies
   a. Loop diuretics: such as furosemide (Lasix) or bumetanide (Bumex); enhance calcium excretion and prevent volume overloading during hydration
   b. Plicamycin (Mithracin): inhibits osteoclastic bone resorption and decreases bone turnover; used selectively with malignant hypercalcemia due to its nephrotoxicity; use cautiously with impaired renal function
   c. Corticosteroids (glucocorticoids): inhibit calcium absorption in intestine, inhibit osteoclastic bone resorption and increase urinary excretion of calcium; give prednisone BID initially, then change to maintenance dose; may not reduce calcium significantly for 5–10 days so use in conjunction with other measures to decrease calcium
   d. Phosphate salts: Phospho-Soda or Neutra-Phos orally for several days or rectally by Fleet retention enema 100 mL twice daily; limit phosphate therapy to clients with phosphate levels < 3.0 mg/dL and normal renal function; a dose of elemental phosphorus (K-Phos) may be given orally three times per day and modestly lowers serum calcium; controversy exists about use of IV phosphates
   e. Bisphosphonate drugs: retard bone turnover by inhibiting activity of osteoclasts; pamidronate disodium (Aredia) is given IV over 24 hours; alendronate (Fosamax), is an oral drug that is taken with water upon arising, 30 minutes before food or other medications (should not be taken with caffeinated products, mineral water, or orange juice)
   f. Calcitonin (salmon) is given IM or subcutaneously every 6–12 hours to temporarily lower serum calcium
   g. Gallium nitrate: inhibits bone resorption; may be given via IV over 24 hours for 5 days along with saline diuresis; do not use if creatinine < 2.5 mg/dL

G. Client education

1. Awareness of predisposing factors associated with hypercalcemia and how to avoid them
   a. Learn causes of hypercalcemia
   b. Take phosphorus agents as prescribed
   c. Correct method of taking prescribed medications
   d. Notify health care provider if flank pain develops (risk of kidney stones)
   e. Check for kidney stones (straining of urine) if indicated (demonstrate to clients as needed)
   f. Notify health care professional if symptoms worsen

2. Dietary education
   a. Instruct client as to which over-the-counter antacids contain high amounts of calcium and to avoid these
   b. Discuss with client foods highest in calcium and offer alternative options; a low calcium diet (< 400 mg/day) is recommended if hypercalcemia is because of vitamin D toxicity
   c. Instruct client to increase fluid intake to 2000–3000 mL in 24 hours, especially fluids high in acid ash such as prune or cranberry juice
   d. Teach client to increase dietary fiber and fluid to prevent constipation
   e. Caution client not to take large doses of vitamin D supplements
   f. Refer client to a dietitian to meet dietary goals

Practice to Pass

A client has hypercalcemia due to milk-alkali syndrome. Which foods and antacids will you teach this client to avoid?

H. Evaluation

1. Total serum calcium is between 8.5 and 10.5 mg/dL
2. Serum-ionized calcium is between 4.0 and 5.0 mg/dL
3. Phosphorus level is between 2.5 and 4.5 mg/dL
4. Twenty-four-hour urine calcium is within normal limits
5. PTH is within normal limits if cause was primary hyperparathyroidism or surgery
6. Signs of heart failure from hydration therapy are absent
7. Serum creatinine and BUN are within normal limits
8. There is resolution of signs and symptoms of hypercalcemia
9. There is an absence of clinical manifestations of hypocalcemia as result of treatment
10. There are no signs of complications of hyper- or hypocalcemia
11. The client demonstrates compliance with therapeutic management regime

Case Study

A 54-year-old male with a diagnosis of multiple myeloma has been admitted to your unit. The client has chief complaints of increasing fatigue, muscle weakness, and bone pain. Lab work indicates pancytopenia, hyperuricemia, hypercalcemia, and elevated creatinine. Bone scans and x-rays have been ordered.

1. What do you suspect is the cause of these signs and symptoms?
2. What is the pathophysiologic mechanism for the calcium imbalance?
3. What immediate medical treatment do you anticipate and why?
4. What are your priority nursing interventions?
5. How will you determine if therapy has been effective?

For suggested responses, see pages 203–204.

POSTTEST

1 A client is admitted with chronic renal failure. The nurse would use which statement to explain the need to monitor for hypocalcemia?

1. "Your kidneys do not eliminate as much calcium, so we need to check for signs of hypocalcemia."
2. "Your calcium level can decrease because it goes down when the creatinine in the bloodstream is high."
3. "Signs of hypocalcemia will appear before you experience pain from renal colic."
4. "Your kidneys are unable to produce calcitriol, which is needed to regulate calcium levels in the bloodstream."

2 A client presents with a mildly elevated calcium level. After completing a nursing history, the nurse identifies which of the following as a contributing factor to the abnormal calcium level?

1. Use of a thiazide diuretic
2. Recent reports of polyuria
3. A high protein diet
4. Ingesting a bisphosphonate weekly

3 A client with hypercalcemia is receiving digoxin (Lanoxin). The nurse plans to incorporate which of the following in client assessments?

1. Checking for Trousseau sign
2. Frequent pulse checks
3. Auscultation of bowel sounds
4. Inspection of skin for signs of bleeding

4 A client returns to the unit following a thyroidectomy. The nurse plans to frequently assess for which of the following? Select all that apply.

1. Signs of laryngospasm
2. Polyuria
3. Hypertension
4. Hypoactive deep tendon reflexes
5. Anxiety

5 Which assessment findings should the nurse expect to see in a client who has a calcium level of 12.2 mg/dL? Select all that apply.

1. Hyperactive reflexes
2. Anxiety
3. Polyuria
4. Constipation
5. Bone pain

6 The nurse notes that a client's total serum calcium level is 7.9 mg/dL. Because the client has no symptoms of imbalance at this time, what interpretation should the nurse make?

1. This level reflects only the ionized calcium.
2. The client's magnesium is high, resulting in false levels of calcium.
3. Phosphorus is low, resulting in low serum calcium levels.
4. This does not reflect the ionized calcium that results in symptomatology.

7 When caring for the client with signs of severe hypocalcemia, the nurse anticipates administration of which of the following?

1. Isotonic normal saline as a rapid infusion
2. 10% calcium gluconate by slow IV push
3. Intravenous phosphorus over six to eight hours
4. 10% calcium chloride by rapid IV push

8 A client who has a serum calcium level of 11.8 mg/dL is receiving a 0.9% sodium chloride infusion. The nurse determines that hydration has been effective after noting which of the following?

1. Chvostek sign is positive.
2. Volume status has been restored.
3. Calcium level is 11.0 mg/dL.
4. Serum creatinine is elevated.

9 The nurse caring for a client with a calcium imbalance places highest priority on nursing interventions that help to manage which of the following?

1. Renal signs and symptoms
2. Cardiac changes
3. Hematologic disorders
4. Neuromuscular clinical manifestations

10 The nurse determines that a client with a serum calcium level of 12 mg/dL understands client teaching when the client makes which statement?

1. "If my stomach becomes upset, I can just take more Tums."
2. "I will need to take my phosphorus supplements once a day."
3. "I will need to be on strict bed rest to help with this problem."
4. "I will need to drink many more fluids than I have been, even up to two to three liters each day."

➤ *See pages 97–99 for Answers and Rationales.*

POSTTEST

ANSWERS & RATIONALES

Pretest

1 **Answer: 1, 3, 4, 2, 5** **Rationale:** Anything other than water will interfere with the absorption of alendronate. It must be given on an empty stomach with a full glass of water. This should be the first step because the drug cannot be given if the client has already eaten or had fluids other than water. Alendronate is contraindicated if client has a history of reflux disease, hiatal hernia, or esophagitis. This should be done before the medication is prepared. After determining that the drug can be administered, the drug should be prepared using three checks. The client must be upright to take the dose and remain in this position for 30 minutes following ingestion of the pill, as it can cause esophagitis. After positioning the client in an upright position, the medication must be administered with at least eight ounces of water. **Cognitive Level:** Applying **Client Need:** Pharmacological and Parenteral Therapies **Integrated Process:** Nursing Process: Implementation **Content Area:** Adult Health **Strategy:** The core concept is the proper steps that must be taken prior to administration of a medication. Recall the assessments that must be done prior to administering alendronate to ensure that it is safe to administer. It is given in such a way as to provide optimum absorption. **Reference:** Adams, M. P., & Holland, L. N. (2011). *Pharmacology for nurses: A pathophysiologic approach* (3rd ed.). Upper Saddle River, NJ: Pearson, p. 737.

2 **Answer: 1, 3** **Rationale:** DiGeorge syndrome is characterized by immature parathyroid glands, causing a deficiency of parathormone production, leading to hypocalcemia. This electrolyte imbalance produces increased excitability of the neuromuscular system and potential seizures. **Cognitive Level:** Analyzing **Client Need:** Reduction of Risk Potential **Integrated Process:** Nursing Process: Implementation **Content Area:** Child Health **Strategy:** To answer this question correctly, it is necessary to understand the risk of hypocalcemia with DiGeorge syndrome. Consider the risks of hypocalcemia to choose correctly. **Reference:** London, M. L., Ladewig, P. W., et al. (2011). *Maternal and child nursing care,* (3rd ed.). Upper Saddle River, NJ: Pearson Education, p. 1411.

3 **Answer: 1** **Rationale:** Prolonged NGT suctioning leads to metabolic alkalosis. Changes in pH will alter the level of ionized calcium. Alkalosis increases calcium binding to albumin, leading to a decrease in ionized calcium. There may be fluid shifts from hypoalbuminemia, but this would not be from NG tube suctioning. Hypomagnesemia can be a cause of hypocalcemia. Metabolic acidosis decreases calcium binding to albumin, leading to more ionized calcium. **Cognitive Level:** Applying **Client Need:** Physiological Adaptation **Integrated Process:** Nursing

Process: Evaluation **Content Area:** Adult Health **Strategy:** Recognize that NG suctioning removes acidic fluids, resulting in an alkalotic state. Recall that calcium salts are bound in alkalosis and serum levels decrease to choose correctly. **Reference:** LeMone, P., & Burke, K. (2008). *Medical surgical nursing: Critical thinking in client care* (4th ed.). Upper Saddle River, NJ: Pearson/ Prentice Hall, pp. 228–231.

4 **Answer: 2** **Rationale:** Many malignant tumors produce chemicals that are carried in the blood to cause release of calcium from the bones, most commonly in association with ovarian cancer, renal cell carcinoma, and breast cancer, among others. Several antineoplastic medications cause hypocalcemia; lack of dairy products and pancreatitis cause hypocalcemia. **Cognitive Level:** Applying **Client Need:** Physiological Adaptation **Integrated Process:** Nursing Process: Evaluation **Content Area:** Adult Health **Strategy:** Recall physiology of malignancy to stimulate release of calcium from the bones to direct you to the correct option. **Reference:** LeMone, P., & Burke, K. (2008). *Medical surgical nursing: Critical thinking in client care* (4th ed.). Upper Saddle River, NJ: Pearson/ Prentice Hall, pp. 231–233.

5 **Answer: 2** **Rationale:** Large doses of corticosteroids decrease calcium absorption in the intestines, leading to a further decrease in serum calcium levels. A positive Chvostek sign indicates hypocalcemia and hypomagnesemia. A positive Trousseau sign would be seen with hypocalcemia. Polyuria and muscle weakness are seen with hypercalcemia. **Cognitive Level:** Applying **Client Need:** Physiological Adaptation **Integrated Process:** Nursing Process: Evaluation **Content Area:** Adult Health **Strategy:** Critical words are *hypocalcemia* and *corticosteroids*. Recall the signs and symptoms of hypocalcemia to direct you to the correct option. **Reference:** LeMone, P., & Burke, K. (2008). *Medical surgical nursing: Critical thinking in client care* (4th ed.). Upper Saddle River, NJ: Pearson/Prentice Hall, pp. 228–231.

6 **Answer: 3** **Rationale:** Elevated serum levels of calcium interfere with nerve conduction and muscle contraction, leading to muscle weakness. Due to greater influx of nerve impulses that occurs with hypocalcemia, tetany can take place. A lack of calcium contributes to the carpo-pedal spasms, indicative of Trousseau sign. Lack of calcium causes an increase in neuromuscular irritability, leading to hyperactive reflexes. **Cognitive Level:** Applying **Client Need:** Physiological Adaptation **Integrated Process:** Nursing Process: Assessment **Content Area:** Adult Health **Strategy:** Recall that excessive calcium results in decreased transmission at the neuromuscular junction to direct you to muscle weakness. **Reference:** LeMone, P., & Burke, K. (2008). Medical surgical nursing: *Critical thinking in* *client care* (4th ed.). Upper Saddle River, NJ: Pearson/Prentice Hall, pp. 231–233.

7 Answer: 2 Rationale: Hypercalcemia causes a shortened plateau phase of the action potential, which in turn causes shortening of the QT interval. Although atrial fibrillation could occur, the nurse is more concerned about the development of heart block, secondary to the slowing of atrioventricular conduction. Because atrial ventricular conduction is slowed with hypercalcemia, the PR interval would be prolonged. Peaked T waves are associated with hyperkalemia, not hypercalcemia. **Cognitive Level:** Applying **Client Need:** Physiological Adaptation **Integrated Process:** Nursing Process: Assessment **Content Area:** Adult Health **Strategy:** This question requires knowledge of ECG interpretation and changes associated with electrolyte abnormalities. Recall ECG changes associated with high calcium levels to direct you to the correct option. **Reference:** Kee, J. (2009). *Laboratory and diagnostic tests with nursing implications* (8th ed.). Upper Saddle River, NJ: Pearson/Prentice Hall, pp. 96–97.

8 Answer: 1 Rationale: The parathyroid glands regulate calcium regulation. The glands lie just underneath the thyroid gland and may be accidentally removed when a thyroidectomy is done, leading to hypocalcemia. An increased release of PTH would result in increased calcium release, not a decrease. Immobility contributes to osteoporosis and calcium resorption from the bones, which leads to elevated calcium levels. Hypophosphatemia is usually seen with hypercalcemia. Calcium gluconate would not be given to treat hypercalcemia. **Cognitive Level:** Applying **Client Need:** Physiological Adaptation **Integrated Process:** Teaching and Learning **Content Area:** Adult Health **Strategy:** The critical words are *post-thyroidectomy*. Recall anatomy and function of the parathyroid gland to choose correctly. **Reference:** LeMone, P., & Burke, K. (2008). *Medical surgical nursing: Critical thinking in client care* (4th ed.). Upper Saddle River, NJ: Pearson/Prentice Hall, pp. 217–218.

9 Answer: 4 Rationale: Symptoms of fatigue, headache, and increasing muscle weakness are clinical manifestations of hypercalcemia. Increased hydration is needed to reduce the serum concentration and aid in elimination. All of the other options will worsen the client's symptoms and increase hypercalcemia. Thiazide diuretics inhibit calcium excretion; vitamin D supplements will increase absorption of vitamin D in the intestine; and fluid restriction will cause hemoconcentration, leading to increased serum calcium. **Cognitive Level:** Analyzing **Client Need:** Physiological Adaptation **Integrated Process:** Nursing Process: Planning **Content Area:** Adult Health **Strategy:** First determine that the symptoms reflect hypercalcemia. Eliminate three options because these would all increase calcium levels even further. Alternatively, note that two options are opposites, which is a clue that one of them may be the correct choice.

Reference: LeMone, P., & Burke, K. (2008). *Medical surgical nursing: Critical thinking in client care* (4th ed.). Upper Saddle River, NJ: Pearson/Prentice Hall, pp. 218–223.

10 Answer: 2 Rationale: Numbness and tingling are signs of hypocalcemia and should be reported to the health care provider. Tums are a good source of calcium and do not need to be avoided. Protein should not be restricted in the presence of hypocalcemia, but encouraged. Kidney stones occur more frequently in the presence of hypercalcemia. **Cognitive Level:** Analyzing **Client Need:** Reduction of Risk Potential **Integrated Process:** Teaching and Learning **Content Area:** Adult Health **Strategy:** Review nursing and medical interventions to increase calcium levels and eliminate the Tums option because Tums are a source of calcium. Recall early warning signs of tetany to direct you to the correct option. **Reference:** LeMone, P., & Burke, K. (2008). *Medical surgical nursing: Critical thinking in client care* (4th ed.). Upper Saddle River, NJ: Pearson/Prentice Hall, pp. 228–231.

Posttest

1 Answer: 4 Rationale: An inability to produce calcitriol explains why the client may experience hypocalcemia and therefore needs to be aware of what symptoms might occur. If the kidneys were not eliminating calcium, the client would experience hypercalcemia, not hypocalcemia. Although the creatinine goes up with renal failure, this does not explain why the calcium is low. The damaged kidneys cannot make calcitriol, which is needed to absorb calcium. Renal colic occurs secondary to elevated calcium levels. **Cognitive Level:** Applying **Client Need:** Reduction of Risk Potential **Integrated Process:** Communication and Documentation **Content Area:** Adult Health **Strategy:** The critical term is *chronic renal failure*. Recall physiology of renal failure to direct you to the correct option. **Reference:** LeMone, P., & Burke, K. (2008). *Medical surgical nursing: Critical thinking in client care* (4th ed.). Upper Saddle River, NJ: Pearson/Prentice Hall, p. 227.

2 Answer: 1 Rationale: Thiazide diuretics cause reabsorption of calcium in the distal tubule, which can contribute to hypercalcemia is some clients. Polyuria is a clinical manifestation of hypercalcemia, not a contributing factor. Eating a high protein diet can contribute to the development of hypocalcemia, not hypercalcemia. Bisphosphonates are used in the treatment of osteoporosis and hypercalcemia. They prevent bone resorption of calcium, thereby helping to lower serum calcium levels and prevent further breakdown of the bone matrix. **Cognitive Level:** Analyzing **Client Need:** Reduction of Risk Potential **Integrated Process:** Nursing Process: Assessment **Content Area:** Adult Health **Strategy:** Systematically evaluate each option for factors that would promote intake or retention of calcium. Eliminate two options that contribute to loss of calcium. Eliminate a third option that is given for treatment of hypercalcemia or osteoporosis. **Reference:** LeMone, P., & Burke, K. (2008). *Medical surgical nursing: Critical thinking in client care* (4th ed.). Upper Saddle River, NJ: Pearson/Prentice Hall, pp. 219–222.

3 Answer: 2 Rationale: Because the elevation of serum calcium levels can affect cardiac conduction, the client is at increased risk for digoxin toxicity, and the heart rate should be checked more frequently to detect dysrhythmias. A Trousseau sign is checked when calcium levels are low, not elevated. Although hypercalcemia can cause a decrease in peristalsis and constipation, this is not related to the use of digoxin. The use of digoxin would not place the client at risk for bleeding; this is more of a concern when hypocalcemia is present. **Cognitive Level:** Applying **Client Need:** Reduction of Risk Potential **Integrated Process:** Nursing Process: Assessment **Content Area:** Adult Health **Strategy:** The core concept is that the client is on digoxin; recall the role of calcium in cardiac contractility and the action of digoxin to direct you to the correct option. **Reference:** LeMone, P., & Burke, K. (2008). *Medical surgical nursing: Critical thinking in client care* (4th ed.). Upper Saddle River, NJ: Pearson/ Prentice Hall, pp. 231–233.

4 Answer: 1, 5 Rationale: Hypocalcemia frequently results from accidental removal or destruction of parathyroid tissue or its blood supply during surgery. Clinical manifestations of tetany include laryngospasm postoperatively. The other options are assessment criteria representative of hypercalcemia. **Cognitive Level:** Applying **Client Need:** Reduction of Risk Potential **Integrated Process:** Nursing Process: Assessment **Content Area:** Adult Health **Strategy:** Recall the parathyroid glands can be accidentally removed during surgery, resulting in hypocalcemia. Eliminate three options because they are related to hypercalcemia. **Reference:** LeMone, P., & Burke, K. (2008). *Medical surgical nursing: Critical thinking in client care* (4th ed.). Upper Saddle River, NJ: Pearson/ Prentice Hall, pp. 228–230.

5 Answer: 3, 4, 5 Rationale: A serum calcium level of 12.2 mg/dL reflects hypercalcemia. Altered renal function is seen with hypercalcemia, causing a decreased ability of the kidneys to concentrate urine, as evidenced by the polyuria. With decreased neuromuscular irritability in hypercalcemia, contractions of the intestinal muscles are decreased, contributing to slowing of peristalsis and constipation. Osteoporosis and bone thinning can occur with hypercalcemia as calcium is resorbed from the bone, leading to bone pain. The excess calcium in cell membranes reduces transmission of neuromuscular impulses, leading to hypoactive reflexes. Clinical manifestations of hypercalcemia are secondary to decreased neuromuscular irritability. Anxiety would be seen with hypocalcemia, which causes increased neuromuscular irritability. **Cognitive Level:** Applying **Client Need:** Physiological Adaptation **Integrated Process:** Nursing

Process: Assessment **Content Area:** Adult Health **Strategy:** First recognize that the calcium level is elevated, indicating hypercalcemia. Recall the effect of elevated calcium levels on the neuromuscular, renal, and skeletal systems to choose correctly. **Reference:** Kozier, B., Erb, G., Berman, A., & Burke, K. (2008). *Fundamentals of nursing: Concepts, process, and practice* (8th ed.). Upper Saddle River, NJ: Prentice-Hall, Inc. pp. 231–233.

6 Answer: 4 Rationale: Ionized calcium is the portion of the serum calcium that is not bound to protein and is physiologically active and clinically important. The level indicated is the total serum calcium level, which is a combination of ionized calcium, which is free and unbound, and the nonionized calcium, which is bound to protein and not physiologically active. Low magnesium levels are associated with low calcium levels, not high magnesium levels. When serum calcium levels are low, the phosphorus level is usually reciprocal, and would be elevated. **Cognitive Level:** Analyzing **Client Need:** Physiological Adaptation **Integrated Process:** Nursing Process: Assessment **Content Area:** Adult Health **Strategy:** The question requires correlation of a hypocalcemic lab value to its cause. Recall factors that influence serum calcium levels to direct you to the correct answer. **Reference:** LeMone, P., & Burke, K. (2008). *Medical surgical nursing: Critical thinking in client care* (4th ed.). Upper Saddle River, NJ: Pearson/Prentice Hall, pp. 227–228.

7 Answer: 2 Rationale: Calcium gluconate is an appropriate treatment for correction of severe hypocalcemia. Saline infusions are given to treat hypercalcemia, not hypocalcemia. When serum calcium levels are low, phosphorus levels are usually high, as calcium and phosphorus have a reciprocal relationship. Phosphorus would not be given to treat low calcium levels. Although calcium chloride can be given to treat severe hypocalcemia, it is given slowly, not by rapid IV push. **Cognitive Level:** Applying **Client Need:** Pharmacological and Parenteral Therapies **Integrated Process:** Nursing Process: Planning **Content Area:** Adult Health **Strategy:** Critical words are *severe hypocalcemia*. Eliminate two options because they would be given to increase calcium. Eliminate a third option, recognizing that calcium should never be given rapidly. **Reference:** LeMone, P., & Burke, K. (2008). *Medical surgical nursing: Critical thinking in client care* (4th ed.). Upper Saddle River, NJ: Pearson/Prentice Hall, pp. 229–231.

8 Answer: 2 Rationale: Hypercalcemia causes polyuria which can lead to volume depletion. Restoration of volume status would be an indicator that the hydration has been effective. A positive Chvostek sign would be indicative of hypocalcemia, indicating the infusion has overcorrected the calcium imbalance. This calcium level is still indicative of an elevated calcium level, indicating that the infusion has not corrected the imbalance. An elevated creatinine level reflects impaired renal function and would not be used to measure effectiveness of the therapy. **Cognitive Level:** Analyzing **Client Need:** Pharmacological and Parenteral Therapies **Integrated Process:** Nursing Process: Evaluation **Content Area:** Adult Health **Strategy:** This question requires you to look for the absence of signs indicative of hypercalcemia and restoration of fluid hydration. Evaluate each option and its association with fluid and electrolyte balance to make a selection. **Reference:** LeMone, P., & Burke, K. (2008). *Medical surgical nursing: Critical thinking in client care* (4th ed.). Upper Saddle River, NJ: Pearson/Prentice Hall, pp. 231–233.

9 **Answer: 4** **Rationale:** Although all systems are impacted by calcium imbalance, the major clinical manifestations of calcium imbalance are due to either increased or decreased neuromuscular irritability. **Cognitive Level:** Applying **Client Need:** Reduction of Risk Potential **Integrated Process:** Nursing Process: Implementation **Content Area:** Adult Health **Strategy:** Note that the question does not specify if calcium is decreased or elevated. Recall the major system affected by calcium to choose correctly. **Reference:** LeMone, P., & Burke, K. (2008).

Medical surgical nursing: Critical thinking in client care (4th ed.). Upper Saddle River, NJ: Pearson/Prentice Hall, p. 227.

10 **Answer: 4** **Rationale:** The client with hypercalcemia (normal 9–11 mg/dL) should increase fluid intake to two to three liters a day. Hydration leads to increased calcium excretion and prevents the development of kidney stones. Tums contain calcium carbonate, which contributes to further increases in the already elevated calcium level. Although phosphorus supplements can help to increase the phosphorus levels and decrease the elevated calcium level, they need to be taken 3–4 times a day. Strict bedrest leads to increased calcium from osteoclastic activity. **Cognitive Level:** Analyzing **Client Need:** Reduction of Risk Potential **Integrated Process:** Teaching and Learning **Content Area:** Adult Health **Strategy:** Recall the treatment modalities for hypercalcemia to answer this question. Eliminate two options that actually increase calcium levels, and recall the role of fluids to choose correctly. **Reference:** LeMone, P., & Burke, K. (2008). *Medical surgical nursing: Critical thinking in client care* (4th ed.). Upper Saddle River, NJ: Pearson/ Prentice Hall, pp. 231–233.

References

Berman, A., & Snyder, S. (2012). *Kozier & Erb's fundamentals of nursing: Concepts, process, and practice* (9th ed.). Upper Saddle River, NJ: Pearson Education.

Dudek, S. (2009). *Nutrition essentials for nursing practice* (6th ed.). Philadelphia: Lippincott Williams & Wilkins, pp. 128–130.

Hockenberry, M. J., & Wilson, D. (2009). *Wong's essentials of pediatric nursing* (8th ed.). St. Louis, MO: Mosby, Elsevier.

Ignatavicius, D., & Workman, M. (2010). *Medical surgical nursing: Patient-centered collaborative care* (6th ed.). St. Louis, MO: Elsevier.

Kee, J. L. (2009). *Laboratory and diagnostic tests with nursing implications* (8th ed.). Upper Saddle River, NJ: Pearson Education.

LeMone, P., Burke, K., & Bauldoff, G. (2011). *Medical-surgical nursing: Critical thinking in client care* (5th ed.). Upper Saddle River, NJ: Pearson Education.

London, M. L., Ladewig, P. W., Ball, J. W., Bindler, R. C., & Cowen, K. J. (2011). *Maternal and child nursing care* (3rd ed.). Upper Saddle River, NJ: Pearson Education.

Osborne, K. S., Wraa, C. E., & Watson, A. B., (2010). *Medical-surgical nursing: Preparation for practice.* Upper Saddle River, NJ: Pearson Education.

Smeltzer, S., Bare, B., Hinkle, J., & Cheever, K. (2010). *Textbook of medical-surgical nursing* (12th ed.). Philadelphia, PA: Lippincott Williams & Wilkins.

Wilson, B. A., Shannon, M. T., & Shields, K. (2011). *Pearson's nurse drug guide 2011.* Upper Saddle River, NJ: Pearson Education.

5 Magnesium Balance and Imbalances

Chapter Outline

Overview of Magnesium
  Regulation

Hypomagnesemia

Hypermagnesemia

NCLEX-RN® Test Prep

Use the accompanying online resource,
NursingReviewsandRationales, to test
yourself with hundreds of NCLEX®-style
practice questions.

Objectives

➤ Review the basic functions of magnesium in the body.
➤ Explain the pathophysiology and etiology of magnesium imbalances.
➤ Identify specific assessment findings in magnesium imbalances.
➤ Identify priority nursing diagnoses for a client experiencing a
  magnesium imbalance.
➤ Describe the therapeutic management of magnesium imbalances.
➤ Describe the nursing management of a client who is experiencing a
  magnesium imbalance.

Review at a Glance

hypermagnesemia an excess of
magnesium in the blood, with a serum
level of greater than 2.1 mEq/L

hypomagnesemia a deficit of magnesium in the blood, with a serum level of
less than 1.4 mEq/L

magnesium the second most abundant cation in the body, found mainly in
bone and within the cells

PRETEST

1 The nurse would expect a client to have a high serum level of magnesium after seeing which health problem listed in the medical history?

1. Malabsorption
2. Anemia
3. Overuse of laxatives
4. Alcoholism

2 The nurse should assess for which classic manifestation in a client with a magnesium level of 2.9 mEq/L?

1. Diarrhea
2. Hyperreflexia
3. Hypertension
4. Diminished deep tendon reflexes

3 The nurse is educating the client who has a magnesium level of 1.2 mEq/L. What information is most important for the nurse to include in discussions with the client?

1. Avoid hazardous activities
2. Weekly laboratory evaluation
3. Diet counseling
4. Moderate alcohol consumption

4 A mother of a child seen in the clinic reports she has been giving the child enemas to treat frequent bouts of constipation. Because the nurse is concerned the child could develop hypermagnesemia, the nurse places priority on asking which question?

1. "When did you last give the child an enema?"
2. "What type of enema are you giving your child?"
3. "When did the child last have a bowel movement?"
4. "Why do think your child is constipated?"

5 A client with chronic renal failure has a magnesium level of 2.8 mEq/L. When reviewing the client's dietary history, the nurse identifies which frequently eaten foods as a possible cause of this laboratory value? Select all that apply.

1. Hot chocolate
2. Apples
3. Pork sausage
4. Spinach salad
5. Swiss cheese

6 A client admitted with a history of alcoholism has a magnesium level of 1.2 mEq/L. The nurse should also plan to check the results of serum laboratory studies for which of the following?

1. Elevated potassium
2. Elevated phosphorus
3. Decreased sodium
4. Decreased calcium

7 The nurse who is teaching a review of basic nutrition is discussing the effects of various electrolytes and minerals in the body. In describing the action of magnesium, the nurse would explain that it has which effect because it diminishes acetylcholine?

1. Nerve stimulant
2. Muscle relaxant
3. Vitamin metabolizer
4. Stimulant for release of blood glucose

8 Following bowel resection surgery, a client's magnesium level is 1.0 mEq/L. Which assessment finding should the nurse report to the physician immediately?

1. Hyperactive reflexes
2. Nausea
3. Anorexia
4. Abdominal pain

9 The nurse is teaching a client with hypomagnesemia to take 600 mg of magnesium oxide with each meal. How many tablets would the nurse administer for the dose if each tablet contains 400 mg?

1. One-half of a tablet
2. One tablet
3. One and one-half tablets
4. Two tablets

PRETEST

⑩ When caring for a client with a magnesium level of 1.1 mEq/L secondary to malabsorption, the nurse encourages the client to increase intake of which of the following foods?

1. Poultry
2. Tomatoes
3. Dairy products
4. Nuts

➤ *See pages 110–112 for Answers and Rationales.*

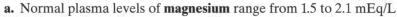

I. OVERVIEW OF MAGNESIUM REGULATION

A. Magnesium balance and function: the second most abundant cation in the human body; absorbed in the small intestine; conserved by the kidney during times of inadequate dietary intake and excreted by the kidneys during times of excessive intake

1. Serum levels

    a. Normal plasma levels of **magnesium** range from 1.5 to 2.1 mEq/L
    b. The maintenance of magnesium levels in the body is mostly a function of dietary intake
    c. Serum concentration of magnesium does not parallel tissue concentration; body stores may be more adequately measured by urinary magnesium excretion

2. Functions in the body

    a. Plays a major role in at least 300 fundamental enzymatic reactions

    b. Powers the sodium-potassium pump in the body
    c. Aids in converting adenosine triphosphate (ATP) to adenosine diphosphate (ADP) for energy release
    d. Transmits electrical impulses across nerves and muscles; is important for skeletal muscle relaxation following contraction

    e. Maintains normal heart rhythm
    f. Is involved in nucleic acid metabolism
    g. Is needed for thiamine activity and for calcium and vitamin B_{12} absorption and utilization
    h. May be involved in stabilization of DNA and RNA
    i. Relaxes smooth muscles of the bronchi and bronchioles
    j. Fights tooth decay by binding calcium to tooth enamel
    k. Decreased magnesium levels may contribute to secondary decreases in potassium, calcium, and phosphate levels
    l. Is involved in fatty acid oxidation and is a cofactor in carbohydrate metabolism and protein synthesis

    m. Decreases or blocks the release of acetylcholine, thereby acting as a smooth muscle relaxant

3. System interactions

    a. Plays a central role in secretion and action of insulin, thereby controlling blood glucose
    b. Is necessary for the release of parathyroid hormone (PTH) and plays a role in preeclampsia
    c. PTH and aldosterone indirectly affect magnesium reabsorption or excretion in the kidney
    d. High amounts of calcium and poorly digested fats and phosphates interfere with magnesium absorption due to the binding mechanism in the small intestine

4. See Table 5-1 for lifespan factors affecting magnesium balance

Table 5-1	Lifespan Considerations for Health Maintenance: Magnesium Balance	
Lifespan Considerations	**Common Risk Factors for Imbalances**	**Nursing Implications**
Infants	*Hypomagnesemia* Chronic diarrhea Malabsorption syndromes Failure to thrive Short bowel syndrome	Teach parents to include magnesium (Mg^{++})-rich foods in diet when diarrhea is present. Teach parents to monitor infant for muscle twitching and increases in deep tendon reflexes (DTRs).
Pediatrics	*Hypomagnesemia* Cardiac surgery Multiple blood transfusions DKA: Mg^{++} lost in urine Prolonged nasogastric suction Cystic fibrosis: Mg^{++} bound to fatty stools and excreted	Assess child for muscle cramping and twitching, hyperactive DTRs, and neuromuscular changes. Teach parents to encourage foods high in Mg^{++}.
Adults	*Hypermagnesemia* Chronic renal failure: Mg^{++} not excreted *Hypomagnesemia* Acute pancreatitis: Mg^{++} binds to fats Chronic alcoholism and malnutrition: lack of dietary intake of Mg^{++}.	Teach client to be alert to signs of hypermagnesemia. Teach client to be alert to signs of signs of hypomagnesemia. Encourage intake of Mg^{++}-rich foods.

B. **Sources of magnesium**
1. Cellular level
    a. More than 50% of magnesium is found in the bone
    b. Much of the remaining magnesium in the body is intracellular (approximately 45%), and the remaining small amount is present in extracellular spaces
    c. Most of the magnesium within the cells is found in the mitochondria and only 5–10% is free in cytosol
    d. Potassium, magnesium, and calcium are tied together intracellularly to maintain a neutral electrical charge; therefore, an altered level of any of these would ultimately affect the others
2. Dietary level
    a. The average diet contains between 168 and 720 mg of magnesium per day
    b. The recommended allowance for magnesium is 300 to 350 mg for young men and women with an extra 150 mg per day during pregnancy and lactation; another way to calculate magnesium need is to base it on 4.5 mg per kilogram of body weight
    c. Sources of magnesium in the diet include green leafy vegetables, nuts, legumes, seafood, whole grains, bananas, oranges, cocoa, and chocolate

II. HYPOMAGNESEMIA: A SERUM MAGNESIUM LEVEL BELOW 1.5 MEQ/L

A. **Etiology and pathophysiology**
1. Cellular level
    a. **Hypomagnesemia** usually occurs with nutritional or metabolic abnormalities; can occur because of altered absorption, increased renal loss, or redistribution of body magnesium
    b. Approximately 50% of dietary magnesium is usually absorbed; absorption is inhibited by phytates, oxalates, and fat

2. Predisposing clinical conditions
   a. Chronic alcoholism is the most common cause
   b. Decreased magnesium intake may be due to dietary factors or prolonged intravenous therapy without magnesium supplementation; in parenteral nutrition therapy, magnesium moves into the cells from the bloodstream, leading to low serum magnesium levels

   c. Decreased absorption may be caused by inflammatory bowel disease, small bowel resection (less surface available to absorb), GI cancer, chronic pancreatitis, or medications such as gentamicin (Garamycin)—an aminoglycoside antibiotic, or cisplatin (Platinol)—an antineoplastic agent
   d. Increased intestinal (lower GI) losses may occur because of prolonged diarrhea, draining intestinal fistulas, and ileostomy
   e. Increased renal excretion may result from diuretic use (furosemide [Lasix] or ethacrynic acid [Edecrin]), hyperaldosteronism that leads to volume expansion, diabetes that leads to osmotic diuresis, and medications such as aminoglycoside antibiotics, amphoteracin B (Fungizone), and cyclosporine (Imuran)
   f. Losses can also occur because of burns and debridement therapy, sepsis, or alkalosis

B. Assessment
1. Clinical manifestations
   a. Do not usually occur until the serum level drops below 1 mEq/L
   b. Muscle twitching, tremors; hyperreactive reflexes occur due to the effect of magnesium on neuromuscular function and hypocalcemic effect
   c. Laryngeal stridor (a life-threatening symptom) can occur
   d. Cardiovascular manifestations include supraventricular tachycardia and ventricular dysrhythmias (premature ventricular contractions and ventricular fibrillation) and increased susceptibility to digitalis toxicity (possibly enhanced by concurrent hypokalemia)
   e. Electrocardiogram (ECG) changes include diminished voltage of P wave; T waves that are broad, flat, or inverted; ST segments that are depressed; and QT intervals that are prolonged; a prominent U wave may be present
   f. Following cardiac surgery in children, watch for ventricular tachycardia and Torsades de Pointes (see Figures 5-1 and 5-2)

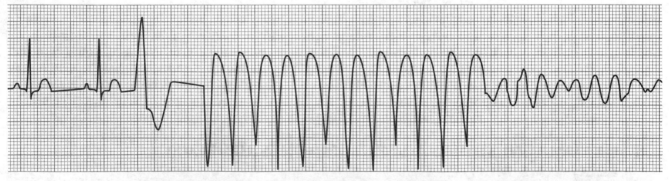

P Wave: Two normal P waves present; PR Interval: Not discernable during dysrhythmia; QRS Complex: Wide and distorted during dysrhythmia; QT Interval: Not discernable during dysrhythmia; Heart Rate: Atrial: Not discernable, Ventricular: Rapid; Rhythm: Both regular and irregular; Ectopic Beats: PVCs, ventricular tachycardia/fibrillation.

Figure 5-1

Ventricular tachycardia deteriorating into ventricular fibrillation.

Source: Osborne, K. S., Wraa, C. E., & Watson, A. B. (2010). *Medical surgical nursing: Preparation for practice.* Upper Saddle River, NJ: Pearson Education.

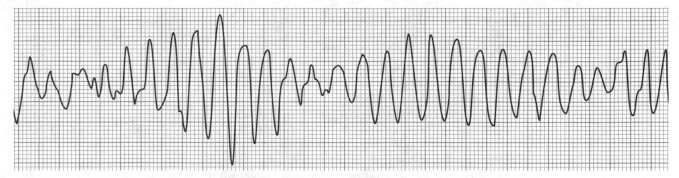

P Waves: Not discernable; PR Interval: Not discernable; QRS Complex: Wide, distorted, and varying heights; QT Interval: not discernable; Rate: Rapid; Rhythm: Both regular and irregular; Ectopic Beats: All.

Figure 5-2

Torsades de Pointes.

Source: Osborne, K. S., Wraa, C. E., & Watson, A. B. (2010). *Medical surgical nursing: Preparation for practice.* Upper Saddle River, NJ: Pearson Education.

g. Central nervous system manifestations include mood changes, such as apathy, depression, and confusion

h. GI manifestations include nausea and vomiting, diarrhea, and anorexia, which occur because of concurrent hypokalemia

i. Growth failure in children can occur

j. Severe deficiency can lead to seizures, hallucinations, or tetany

k. Signs and symptoms are somewhat similar to those of hypokalemia or hypocalcemia because they are all cations; positive Chvostek sign and Trousseau sign can occur

2. Diagnostic and laboratory findings

a. Plasma magnesium levels < 1.5 mEq/L

b. Associated electrolyte levels: concurrent decreases in calcium, potassium, and phosphate levels

c. Trending of results

1) Because most magnesium is stored in the cells, serum plasma levels may be normal despite an overall body depletion of magnesium

2) Hypomagnesemia should be considered with reference to presenting clinical manifestations or in the presence of other electrolyte imbalances, such as hypocalcemia or hypokalemia

3. Identification of risk factors: dietary insufficiency or previously identified coexisting medical conditions that lead to or exacerbate hypomagnesemia

C. Priority nursing diagnoses

1. Imbalanced Nutrition: Less Than Body Requirements related to decreased magnesium intake

2. Deficient Knowledge related to magnesium content in food and alternative food choices

3. Risk for Injury related to neuromuscular manifestations

4. Risk for Decreased Cardiac Output related to increased risk of cardiac arrhythmias

D. Therapeutic management

1. Replacement therapies

a. Vary depending on presenting signs and symptoms and severity of condition

b. Include any of the following:

1) Intravenous infusion of magnesium sulfate

2) Oral magnesium salts

3) Dietary interventions

Practice to Pass

By what mechanism does hypokalemia occur with hypomagnesemia?

2. Continued monitoring of client
   a. Serum magnesium levels
   b. Neuromuscular manifestations
   c. Altered GI function
   d. Cardiovascular changes/dysrhythmias
   e. Other electrolyte imbalances
   f. Unresolved signs and symptoms after therapy
   g. ECG for T waves that are broad, flat, or inverted; ST segments that are depressed; and QT intervals that are prolonged
3. Restoration of balance
   a. Promote dietary changes to increase magnesium intake
   b. Administer magnesium supplements as ordered
   c. Continue to assess those clients at risk
   d. Provide parenteral administration if warranted
   e. Monitor the client taking digoxin (Lanoxin), as there is increased susceptibility to digitalis toxicity with hypomagnesemia

E. **Planning and implementation**
   1. Identify risk factors: malabsorption and/or GI dysfunction, renal disease, diabetes, alcohol intake, and medications such as diuretics
   2. Monitor the diabetic client for hyperglycemia leading to osmotic diuresis, resulting in decreased magnesium
   3. Monitor the client with continuous IV fluid therapy; this client may need addition of magnesium in fluid solution
   4. Monitor the client with hyperaldosteronism because volume expansion may result in decreased magnesium
   5. Monitor the client taking a diuretic for increased renal excretion of magnesium
   6. Institute ECG monitoring and seizure precautions
   7. Monitor for stridor and/or difficulty swallowing
   8. Keep bed rails raised if client is confused; take other safety precautions as needed
   9. Maintain accurate intake and output (I&O) records
   10. Monitor deep tendon reflexes (DTRs) in clients receiving IV magnesium solutions; depressed DTRs indicate an elevated magnesium level
   11. Monitor for hypotension in clients receiving IV magnesium replacements, which could be a sign of **hypermagnesemia**

F. **Medication therapy**
   1. Oral replacement therapy
      a. Magnesium-containing antacids
      b. Magnesium oxide 300 mg/day in divided doses
      c. Use caution because oral administration may cause diarrhea, leading to decreased absorption
   2. Parenteral replacement therapy
      a. Magnesium sulfate 2 grams (16 mEq) in 50% solution IV as prescribed; infuse slowly per order and manufacturer's recommendations; giving too rapidly could cause respiratory or cardiac arrest
      b. Magnesium chloride 48 mEq/day by continuous IV infusion; give slowly as per manufacturer's recommendations for reason described above
      c. Ensure that client maintains a urine output of at least 30 mL/hr or 120 mL every four hours during therapy to avoid rebound hypermagnesemia if renal insufficiency is present
      d. Monitor deep tendon reflexes (such as patellar reflex) before each dose of parenteral magnesium; if reflex is present, hypermagnesemia from previous doses has not occurred
      e. Watch for signs of rebound hypermagnesemia

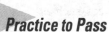

Practice to Pass

What commonly used antacids are high in magnesium?

3. Dietary therapy: for mild hypomagnesemia, encourage foods high in magnesium, such as legumes, whole grain cereals, nuts, dark green vegetables, and cocoa

G. Client education

1. Teach awareness of predisposing factors, including the following:
   a. Diabetes mellitus
   b. Anorexia, nausea, and vomiting
   c. Chronic diarrhea or chronic aluminum-based laxative abuse
   d. Alcoholism
   e. Hyperaldosteronism
   f. Renal tubular disorders
   g. Chronic diuretic therapy
   h. Hypokalemia or hypocalcemia
   i. Metabolic alkalosis
2. Dietary education
   a. Review foods high in magnesium
   b. Increase intake of hard water or mineral water as these are high in magnesium

   c. Recommend 300 to 350 mg magnesium intake daily with an extra 150 mg for pregnant or lactating women
   d. Collaborate with dietitian as necessary

H. Evaluation

1. Serum magnesium, calcium, and other electrolyte levels are within normal limits
2. Client remains safe and free from injury
3. Manifestations of hypomagnesemia resolve

III. HYPERMAGNESEMIA: A SERUM MAGNESIUM LEVEL ABOVE 2.1 MEQ/L

A. Etiology and pathophysiology

1. Cellular level: is usually due to iatrogenic causes
   a. Decreased renal excretion of magnesium, such as with decreased urine output or renal failure
   b. Increased magnesium intake, such as with overuse of magnesium-containing antacids, cathartics, or enemas; total parenteral nutrition; or hemodialysis using hard water dialysate
2. Predisposing clinical conditions
   a. Untreated diabetic ketoacidosis (glucose carries cations across cell membranes)
   b. Adrenal insufficiency (Addison's disease): causes fluid and electrolyte shifts
   c. Magnesium treatment in preeclampsia of pregnancy
   d. Lithium ingestion
   e. Volume depletion

B. Assessment

1. Clinical manifestations
   a. Neuromuscular symptoms are the most common, including decreased deep tendon reflexes and depressed neuromuscular activity; these are similar to those seen in hyperkalemia
   b. Cardiovascular manifestations include hypotension, bradycardia, bradyarrhythmias, flushing and sensation of warmth, possible cardiac arrest
   c. ECG may show prolonged PR interval, widened QRS complex, and elevated T wave
   d. CNS depression may include somnolence, weakness and lethargy, respiratory depression, and coma

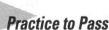

Practice to Pass

What cardiovascular symptoms may occur with hypermagnesemia?

Box 5-1	**Antacids**	**Laxatives**
Medications Containing Magnesium	• Maalox • Riopan • Milk of Magnesia • Mylanta • Gaviscon • Gelusil • Rolaids	• Milk of Magnesia • SloMag • MagOx • Epsom Salt • Maalox • Magnesium citrate

2. Diagnostic and laboratory findings
  a. Plasma magnesium levels are >2.5 mEq/L
  b. Associated electrolyte levels: none
  c. Trending of results: the degree of elevation of magnesium is proportionate to the severity of the symptoms

C. Priority nursing diagnoses
  1. Decreased Cardiac Output related to altered cardiac conduction
  2. Risk for Injury
  3. Risk for Ineffective Breathing Pattern
  4. Deficient Knowledge related to causes of elevated magnesium levels

D. Therapeutic management
  1. Decrease magnesium intake; withdraw all magnesium-containing agents including antacids and laxatives (see Box 5-1)
  2. Promote magnesium excretion using diuretics (in stable renal function)
  3. Continued monitoring of client
    a. Overhydration, magnesium toxicity
    b. Cardiac status and ECG changes
    c. Symptoms of CNS depression
    d. Respiratory status and changes
  4. Restoration of balance
    a. Correct diabetic ketoacidosis by administration of insulin and IV dextrose to halt cellular catabolism
    b. Provide rehydration to promote increased urinary output and magnesium excretion
    c. Emergency treatment includes IV calcium gluconate to antagonize the effect of magnesium and counteract cardiac and respiratory symptoms
    d. Dialysis: in clients with renal failure, dialysis may be necessary for magnesium removal; if hemodialysis is not feasible, peritoneal dialysis is an option

E. Planning and implementation
  1. Monitor I&O
  2. Identify risk factors such as antacid use, laxative use, diabetic instability, and renal failure
  3. Monitor for potential complications
  4. Promote client safety

F. Medication therapy

Practice to Pass

What role does calcium gluconate have in the treatment of hypermagnesemia?

  1. Parenteral administration
    a. IV calcium gluconate 10% for emergency situations
    b. IV diuretics to promote urinary excretion and output
    c. Rehydration to increase urinary output
  2. Specific drug therapies: as above

G. Client education
1. Awareness of predisposing factors
   a. Avoid medications and supplements high in magnesium
   b. Risks of chronic antacid and enema use
   c. Diabetic control measures
   d. Signs and symptoms of high or low magnesium levels
2. Dietary education: avoid high magnesium foods such as legumes, whole grain cereals, nuts, dark green vegetables, and cocoa

H. Evaluation
1. Manifestations of hypermagnesemia resolve and serum levels return to normal
2. Client verbalizes an understanding of importance of diet, follow-up visits, and laboratory testing

Case Study

A 32-year-old female tells the nurse she feels her heart is racing and she has been getting frequent cramps in her legs and hands for the past week or so. She has had no recent illness or injury. She has no known allergies and denies any medication or drug use. Her review of systems is negative except for constipation. Intake information for this visit is as follows: height 5'8'', weight 120 lbs, B/P 110/72, pulse 98, respirations 18.

1. What data from the above may indicate a risk factor for hypomagnesemia?

2. What other subjective data is necessary to gather?

3. What diagnostic evaluation measures would be helpful?

4. What collaborative measures should be considered?

5. What instructions would you give this client to avoid fluctuating magnesium levels?

For suggested responses, see page 204.

POSTTEST

POSTTEST

1 When caring for a client receiving intravenous (IV) replacement of magnesium sulfate, the nurse should plan to monitor the client for which potential complication?
1. Rebound hypermagnesemia
2. Abdominal cramping
3. Tachypnea
4. Headaches

2 The nurse should plan to assess a client for hypotension and diminished deep tendon reflexes when laboratory values reflect which level of magnesium?
1. 1.2 mEq/L
2. 1.4 mEq/L
3. 2.3 mEq/L
4. 2.8 mEq/L

3 The nurse would recommend to a client who has hypomagnesemia that the client should increase intake of which foods? Select all that apply.
1. Rice
2. Seafood
3. Legumes
4. Fresh fruit
5. Whole grains

4 The nurse anticipates that which treatment would be used for a client who has a magnesium level of 2.9 mEq/L?

1. Magnesium oxide (MagOx)
2. Furosemide (Lasix)
3. Calcium carbonate (Tums)
4. Fluid restriction

5 The nurse anticipates that which client is at risk for hypermagnesemia?

1. An anorexic 16-year-old female
2. A 57-year-old male who has alcoholism
3. A 47-year-old female with a history of partial gastrectomy
4. A 62-year-old male with chronic renal failure

6 The nurse explains to a new nurse orientee that a hyperglycemic diabetic client may experience magnesium imbalances secondary to the osmotic diuresis that occurs. The nurse instructs the orientee to observe the client for which finding?

1. Elevated liver enzymes
2. Muscle twitching
3. Bradycardia
4. Hypotension

7 The nurse would assess for which common side effect when administering oral magnesium to a client?

1. Decreased appetite
2. Decreased urine output
3. Increased thirst
4. Diarrhea

8 The nurse would assess for signs of hypomagnesemia in which of the following clients? Select all that apply.

1. A client with a history of laxative abuse
2. A client who is noncompliant with diuretic therapy
3. A client who takes magnesium-containing antacids
4. A client who is taking gentamicin (Garamycin)
5. A client with a history of alcoholism

9 A client is admitted with new onset renal failure. The nurse would observe for which of the following as the most common clinical manifestation of hypermagnesemia?

1. Palpitations
2. Decreased deep tendon reflexes
3. Decreased respirations
4. Hypertension

10 After treating hypomagnesemia with IV fluids, a repeat serum magnesium level is 4.0 mEq/L. The nurse anticipates receiving an order for which medication?

1. Dextrose
2. Calcium gluconate
3. Potassium chloride
4. Sodium chloride

➤ *See pages 112–113 for Answers and Rationales.*

ANSWERS & RATIONALES

Pretest

1 **Answer: 3** **Rationale:** Many laxatives are magnesium-based compounds. Overuse could result in increased absorption of magnesium and decreased kidney excretion. The other problems listed do not elevate magnesium levels. **Cognitive Level:** Applying **Client Need:** Physiological Adaptation **Integrated Process:** Nursing Process: Diagnosis **Content Area:** Adult Health

Strategy: The question requires you to correlate a high magnesium level to a cause. Eliminate malabsorption and alcoholism because they would contribute to lowering magnesium. Recall content of many laxatives to choose the correct option. **Reference:** LeMone, P., & Burke, K. (2008). *Medical surgical nursing: Critical thinking in client care* (4th ed.). Upper Saddle River, NJ: Pearson/Prentice Hall, pp. 235–236.

2 **Answer: 4** **Rationale:** Deep tendon reflexes (DTRs) may be diminished or absent when magnesium levels are high (normal 1.4 to 2.1 mEq/L). This is because magnesium diminishes acetylcholine activity at the myoneural junction, thus impairing impulse transmission. **Cognitive Level:** Analyzing **Client Need:** Reduction of Risk Potential **Integrated Process:** Nursing Process: Assessment **Content Area:** Adult Health **Strategy:** First recognize that the magnesium level is elevated. The critical word is *manifestations* and the core concept is *hypermagnesemia*. Recall the role of magnesium in regulating the neuromuscular conduction to direct you to the correct option. **Reference:** LeMone, P., & Burke, K. (2008). *Medical surgical nursing: Critical thinking in client care* (4th ed.). Upper Saddle River, NJ: Pearson/Prentice Hall, pp. 233–236.

3 **Answer: 3** **Rationale:** A magnesium level of 1.2 mEq/L reflects hypomagnesemia. The client needs diet counseling to learn what foods are high in magnesium so they can be increased in the diet. Although clients should always avoid hazardous activities and reflexes may be hyperactive, this is not the most important action for the nurse to take. Weekly laboratory evaluations would not be sufficient to monitor the magnesium level. The client needs to have measures that will increase the magnesium and then have the level rechecked. A magnesium level of 1.2 mEq/L reflects hypomagnesemia. Alcohol intake may interfere with adequate intake of dietary sources of magnesium and would not be suggested. **Cognitive Level:** Analyzing **Client Need:** Reduction of Risk Potential **Integrated Process:** Teaching and Learning **Content Area:** Adult Health **Strategy:** First recognize that the magnesium level is low and recall that food supplies the electrolytes needed by the body. Use this concept to focus on diet counseling as the correct option. **Reference:** LeMone, P., & Burke, K. (2008). *Medical surgical nursing: Critical thinking in client care* (4th ed.). Upper Saddle River, NJ: Pearson/Prentice Hall, pp. 233–235.

4 **Answer: 2** **Rationale:** It is important to determine what type of enema the mother is using. Epsom salt contains magnesium and if used excessively, it can be absorbed through the bowel, contributing to hypermagnesemia. Although it would be important to know how frequently the child is being given enemas, the nurse wants to determine if the child is at risk for hypermagnesemia, which would be caused by absorption of the electrolyte in the enema solution. Timing of last bowel movement will not help the nurse to know if the child has received enema solutions containing magnesium. Although a discussion of constipation and alternatives to frequent enemas should be discussed, this is the not the best question to ask to determine if the child is at risk for hypermagnesemia. **Cognitive Level:** Applying **Client Need:** Reduction of Risk Potential **Integrated Process:** Nursing Process: Evaluation **Content Area:** Child Health **Strategy:** The key words are *children*, *enema*, and

hypermagnesemia. Recall the dangers of excessive use of enemas and cause of hypermagnesemia to choose correctly. **Reference:** London, M. L., Ladewig, P. W., et al. (2011). *Maternal and child nursing care* (3rd ed.). Upper Saddle River, NJ: Pearson/Prentice Hall, pp. 1232–1260.

5 **Answer: 1, 4** **Rationale:** A magnesium level of 2.8 is elevated (normal 1.4 to 2.1 mEq/L), most likely as a result of inadequate renal secretion secondary to the chronic renal failure. Foods high in magnesium include whole grains, legumes, oranges, bananas, green leafy vegetables, and chocolate. **Cognitive Level:** Applying **Client Need:** Reduction of Risk Potential **Integrated Process:** Nursing Process: Assessment **Content Area:** Adult Health **Strategy:** First recognize that the magnesium level is elevated. Recall foods high in magnesium to choose correctly. **Reference:** Dudek, S. (2010). *Nutrition essentials for nursing practice* (6th ed.). Philadelphia: Lippincott Williams & Wilkins, pp. 128, 131.

6 **Answer: 4** **Rationale:** Decreased magnesium levels also contribute to reductions in potassium, calcium, and phosphate because these electrolytes are also involved in cellular metabolisms and are frequently low in the client with alcoholism. **Cognitive Level:** Applying **Client Need:** Reduction of Risk Potential **Integrated Process:** Nursing Process: Planning **Content Area:** Adult Health **Strategy:** First recognize that the magnesium level is decreased. Then recall which electrolyte may be abnormal in the presence of low magnesium to direct you to choose decreased calcium. **Reference:** LeMone, P., & Burke, K. (2008). *Medical surgical nursing: Critical thinking in client care* (4th ed.). Upper Saddle River, NJ: Pearson/Prentice Hall, pp. 233–236.

7 **Answer: 2** **Rationale:** Transmission of impulses is decreased through magnesium's regulation of acetylcholine in the neuromuscular synapse, producing muscle relaxation. Because magnesium acts to regulate and diminish acetylcholine, neuromuscular transmissions are decreased, not stimulated. Acetylcholine is not involved in vitamin metabolism. Magnesium and acetylcholine are not involved in blood glucose regulation. **Cognitive Level:** Comprehension **Client Need:** Physiological Adaptation **Integrated Process:** Teaching and Learning **Content Area:** Adult Health **Strategy:** This question requires you to translate the chemical action of magnesium to its physiological effect in the body. Recall the action of acetylcholine on neuromuscular function to direct you to choose correctly. **Reference:** LeMone, P., & Burke, K. (2008). *Medical surgical nursing: Critical thinking in client care* (4th ed.). Upper Saddle River, NJ: Pearson/Prentice Hall, p. 233.

8 **Answer: 1** **Rationale:** A magnesium level of 1.0 meq/L reflects hypomagnesemia (normal 1.4 to 2.1 mEq/L), which can lead to tetany if levels continue to decrease. Hyperactive reflexes are early signs of tetany. Although the client's nausea needs to be addressed, it may be related to effects of the anesthesia, postoperative medications, or an electrolyte imbalance, and is not of as high a priority as hyperactive reflexes. Anorexia may be related to the client's postoperative status and is of lesser priority. Although it needs to be addressed, abdominal pain is an expected finding in the client who has just had a bowel resection. **Cognitive Level:** Analyzing **Client Need:** Reduction of Risk Potential **Integrated Process:** Nursing Process: Diagnosis **Content Area:** Adult Health **Strategy:** Recognize the critical level of the magnesium. Recall that this imbalance can lead to seizures to direct you to hyperactive reflexes. **Reference:** LeMone, P., & Burke, K. (2008). *Medical surgical nursing: Critical thinking in client care* (4th ed.). Upper Saddle River, NJ: Pearson/Prentice Hall, pp. 235–237.

9 **Answer: 3** **Rationale:** The question is set up with the desired dose as the numerator and the dose on hand as the denominator. Multiply that by the quantity (which is one tablet) to obtain the correct result.
600/400 × 1 tab = 1.5 = 1.5 tabs **Cognitive Level:** Applying **Client Need:** Pharmacological and Parenteral Therapies **Integrated Process:** Nursing Process: Implementation **Content Area:** Adult Health **Strategy:** Recognize that only 400 mg is contained in each pill. Divide the desired amount (600 mg) over what you have (400 mg) to calculate the correct dose. **Reference:** Olsen, J., Giangrasso, A., Shrimpton, D., & Dillon, P. (2008). *Medical dosage calculations* (9th ed.). Upper Saddle River, NJ: Pearson Education, Inc., p. 105. http://www.google.com/imgres?imgurl=http://www.healthsquare.com/common/images/c/

10 **Answer: 4** **Rationale:** Sources of magnesium in the diet include green leafy vegetables, nuts, legumes, whole grains, seafood, bananas, oranges, and chocolate. Poultry is not high in magnesium. Tomatoes are lower in magnesium than green leafy vegetables. Dairy products are not rich in magnesium. **Cognitive Level:** Application **Client Need:** Reduction of Risk Potential **Integrated Process:** Nursing Process: Implementation **Content Area:** Adult Health **Strategy:** Specific knowledge of the mineral content of various types of foods is needed to answer the question. Recall foods high in magnesium to choose correctly. **Reference:** LeMone, P., & Burke, K. (2008). *Medical surgical nursing: Critical thinking in client care* (4th ed.). Upper Saddle River, NJ: Pearson/Prentice Hall, pp. 235–237.

Posttest

1 **Answer: 1** **Rationale:** Replacement of any electrolyte solution can lead to elevated levels of that electrolyte if the infusion is given too quickly or excessive replacement is given. Abdominal cramping and diarrhea are seen more often with oral magnesium replacements. Replacement of magnesium can lead to hypermagnesemia, which would be reflected by respiratory depression, not tachypnea. Replacement of magnesium can lead to hypermagnesemia; headaches are not associated with this imbalance. **Cognitive Level:** Applying

Client Need: Physiological Adaptation **Integrated Process:** Nursing Process: Planning **Content Area:** Adult Health **Strategy:** The critical words in the question are *IV*, *magnesium sulfate*, and *complication*. Recall the need to infuse magnesium slowly to prevent rapid increases in plasma levels to direct you to the correct option. **Reference:** LeMone, P., & Burke, K. (2008). *Medical surgical nursing: Critical thinking in client care* (4th ed.). Upper Saddle River, NJ: Pearson/Prentice Hall, pp. 235–236.

2 **Answer: 4** **Rationale:** A level of 2.8 mEq/L is elevated. Symptoms of hypermagnesemia include hypotension, bradycardia and heart block, decreased or absent deep tendon reflexes, and muscle weakness. A magnesium level of 1.2 mEq/L is below normal and symptoms would include hypertension, bradycardia, and increased deep tendon reflexes. A magnesium level of 1.4 mEq/L is below normal, and symptoms would include hypertension, prolonged PR and QT intervals, and increased deep tendon reflexes. A level of 2.3 mEq/L is within normal limits. **Cognitive Level:** Analyzing **Client Need:** Physiological Adaptation **Integrated Process:** Nursing Process: Assessment **Content Area:** Adult Health **Strategy:** The critical words are *hypotension* and *diminished deep tendon reflexes*. Recall that these are symptoms associated with hypermagnesemia to choose correctly. **Reference:** LeMone, P., & Burke, K. (2008). *Medical surgical nursing: Critical thinking in client care* (4th ed.). Upper Saddle River, NJ: Pearson/Prentice Hall, pp. 235–236.

3 **Answer: 2, 3, 5** **Rationale:** Legumes, seafood, and whole grains are high in magnesium. Rice and fresh fruit contain either low or trace amounts of magnesium. **Cognitive Level:** Applying **Client Need:** Physiological Adaptation **Integrated Process:** Teaching and Learning **Content Area:** Foundational Sciences **Strategy:** This question requires specific knowledge to make the correct choices. Recall food sources high in magnesium to choose correctly. **Reference:** Dudek, S. (2010). *Nutrition essentials for nursing practice* (6th ed.). Philadelphia: Lippincott Williams & Wilkins, pp. 128–131.

4 **Answer: 2** **Rationale:** Treatment for hypermagnesemia is to promote urinary excretion of magnesium to decrease serum levels, so a diuretic may be indicated. Laxatives and antacids often contain magnesium, which could worsen the imbalance. Fluid restriction would be contraindicated because it would prevent flushing of excess magnesium from the body. **Cognitive Level:** Analyzing **Client Need:** Reduction of Risk Potential **Integrated Process:** Nursing Process: Planning **Content Area:** Adult Health **Strategy:** First determine that the magnesium level is elevated. Eliminate the magnesium source, the option that would inhibit magnesium excretion, and the option that is not useful. **Reference:** LeMone, P., & Burke, K. (2008). *Medical surgical nursing: Critical thinking in client care* (4th ed.). Upper Saddle River, NJ: Pearson/Prentice Hall, pp. 235–236.

5 **Answer: 4** **Rationale:** Clients with chronic renal failure have difficulty excreting magnesium and are at risk to develop hypermagnesemia. Clients with anorexia restrict intake of nutrients and so would be at risk to develop hypomagnesemia. Clients with alcoholism often do have adequate dietary intake of foods high in magnesium. Hypomagnesemia is often seen with alcoholism. A partial gastrectomy may cause faster gastric emptying and transit through the small intestine, which would reduce absorption of magnesium. **Cognitive Level:** Analyzing **Client Need:** Physiological Adaptation **Integrated Process:** Nursing Process: Assessment **Content Area:** Adult Health **Strategy:** Critical words are *hypermagnesemia* and *risk*. Eliminate two options because intake of magnesium is reduced in these conditions. Recall that magnesium is absorbed in the small intestine and eliminate a third option. **Reference:** LeMone, P., & Burke, K. (2008). *Medical surgical nursing: Critical thinking in client care* (4th ed.). Upper Saddle River, NJ: Pearson/Prentice Hall, pp. 235–236.

6 **Answer: 2** **Rationale:** The osmotic diuresis that occurs with hyperglycemia can lead to urinary losses of magnesium and hypomagnesemia. Symptoms include hyperactive reflexes and neuromuscular irritability (muscle twitching), cardiac dysrhythmias, mood changes, depression, and confusion. Elevated liver enzymes are not seen with hypomagnesemia. Bradycardia would be seen with hypermagnesemia. Hypotension can occur with hypermagnesemia. **Cognitive Level:** Analyzing **Client Need:** Physiological Adaptation **Integrated Process:** Teaching and Learning **Content Area:** Adult Health **Strategy:** First recognize the electrolyte imbalance that will occur is hypomagnesemia, secondary to hyperglycemia, producing a hyperosmotic state in the blood leading to diuresis. Recall signs of low magnesium to be directed to the correct option. **Reference:** LeMone, P., & Burke, K. (2008). *Medical surgical nursing: Critical thinking in client care* (4th ed.). Upper Saddle River, NJ: Pearson/Prentice Hall, pp. 234–235.

7 **Answer: 4** **Rationale:** Oral magnesium supplements frequently cause diarrhea, which can decrease the absorption of the magnesium. Oral magnesium supplements should not cause a decrease in appetite. Oral magnesium supplements do not reduce urine output. Oral magnesium supplements do not result in increased thirst. **Cognitive Level:** Applying **Client Need:** Pharmacological and Parenteral Therapies **Integrated Process:** Nursing Process: Assessment **Content Area:** Adult Health **Strategy:** The critical word is *oral*. Recall magnesium is a common ingredient in laxatives to direct you to the correct option. **Reference:** LeMone, P., & Burke, K. (2008). *Medical surgical nursing: Critical thinking in client care* (4th ed.). Upper Saddle River, NJ: Pearson/Prentice Hall, p. 235.

8 **Answer: 4, 5** **Rationale:** A side effect of gentamicin is hypomagnesemia, which is excreted through the kidneys. Clients with alcoholism often do not consume sufficient nutrients with magnesium and experience hypomagnesemia. Many laxatives contain magnesium, which will be absorbed in the small intestines. Loop diuretics can contribute to magnesium losses. If a client is noncompliant with the diuretic therapy, the risk for magnesium losses is reduced. Use of magnesium antacids would place the client at risk for hypermagnesemia. **Cognitive Level:** Analyzing **Client Need:** Physiological Adaptation **Integrated Process:** Nursing Process: Assessment **Content Area:** Adult Health **Strategy:** Eliminate laxative abuse and antacid use because these conditions would contribute to an increase of magnesium. Eliminate noncompliance with diuretic therapy because this would reduce the amount of magnesium lost in the urine. **Reference:** LeMone, P., & Burke, K. (2008). *Medical surgical nursing: Critical thinking in client care* (4th ed.). Upper Saddle River, NJ: Pearson/Prentice Hall, pp. 235–237.

9 **Answer: 2** **Rationale:** Neuromuscular symptoms such as depressed deep tendon reflexes are among the most common clinical manifestations of hypermagnesemia. Decreased respirations, hypotension, and ventricular arrhythmias may also occur in some clients, but are not the most common signs. **Cognitive Level:** Applying **Client Need:** Reduction of Risk Potential **Integrated Process:** Nursing Process: Assessment **Content Area:** Adult Health **Strategy:** Recall magnesium's role in the regulation of acetylcholine at the neuromuscular junction to direct you to decreased deep tendon reflexes. **Reference:** LeMone, P., & Burke, K. (2008). *Medical surgical nursing: Critical thinking in client care* (4th ed.). Upper Saddle River, NJ: Pearson/Prentice Hall, pp. 235–237.

10 **Answer: 2** **Rationale:** A magnesium level of 4.0 mEq/L is elevated. Calcium gluconate is the antagonist given to counteract the effect of excess magnesium on cardiac and muscular tissues. Dextrose would not help to counteract the effects of the elevated magnesium level. Potassium chloride is not given to treat high magnesium levels. Sodium chloride is a salt and is not useful in treating elevated magnesium levels. **Cognitive Level:** Analyzing **Client Need:** Reduction of Risk Potential **Integrated Process:** Nursing Process: Planning **Content Area:** Adult Health **Strategy:** Recognize that the magnesium level is dangerously elevated. Recall the need to antagonize the cardiac and muscular effects of excessive magnesium to choose correctly. **Reference:** LeMone, P., & Burke, K. (2008). *Medical surgical nursing: Critical thinking in client care* (4th ed.). Upper Saddle River, NJ: Pearson/Prentice Hall, pp. 233–235.

ANSWERS & RATIONALES

References

Adams, M. P., Josephson, D. L., & Holland, L. N. (2011). *Pharmacology for nurses: A pathophysiologic approach* (3rd ed.). Upper Saddle River, NJ: Pearson Education.

Berman, A., & Snyder, S. (2012). *Kozier & Erb's fundamentals of nursing: Concepts, process, and practice* (9th ed.). Upper Saddle River, NJ: Pearson Education.

Dudek, S. (2009). *Nutrition essentials for nursing practice* (6th ed.). Philadelphia: Lippincott Williams & Wilkins.

Hockenberry, M. J., & Wilson, D. (2008). *Wong's essentials of pediatric nursing* (8th ed.). St. Louis, MO: Mosby, Elsevier.

Ignatavicius, D., & Workman, M. (2009). *Medical-surgical nursing: Critical thinking in collaborative care* (6th ed.). St. Louis, MO: Elsevier Saunders.

Kee, J. L. (2009). *Handbook of laboratory and diagnostic tests with nursing implications* (6th ed.). Upper Saddle River, NJ: Pearson Education.

LeMone, P., & Burke, K. (2011). *Medical-surgical nursing: Critical thinking in client care* (5th ed.). Upper Saddle River: NJ: Pearson Education.

London, M. L., Ladewig, P. W., Ball, J. W., Bindler, R. C., & Cowen, K. J. (2011). *Maternal and child nursing care* (3rd ed.). Upper Saddle River, NJ: Pearson Education.

Osborne, K. S., Wraa, C. E., & Watson, A. B., (2010). *Medical-surgical nursing: Preparation for practice.* Upper Saddle River, NJ: Pearson Education.

Chloride Balance and Imbalances

6

Chapter Outline

Overview of Chloride Regulation   Hypochloremia   Hyperchloremia

Objectives

➤ Review the basic functions of chloride in the body.
➤ Explain the pathophysiology and etiology of chloride imbalances.
➤ Identify specific assessment findings in chloride imbalances.
➤ Identify priority nursing diagnoses for a client experiencing a chloride imbalance.
➤ Describe the therapeutic management of chloride imbalances.
➤ Describe the nursing management of a client who is experiencing a chloride imbalance.

NCLEX-RN® Test Prep

Use the accompanying online resource, NursingReviewsandRationales, to test yourself with hundreds of NCLEX®-style practice questions.

Review at a Glance

halogen a nonionized form of a halide that combines with alkali metals in the body to form salts such as sodium chloride or potassium chloride

hyperchloremia a serum chloride level greater than 108 mEq/L

hypochloremia a serum chloride level less than 95 mEq/L

PRETEST

1 A client is being discharged with a prescription for prednisone (Deltasone). Which statement would indicate the client understands the side effects that affect the client's serum sodium and chloride levels?

1. "I should limit my salt intake."
2. "I will not need to take my diuretic now."
3. "It will be important to eat more vegetables."
4. "I should increase my intake of spinach and celery, which I enjoy."

2 Which intervention should the nurse include in the plan of care for a client who received multiple ampules of sodium bicarbonate over several days time?

1. Administer dextrose 5% in water infusion at 125 mL/hour for five days.
2. Closely monitor serum chloride level.
3. Check serum magnesium level daily.
4. Administer diuretics to prevent metabolic acidosis.

3 Which laboratory test result would the nurse expect to see in a client admitted with Cushing's syndrome?

1. Serum chloride level of 111 mEq/L
2. Serum sodium level of 130 mEq/L
3. Serum potassium level of 5.0 mEq/L
4. Serum bicarbonate of 28 mEq/L

4 Which of the following interventions should the nurse complete when preparing to draw a serum chloride level on a client? Select all that apply.

1. Draw the blood from an implanted port used for chemotherapy, if necessary.
2. Do not ask the client to clench and unclench the hand prior to drawing the blood.
3. Draw a three to five mL blood sample without a tourniquet if possible.
4. Ensure that the specimen is not hemolyzed.
5. Ensure that the client has been NPO for at least six hours prior to drawing a blood sample.

5 Which of the following clients does the nurse identify as being the least likely to benefit from the administration of 3% saline solution for hypochloremia?

1. A client diagnosed with Addison's disease
2. A client who has been NPO for several days
3. A client diagnosed with congestive heart failure (CHF)
4. A client experiencing metabolic alkalosis

6 A client has developed weakness, lethargy, and fatigue because of a chloride imbalance. Which statement made by the nurse to the client is most accurate?

1. "Your symptoms are permanent but you can learn to live with them."
2. "If you increase your exercise routine, your chloride level will return to normal."
3. "You will have to increase your salt intake in order to eliminate your symptoms."
4. "Your symptoms will disappear after your chloride level decreases to normal."

7 The nurse should place highest priority on which intervention when caring for a client admitted with symptoms related to a chloride level of 70 mEq/L and extracellular fluid (ECF) loss?

1. Monitoring blood pressure for decrease in value
2. Assisting client to the restroom to prevent injury
3. Starting an IV with dextrose in water
4. Monitoring pulse for pounding slow rate

8 Which nursing diagnosis would the nurse place as a priority when caring for a client experiencing neuromuscular abnormalities related to a chloride imbalance?

1. Excess fluid volume
2. Deficient fluid volume
3. Risk for injury
4. Interrupted thought processes

9 An alert client is admitted with a diagnosis of hyperchloremia. The nurse should implement which of the following as a priority intervention?

1. Place the client on isolation precautions.
2. Document the client's history.
3. Allow the client to ambulate unassisted.
4. Start an IV of 0.9% sodium chloride infusion.

10 A client with anorexia nervosa has been taught to increase foods high in chloride. The nurse determines teaching has been effective when the client identifies to increase intake of which foods? Select all that apply.

1. Bananas
2. Canned soups
3. Apples
4. Beef
5. Pasta

➤ *See pages 128–130 for Answers and Rationales.*

I. OVERVIEW OF CHLORIDE REGULATION

    A. Chloride balance and function: major extracellular anion (average level 104 mEq/L) that also exists in a lesser concentration in the cell (average 4 mEq/L); it is closely associated with serum sodium levels and affects acid–base balance

      1. Chloride levels

        a. Adult norm 95 to 108 mEq/L

        b. Child norm 98 to 105 mEq/L

        c. Newborn norm 96 to 106 mEq/L

        d. Normal urinary chloride level ranges from 110 to 254 mEq/24 hours in adults and varies significantly in children depending on age (see Table 6-1)

        e. Chloride sweat levels: 10 to 70 mEq/L in adults and 5 to 45 mEq/L in children

      2. Functions in the body

        a. Chloride is a **halogen** (nonionized form of a halide) that combines with alkali metals to form salts in the body, such as sodium chloride or potassium chloride

        b. Chloride circulates primarily with sodium and water and aids cellular integrity by maintaining a balance between intracellular and extracellular fluids; it also helps to control osmotic pressure

        c. In addition to its function as a passive transport companion for sodium and potassium in the body, active transport mechanisms may also be involved

Table 6-1	Normal Urine Chloride Levels	
Age		**Normal Range**
24-Hour Urine		
Adult	Age 18–59	110–254 mEq/24h
	Age 60 and older	95–195 mEq/24h
Child		2–10 mEq/24h
Infant		15–40 mEq/24h

> **d.** Chloride is essential for maintaining acid–base and electrolyte balance and is an enzyme activator; it serves as a buffer in the exchange of oxygen and carbon dioxide in red blood cells
>
> **e.** When joined with hydrogen (a cation), the chloride anion plays an important role in digestion by forming hydrochloric acid (HCl) in the stomach; chloride regulates the pH of the stomach and helps in digestion of protein
>
> **f.** In conjunction with calcium and magnesium, chloride helps to maintain nerve transmission and normal muscle contraction and relaxation
>
> **g.** The kidneys eliminate or retain chloride mainly as sodium chloride to regulate acid–base levels
>
> **h.** Chloride may also assist the liver in clearing waste products
>
> **i.** Chloride is also found in significant amounts in sweat
>
> **j.** Refer to Table 6-2 for a listing of chloride concentration in body fluids

3. System interactions
    a. There is a correlation between chloride levels and serum osmolality and sodium levels
        1) When serum osmolality is increased to > 295 mOsm/kg, there are a greater number of sodium and chloride ions in proportion to body water, leading to elevated serum chloride levels
        2) When serum osmolality is decreased to < 280 mOsm/kg, there are relatively fewer sodium and chloride ions in proportion to body water, leading to decreased serum chloride levels
        3) Chloride is frequently retained when sodium is retained; sodium retention leads to water retention
    b. The kidneys excrete the chloride anion or bicarbonate, and sodium reabsorbs either chloride or bicarbonate to maintain acid–base balance
    c. Chloride combines with hydrogen ion in the stomach to form hydrochloric acid
4. See Table 6-3 for lifespan factors affecting chloride balance

B. **Sources of chloride**
1. Cellular level
    a. Chloride passively diffuses from the tubule to the capillary; reabsorption depends on active reabsorption of sodium into the cell
    b. Chloride is absorbed from the small intestine and is primarily found in the extracellular fluid
    c. It is secreted in the gastric juice as hydrochloric acid
    d. The kidneys play a role in chloride regulation that affects acid–base balance in the body

Table 6-2 **Concentration of Chloride in Body Fluids**

Fluid	Chloride (mEq/L)
Saliva	34
Cecal fluid	48
Sweat	< 60 adults; < 50 children
Pancreatic juice	77
Gastric juice	84
Bile	101
Ileal fluid	116
Cerebrospinal fluid	127

Table 6-3	Lifespan Considerations for Health Maintenance: Chloride Balance	
Lifespan Considerations	**Common Risk Factors for Imbalances**	**Nursing Implications**
Infants	*Hypochloremia* Severe diarrhea, tube-feedings, failure to thrive, burns	Prolonged diarrhea/vomiting can quickly lead to dehydration and arrhythmias. Electrolyte solution replacements are needed.
	Hyperchloremia Renal tubular acidosis, ileal loops, dehydration	Administer hypotonic IV solutions as prescribed.
Pediatrics	*Hypochloremia* Diarrhea, poor dietary intake, cystic fibrosis, excessive sweating/fever, gastroenteritis, congenital chloride-losing diarrhea, burns	Close assessment for manifestations of electrolyte imbalance. Electrolyte solution replacements are needed.
	Hyperchloremia Renal failure, loss of pancreatic secretions, renal compromise, prolonged diarrhea	Administer hypotonic IV solutions or diuretics as prescribed; dialysis is needed for renal failure.
Adults	*Hypochloremia* Increased use of diuretics, heart failure, poor dietary intake, laxative abuse, renal tubular acidosis, Addison's disease, SIADH, thiazide diuretics	Educate client on manifestations of low chloride and sources of chloride as well as sodium supplements.
	Hyperchloremia Hyperparathyroidism, metabolic acidosis, hypernatremia, ureteral colonic anastomosis, bromide intoxication, acetazolamide, boric acid, ammonium chloride	Monitor for manifestations of hyperchloremia. Provide hypotonic IV solutions as prescribed. Educate client on proper use of medications.

2. Dietary level
   a. Chloride is obtained primarily from salt, such as standard table salt or sea salt
   b. Foods with high chloride levels include canned vegetables, dates, bananas, cheese, spinach, milk, eggs, celery, crabs, fish, olives, and rye (refer to Table 6-4 for a list of foods high in chloride)
   c. Processed foods are high in chloride content
   d. Chloride is a constituent part of sodium chloride as well as other dietary salts
   e. There is no RDA for this micronutrient, but there is an adult estimated minimum requirement of 750 mg/day

Table 6-4	Foods High in Chloride
Food Group	**Examples**
Fruits	Dates and bananas only
Dairy products	Cheese, milk
Vegetables	Canned vegetables and soup, spinach, celery, olives, and rye
Meat, fish, and poultry	Eggs, crabs, fish, turkey

II. HYPOCHLOREMIA: A SERUM CHLORIDE LEVEL BELOW 95 MEQ/L

A. Etiology and pathophysiology

1. Cellular level
   a. Decreases in chloride usually are accompanied by decreases in sodium and potassium
   b. A reduction in hydrochloric acid decreases chloride
   c. Chloride is excreted with cations during massive diuresis and when the bicarbonate level is elevated
   d. When the serum level falls, the urinary excretion of chloride is decreased in an attempt to retain more of the electrolyte
2. Predisposing clinical conditions (see Table 6-5)
   a. Fluid and electrolyte imbalances
      1) Hyponatremia
      2) Metabolic alkalosis (due to ingestion of alkaline substances such as antacids or as a consequence of elevated bicarbonate concentration due to disease processes—can be chloride responsive or chloride resistant depending on urinary chloride levels)
      3) Hypokalemia
      4) Prolonged administration of D_5W IV therapy
   b. Chronic respiratory acidosis
   c. Clients with chronic lung disease have high pCO_2 levels with chronic elevation of bicarbonate levels, which results in a decreased serum chloride
   d. Diabetic acidosis because of increased anion gap
   e. Acute infections, although the mechanism by which they lower serum chloride level is unclear
   f. Vomiting (loss of HCl), GI suctioning, perspiration, diarrhea, and presence of fistulas, bulimia, and tap water enemas
   g. Metabolic stress conditions, such as severe burns, fever, and heat and exhaustion states

Table 6-5   **Chloride Imbalances with Abnormal Values and Etiologies**

Etiology	Hypochloremia (serum level < 95 mEq/L adults)	Hyperchloremia (serum level > 108 mEq/L adults)
Metabolic imbalance	Metabolic alkalosis	Metabolic acidosis
Gastrointestinal disorders and dietary changes	GI suctioning, vomiting, diarrhea, GI surgery, hypokalemia, excessive ingestion of alkaline substances	Increased retention or intake, hyperkalemia, hypernatremia, severe vomiting, salicylate intoxication, stomach cancer, dehydration
Renal disorders	Advanced renal disorders, diuretics	Reduced glomerular filtration, renal failure
Hormonal influences	SIADH, Addison's disease, diabetic ketoacidosis	Excess adrenocortical hormone production (Cushing's syndrome), IV or oral cortisone therapy
Altered cellular function	Hypervolemic CHF and cirrhosis	
Skin/environmental changes	Burns, fever, large skin wounds, profuse perspiration	
Head injury		Head trauma

Table 6-6 | Pharmacologic Agents Affecting Chloride Balance

Decrease Serum Chloride Levels	Increase Serum Chloride Levels
Aldosterone	Acetazolamide (Diamox)
Amiloride (Midamor)	Ammonium chloride
Bumetanide (Bumex)	Boric acid
Corticotropin (ACTH)	Chlorothiazide (Diuril)
Dextrose infusion (prolonged)	Cyclosporine (Neoral)
Furosemide (Lasix)	Glucocorticoids
Mercurial diuretics	Phenylbutazone
Prednisolone (Delta-Cortef)	Sodium bromide
Sodium bicarbonate (Citrocarbonate)	0.9% Sodium chloride solution
Thiazide diuretics	3% Sodium chloride solution
	Triamterene (Dyrenium)

    h. Disease states such as Addison's disease, anorexia, salt-wasting renal nephropathy, syndrome of inappropriate antidiuretic hormone (SIADH), and hypervolemic states such as congestive heart failure (CHF) and cirrhosis

    i. Various medications that promote electrolyte loss, have diuretic activity, or promote alkalosis (see Table 6-6 for a listing of medications that contribute to hypochloremia)

    j. Low sodium diet, anorexia nervosa

B. Assessment

  1. Clinical manifestations (refer to Table 6-7)

    a. Hyperexcitability of nerves and muscles leads to tremors and twitching

    b. Respiratory abnormalities include slow and shallow breathing

    c. Cardiac abnormalities include hypotension when there are severe chloride and extracellular fluid (ECF) losses

    d. Alterations in serum chloride levels are seldom a primary problem; there are usually associated electrolyte imbalances (such as hyponatremia or hypokalemia) and acid–base disturbances such as metabolic alkalosis and hypokalemic alkalosis

    e. Decreased levels are associated with diarrhea, emphysema, gastric suction, fluid volume excess states (such as CHF, hyponatremia, and SIADH), pyloric obstruction, malabsorption syndrome, diabetes with ketoacidosis, excess of mineralocorticoids, and salt-wasting renal disease

    f. Decreased chloride sweat levels are seen in hypoaldosteronism, sodium depletion, and the administration of mineralocorticoids

Table 6-7 | Clinical Manifestations of Chloride Imbalances

System Alteration	Hypochloremia	Hyperchloremia
Respiratory	Slow and shallow respirations (signs of metabolic alkalosis due to bicarbonate retention)	Deep rapid respirations (signs of metabolic acidosis due to loss of bicarbonate)
Cardiac	Hypotension with severe chloride and extracellular fluid loss	
Neurological	Muscle tremors and twitching	Weakness, lethargy, stupor, unconsciousness
Serum laboratory value	< 95 mEq/L	> 108 mEq/L

Box 6-1	Laboratory Values: < 80 or > 115 mEq/L
Severe Serum Chloride Imbalance (Panic Level)	Manifestations
	• Impaired mentation
	• Hypotension or hypertension
	• Cardiac dysrhythmias
	Treatment: correct the underlying disorder

2. Diagnostic and laboratory findings

a. Serum chloride level is < 95 mEq/L
b. Panic value for serum chloride level is < 80 mEq/L (see Box 6-1)
c. Urinary chloride concentration varies with salt intake and urine volume and is helpful when discriminating between chloride responsive (< 10 mEq/L) and chloride resistant (> 10 mEq/L) metabolic alkalosis disturbances
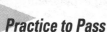
d. Obtaining ABG results and serum sodium and potassium levels may provide information necessary for the management of clients with chloride deficit
e. Trending of results
 1) Helpful in differentiating between types of metabolic alkalosis
 2) Hypochloremia should be considered with reference to presenting clinical manifestations or the presence of other electrolyte imbalances, such as hyponatremia or hypokalemia

Practice to Pass

A client is being treated for metabolic alkalosis and is at risk for altered serum chloride level, which can occur concurrently with this condition. Would you expect the serum chloride level to be increased or decreased? Why?

3. Identification of risk factors: dietary insufficiency or previously identified coexisting medical conditions that lead to or exacerbate hypochloremia

C. Priority nursing diagnoses
1. Imbalanced Nutrition: Less Than Body Requirements related to decreased chloride intake or increased loss
2. Excess Fluid Volume related to disease process
3. Risk for Impaired Sensory/Perception related to neurological changes
4. Fatigue related to muscle weakness
5. Risk for Injury related to weakness and lethargy
6. Self-Care Deficit related to altered respiratory status
7. Anxiety related to increased muscle irritability

D. Therapeutic management
1. Replacement therapies
 a. If chloride levels are slightly low and client is able to tolerate PO feedings, then administer oral salt tablets or increase chloride dietary sources
 b. Provide IV infusion of chloride if levels are critical or if client is unable to tolerate PO administration
2. Continued monitoring of client
 a. Serum and urinary chloride levels

 b. I&O (intake and output) because excess water administration can cause dilutional hypochloremia and hyponatremia
 c. Blood pressure because a drop in blood pressure can occur if hypochloremia is due to ECF volume loss
 d. ABG results if client's clinical presentation or underlying medical history suggests accompanying acid–base imbalance
 e. When drawing a serum chloride specimen:

1) Client should be NPO (8 to 12 hours) prior to test to obtain most accurate result
2) Do not draw specimen from hemodialysis access because this can lead to unreliable results due to coagulation factors
3) Draw specimen from an extremity that does not have saline infusing into it because this can affect results
4) When possible, do not use a tourniquet and prevent the client from pumping the fist, because this can lead to hemolysis of blood specimen and yield inaccurate results

3. Restoration of balance
   a. Promote dietary changes to increase chloride intake
   b. Administer chloride supplements as ordered
   c. Continue to assess those clients at risk
   d. Provide parenteral administration if warranted
   e. Monitor the client with underlying or contributory disease processes and/or medication therapy that would lead to chloride deficiencies

E. **Planning and implementation**
   1. Identify risk factors specific to development of chloride loss, such as dietary factors, GI losses, renal losses, altered hormone secretion, altered cellular states, and metabolic alkalosis
   2. Monitor the client during the course of therapy, looking at pertinent lab values and clinical manifestations
   3. Monitor vital signs (VS) and I&O parameters
   4. Maintain safety precautions by keeping bedrails up and assisting client with ambulation if client presents with muscle tremors and/or decreased blood pressure

F. **Medication therapy**
   1. Oral replacement therapy
      a. Utilize salt tablets or potassium chloride salts to raise serum chloride levels
      b. Chloride is usually not administered as a separate medication but rather is found in combination with other elements in salt formation products or as an additive/buffer
   2. Parenteral replacement therapy
      a. Chloride can be given parenterally as a constituent part of a medication such as potassium chloride or sodium chloride in the clinical setting
      b. Monitoring of IV solutions containing chloride depends on concentration of overall solution and may require the use of IV administration pumps
   3. Dietary therapy: include foods that are high in chloride, such as salt, processed foods, canned vegetables, dates, bananas, cheese, spinach, milk, eggs, celery, crabs, fish, olives, and rye (refer back to Table 6-4)

G. **Client education**
   1. Teach awareness of predisposing factors, including contributory conditions
      a. Endocrine states that result in adrenocortical insufficiency or primary aldosteronism
      b. Acid–base imbalances that result in metabolic acidosis (high anion gap), such as diabetic ketoacidosis, Addison's disease, and nephritis
      c. Acid–base imbalances that result in metabolic alkalosis, such as pyloric obstruction
      d. Acid–base imbalances that result in chronic respiratory acidosis
      e. Use of medications that would likely increase chloride loss (refer back to Table 6-6)
      f. Recognition of fluid volume states that would cause fluid shifting and electrolyte deficit

2. Dietary education
   a. Review foods that are high in chloride
   b. Advise client to include in the diet sodium and processed foods that are also high in chloride
   c. Advise client that electrolyte replacement as well as fluid replacement is important if activity level is increased and client has excessive perspiration
   d. Collaborate with dietitian as needed

H. **Evaluation**
   1. Chloride serum levels and other pertinent electrolyte levels return to normal baseline
   2. Acid–base balance returns to normal baseline
   3. Clinical manifestations resolve

Practice to Pass

A client is diagnosed with hypochloremia. How would you explain the disorder? What strategies can be used to correct the problem?

III. HYPERCHLOREMIA: A SERUM CHLORIDE LEVEL ABOVE 108 MEQ/L

A. **Etiology and pathophysiology**
   1. Cellular level
      a. Cellular chloride shifts are seen in response to acid–base changes and volume disturbances in the body
      b. Increases in serum chloride are seen in conjunction with other electrolyte imbalances and are usually assessed with sodium, potassium, water, and CO_2 levels in the body

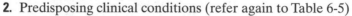

   2. Predisposing clinical conditions (refer again to Table 6-5)
      a. Fluid and electrolyte imbalances
         1) Hypernatremia
         2) Metabolic acidosis (loss of sodium bicarbonate because of prolonged diarrhea), hyperchloremic metabolic acidosis (renal disease that causes decreased excretion of hydrogen ions and prevents reabsorption of bicarbonate), or respiratory alkalosis (hyperventilation)
      b. Ingestion or administration of drugs that promote chloride retention, such as IV saline, certain diuretics, salicylate intoxication, and corticosteroids (refer back to Table 6-5)
      c. Fluid volume disturbances that result in dehydration states
      d. Endocrine disturbances that result in diabetes insipidus (DI) and certain cases of hyperparathyroidism (seen in association with hypercalcemia)
      e. Renal changes that manifest as renal tubular acidosis or acute renal failure can result in elevated serum chloride levels

Practice to Pass

A client is taking both furosemide (Lasix) for treatment of hypertension and a steroid Medrol dose pack for an allergic reaction. Which of these medications would intensify hyperchloremia?

B. **Assessment**
   1. Clinical manifestations (refer again to Table 6-7)
      a. Neuromuscular symptoms include weakness and lethargy and can progress to significant CNS damage
      b. Respiratory abnormalities include deep, rapid, vigorous breathing that can lead to unconsciousness as the client attempts to compensate for acidotic state due to loss of bicarbonate
      c. Cardiac abnormalities include risk of dysrhythmias due to retained chloride levels and accompanying acid–base disturbances
      d. Alterations in hormonal response as a result of increased aldosterone levels can lead to elevations of both sodium and chloride due to greater reabsorption
      e. Fluid volume disturbances can lead to increased chloride levels, including dehydration, retention of salt and water due to drug administration, and a greater sodium loss than chloride loss, leading to imbalance

Practice to Pass

A client diagnosed with hyperchloremia should be monitored for respiratory abnormalities. Which symptoms should the nurse assess for?

        f. Presence of disease states such as DI, certain types of hyperparathyroidism, and renal tubular diseases result in hydrogen ion retention and decreased reabsorption of bicarbonate

        g. Increased chloride sweat levels are seen in DI, hypothyroidism, malnutrition, acute renal failure, and certain genetic disorders such as cystic fibrosis and glucose-6-phosphate-dehydrogenase (G6PD) deficiency

    2. Diagnostic and laboratory findings

        a. Panic value for serum chloride is > 115 mEq/L (refer again to Box 6-1)

        b. Urine chloride level > 250 mEq/L in 24 hours is significant and is associated with sodium and fluid imbalances

        c. In dehydration states, serum chloride levels are increased due to hemoconcentration

        d. Increased chloride sweat levels are seen in many disease states and can be used as a diagnostic tool in the workup for cystic fibrosis

        e. Associated electrolyte imbalances that usually occur with elevated chloride levels are elevated potassium and sodium levels and decreased bicarbonate levels

        f. Trending of results

           1) It is important to monitor the client with attention to acid–base values and trend results by examining anion gap

           2) Hyperchloremic acidosis is associated with a normal anion gap

           3) Because there can be artifact disturbances in acid–base imbalances resulting in falsely elevated chloride levels, trend results and evaluate the client using complete assessment parameters and not merely one lab value

C. Priority nursing diagnoses

    1. Ineffective Breathing Pattern related to tachypnea

    2. Imbalanced Nutrition: Greater Than Body Requirements related to increased chloride intake or decreased loss

    3. Impaired Skin Integrity related to dehydration

    4. Ineffective Health Maintenance related to weakness

    5. Risk for Impaired Sensory/Perception related to lethargy

    6. Risk for Injury related to weakness and lethargy

    7. Self-Care Deficit related to altered respiratory status

    8. Anxiety related to increased lethargy

D. Therapeutic management

    1. Decrease chloride intake; withdraw all chloride-containing agents used as treatment measures

    2. Promote chloride excretion by administering diuretics

    3. Continue monitoring client, including acid–base, respiratory, and cardiac status

    4. Restoration of balance

        a. Administer appropriate IV therapy to restore fluid and electrolyte balance

        b. Correct dehydration states with oral and parenteral fluids as needed to restore serum chloride levels

        c. Promote dietary changes to decrease chloride intake

        d. Increase water intake

        e. Continue to assess those clients at risk due to underlying or contributory disease and implement appropriate therapies to decrease serum chloride levels

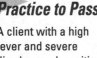

Practice to Pass

A client with a high fever and severe diarrhea and vomiting is admitted to the hospital. Which chloride imbalance is occurring and what are the most likely etiologies for the suspected imbalance?

E. Planning and implementation

    1. Identify risk factors specific to the development of chloride excess, such as dietary factors, specific disease states, medical therapies, and acidotic states

    2. Monitor the client during the course of therapy, trending pertinent laboratory test results and response to treatment

   3. Monitor VS and I&O parameters
   4. Promote client safety
F. **Medication therapy**
   1. Parenteral administration
      a. Hypotonic solutions such as 0.45% NaCl or D_5W to restore balance
      b. IV administration of diuretics may be utilized to restore acid–base disturbances
   2. Additional drug therapies may be indicated based on underlying clinical conditions and presence of contributory disease
G. **Client education**
   1. Awareness of predisposing factors
      a. Educate the client to avoid medications and supplements containing chloride
      b. If the client is experiencing other electrolyte imbalances (sodium, potassium, and water), have a high index of suspicion for possible development of hyperchloremia
   2. Dietary education
      a. Avoid foods that are high in chloride levels and restrict use of processed foods because they are high in both sodium and chloride content
      b. Maintain adequate hydration status
      c. Collaborate with dietitian as needed
H. **Evaluation**
   1. Chloride serum levels and other pertinent electrolyte levels return to normal baseline
   2. Client is able to identify restricted foods, medications, and therapies that would cause serum chloride elevations
   3. Correction of underlying disease states and contributory clinical conditions that will assist in returning chloride levels to normal
   4. Resolution of symptoms relative to hyperchloremia

Case Study

A 38-year-old male client is being admitted to the hospital with a diagnosis of vomiting related to a gastrointestinal virus. Vital signs reveal BP 100/70, pulse 88, and respirations 18. Client has been unable to keep solid food down for two days and has been drinking liquids (water, soda, and tea) during that time period.

1. What questions will you ask the client on admission?
2. What assessments will you make before starting interventions?
3. What nursing diagnoses are applicable for this client?
4. What nursing interventions would you implement?
5. What discharge instructions will you include in your plan of care?

For suggested responses, see page 204.

POSTTEST

1 A client's laboratory test results indicate that the client has a serum chloride level of 114 mEq/L. The nurse would assess the client for which anticipated manifestations?

1. Tremors and flaccid muscles
2. Twitching and spastic reflexes
3. Hyperreflexia and tremors
4. Weakness and lethargy

2 Which of the following should be included as a priority intervention for a client diagnosed with metabolic alkalosis associated with hypochloremia?

1. Assess for muscle tremors and slow deep respirations.
2. Assess for rapid deep respirations and stupor.
3. Restrict salt in the diet.
4. Administer diuretics.

3 When a client is admitted with a chloride level of 80 mEq/L, the nurse anticipates administration of which intravenous solution?

1. 5% dextrose and water
2. 0.9% sodium chloride
3. 0.45% sodium chloride with 20 mEq of potassium
4. 3% sodium chloride with 10 mEq of potassium

4 Which statement would the nurse make during dietary teaching for a client who has a serum chloride level of 86 mEq/L?

1. "Avoid eating foods containing rye."
2. "Take your prescribed diuretic daily."
3. "Increase the amount of citrus fruit in your diet."
4. "Increase intake of dates and bananas in your diet."

5 After checking the medical record of a client admitted with shortness of breath and lethargy, the nurse noted a chloride level of 110 mEq/L. Which coexisting health problems would the nurse suspect? Select all that apply.

1. Addison's disease
2. Cushing's syndrome
3. Metabolic alkalosis
4. Syndrome of inappropriate antidiuretic hormone (SIADH)
5. Renal disease

6 Which nursing diagnosis would the nurse most likely identify for a client with a serum chloride level of 112 mEq/L?

1. Ineffective Health Maintenance related to nasogastric (NG) suctioning
2. Pain related to muscle spasms
3. Imbalanced Nutrition: More than Body Requirements related to excess intake of foods rich in salt
4. Anxiety related to excessive neuromuscular stimulation

7 A client who is experiencing hypochloremia is scheduled to have blood drawn for a chloride level. In preparation for the blood work, the nurse instructs the client to do which of the following?

1. Eat a typical diet with ordinary or typical salt intake.
2. Restrict intake of caffeine-containing beverages the day before blood is drawn.
3. Fast for eight hours before the blood is to be drawn.
4. Stop taking any hormone medications for 24 hours.

8 A client is admitted to the intensive care unit (ICU) with metabolic alkalosis, hypokalemia, and hyponatremia. The nurse should look at the results of serum laboratory studies to detect which additional test that likely has an abnormal result?

1. Ammonia
2. Uric acid
3. Creatinine
4. Chloride

9 Which of the following items in a client's recent history does the nurse identify as contributing to a state of hyperchloremic acidosis?

1. Administration of acetazolamide (Diamox)
2. Administration of antacids
3. Administration of thiazide diuretics
4. Chronic laxative use

10 Which of the following changes in urine electrolyte levels would be expected in a client with cardiac disease who is experiencing pitting edema? Select all that apply.

1. Decreased sodium
2. Decreased chloride
3. Increased magnesium
4. Decreased calcium
5. Increased phosphorus

➤ *See pages 130–131 for Answers and Rationales.*

ANSWERS & RATIONALES

Pretest

1 **Answer: 1** **Rationale:** Glucocorticoids cause retention of chloride and sodium leading to fluid retention. All of the other options, such as decreasing diuretic intake, eating more vegetables, and eating foods such as spinach and celery (high in chloride content), will increase the serum chloride level. **Cognitive Level:** Application **Client Need:** Pharmacological and Parenteral Therapies **Integrated Process:** Teaching and Learning **Content Area:** Adult Health **Strategy:** The critical words are *prednisone* and *side effects*. Recall that this drug is a corticosteroid, and that this type of drug causes retention of sodium and chloride to direct you to the correct option. **Reference:** Adams, M., Josephson, D., & Holland, L. (2011). *Pharmacology for nurses: A pathophysiologic approach* (3rd ed.). Upper Saddle River, NJ: Pearson/Prentice Hall, pp. 441–445.

2 **Answer: 2** **Rationale:** Increased use of sodium bicarbonate causes excretion of chloride or hypochloremia; therefore, it would be appropriate to have serum chloride levels monitored for potential deficits. A D_5W infusion is hypotonic and will cause further fluid shifting and more potential electrolyte imbalances given the high rate. This will decrease chloride levels if administered over a prolonged time. Checking a magnesium value will not give any additional information and is, therefore, unnecessary. Administration of diuretics will decrease chloride levels. **Cognitive Level:** Analyzing **Client Need:** Pharmacological and Parenteral Therapies **Integrated Process:** Nursing Process: Implementation **Content Area:** Adult Health **Strategy:** Critical words are *multiple ampules* and *sodium bicarbonate*. Recall chloride losses occur with bicarbonate use or retention to choose correctly. **Reference:** LeMone, P., & Burke, K. (2008.). *Medical surgical nursing: Critical thinking in client care* (4th ed.). Upper Saddle River, NJ: Pearson/Prentice Hall, p. 218.

3 **Answer: 1** **Rationale:** In a client who has Cushing's syndrome, one would expect to see elevated serum chloride because of sodium retention. A sodium level of 130 mEq/L is below normal and is not expected. In a client who has Cushing's syndrome, one would expect to see a decreased potassium level because of higher sodium; a potassium level of 5.0 mEq/L is at the high end of normal. An elevated chloride level would not be associated with an elevated bicarbonate level, because both of these are anions. **Cognitive Level:** Analyzing **Client Need:** Physiological Adaptation **Integrated Process:** Nursing Process: Assessment **Content Area:** Adult Health **Strategy:** Critical words are *Cushing's syndrome*. Recognize that the electrolytes that are retained are sodium and chloride. Recall normal lab values for these electrolytes and choose the option that shows elevated sodium chloride. **Reference:** Corbett, J. (2008). *Laboratory tests and diagnostic procedures with nursing diagnoses* (7th ed.). Upper Saddle River, NJ: Pearson Education, pp. 131–132.

4 **Answer: 2, 3, 4** **Rationale:** The action of clenching and unclenching the fist can lead to hemolysis of RBCs and cause altered test results. A tourniquet can potentially cause turbulence in blood flow and alter results by hemolyzing erythrocytes. If possible, blood should be drawn without the use of a tourniquet. It is important for accurate results that the blood sample not be hemolyzed. Drawing blood from an implanted port used for chemotherapy is not a recommended procedure. The client does not need to be NPO prior to drawing any electrolyte sample. **Cognitive Level:** Applying **Client Need:** Reduction of Risk Potential **Integrated Process:** Nursing Process: Implementation **Content Area:** Adult Health **Strategy:** Recall knowledge of the effect of hemolysis on blood samples to aid in making the correct selections. Recall that many routine labs such as electrolytes do not require NPO status. **Reference:** Kee, J. (2009).

Laboratory and diagnostic tests with nursing implications (8th ed.). Upper Saddle River, NJ: Pearson/Prentice Hall, p. 120.

5 **Answer: 3** **Rationale:** In CHF, chloride is increased, and the administration of hypertonic saline may cause a lethal hypervolemia. In addition, mechanisms for excreting sodium, chloride, and water are compromised in CHF, causing significant fluid and electrolyte alterations if such a therapy were to be utilized. A client with Addison's disease would benefit from administration of a hypertonic solution in a closely monitored situation because this client loses sodium and chloride. A client who has been NPO for several days would benefit from administration of a hypertonic solution in a closely monitored situation. A client diagnosed with alkalosis would benefit from administration of a hypertonic solution, because the client would most likely be experiencing chloride and sodium deficits. **Cognitive Level:** Analyzing **Client Need:** Physiological Adaptation **Integrated Process:** Nursing Process: Planning **Content Area:** Adult Health **Strategy:** This question requires you analyze each option for the effect of additional sodium and its ability to improve chloride level. Eliminate incorrect options because sodium may improve these conditions. **Reference:** LeMone, P., & Burke, K. (2008). *Medical surgical nursing: Critical thinking in client care* (4th ed.). Upper Saddle River, NJ: Pearson/Prentice Hall, pp. 213–215.

6 **Answer: 4** **Rationale:** The clinical symptoms of weakness, lethargy, and fatigue are associated with hyperchloremia and will diminish as the chloride level decreases. The symptoms related to chloride deficiency can be reversed with clinical treatment that restores serum chloride levels to normal. There is no correlation between exercise and increase in serum chloride level. It is likely that increased exercise would lead to a chloride deficiency through sweat and perspiration losses. Increasing salt intake will worsen the serum chloride level. **Cognitive Level:** Applying **Client Need:** Physiological Adaptation **Integrated Process:** Communication and Documentation **Content Area:** Adult Health **Strategy:** Note that this question does not identify the type of chloride imbalance. Recognize the symptoms reflect hyperchloremia to direct you to the correct option. **Reference:** LeMone, P., & Burke, K. (2008). *Medical surgical nursing: Critical thinking in client care* (4th ed.). Upper Saddle River, NJ: Pearson Education, pp. 213–217.

7 **Answer: 1** **Rationale:** With severe chloride and ECF losses, the blood pressure drops, potentially leading to shock if not corrected. The nurse should place the highest priority on monitoring the client to prevent development of potential complications and to maintain client safety. Although it may be necessary to assist the client to the bathroom, this is not the priority intervention. If there is sufficient ECF loss, then the client would more likely be too weak to ambulate and bedrest would be indicated. Starting IV therapy with a hypotonic solution may further exacerbate the client's clinical condition.

Although it would be important to monitor the client's pulse, this again is not the priority intervention at this point in time because it is an assessment rather than an action. **Cognitive Level:** Analyzing **Client Need:** Reduction of Risk Potential **Integrated Process:** Nursing Process: Implementation **Content Area:** Adult Health **Strategy:** The critical words are *highest priority*. Recognize the level reflects a critically low chloride level and that a fluid loss is also present to direct you to the correct option. **Reference:** LeMone, P., & Burke, K. (2008). *Medical surgical nursing: Critical thinking in client care* (4th ed.). Upper Saddle River, NJ: Pearson Education, pp. 213–217.

8 **Answer: 3** **Rationale:** Neurological alteration related to chloride imbalance includes tremors and twitching of the muscles with hypochloremia or weakness and lethargy with hyperchloremia. These manifestations place the client at risk for injury. It is not clear that the client has an excess fluid volume. There is not enough information to determine whether the client is dehydrated. There is insufficient data to support a nursing diagnosis of interrupted thought processes. **Cognitive Level:** Application **Client Need:** Reduction of Risk Potential **Integrated Process:** Nursing Process: Diagnosis **Content Area:** Adult Health **Strategy:** The critical word in the question is *neuromuscular*. Eliminate two options because these are related to fluid imbalances, and eliminate a third option because this may or may not be a related diagnosis. **Reference:** LeMone, P., & Burke, K. (2008). *Medical surgical nursing: Critical thinking in client care* (4th ed.). Upper Saddle River, NJ: Pearson Education, pp. 213–217.

9 **Answer: 2** **Rationale:** Documenting the history can assist in determining the cause of the elevated chloride level. This should occur, if possible, prior to intervention. Isolation is not indicated for hyperchloremia. Ambulating independently without assessment is unsafe because the client will probably have weakness and lethargy. Infusing saline is an unsafe intervention that would lead to increased chloride levels. **Cognitive Level:** Analyzing **Client Need:** Reduction of Risk Potential **Integrated Process:** Nursing Process: Implementation **Content Area:** Adult Health **Strategy:** The critical words in the question are *alert*, *hyperchloremia*, and *priority*. Eliminate options that are unwarranted, unsafe, or that would worsen the problem. **Reference:** LeMone, P., & Burke, K. (2008). *Medical surgical nursing: Critical thinking in client care* (4th ed.). Upper Saddle River, NJ: Pearson Education, pp. 213–217.

10 **Answer: 1, 2** **Rationale:** Foods high in chloride include bananas and dates, green leafy vegetables, seafood, poultry, and dairy products. Canned soups tend to be higher in sodium and chloride is combined with sodium as salt. **Cognitive Level:** Applying **Client Need:** Physiological Adaptation **Integrated Process:** Teaching and Learning **Content Area:** Adult Health **Strategy:** Clients with anorexia nervosa usually have electrolyte deficiencies. Foods high in chloride are also foods generally high in sodium.

ANSWERS & RATIONALES

Reference: Dudek, S. (2010). *Nutrition essentials for nursing practice* (6th ed.). Philadelphia: Lippincott Williams & Wilkins, pp. 123–125.

Posttest

1 **Answer: 4** **Rationale:** Weakness and lethargy occur with hyperchloremia (normal 95 to 108 mEq/L). All of the other options reflect manifestations that are associated with hypochloremia. **Cognitive Level:** Applying **Client Need:** Physiological Adaptation **Integrated Process:** Nursing Process: Assessment **Content Area:** Adult Health **Strategy:** The core issue of the question is that the client has hyperchloremia. Recognize the similarities in the incorrect options to eliminate them. **Reference:** LeMone, P., & Burke, K. (2008). *Medical surgical nursing: Critical thinking in client care* (4th ed.). Upper Saddle River, NJ: Pearson/Prentice Hall, pp. 213–217.

2 **Answer: 1** **Rationale:** In metabolic alkalosis, bicarbonate ions are retained, and the kidneys respond by excreting chloride ions, which in turn causes reciprocal hypochloremia. Hypochloremia is manifested by muscle tremors and slow deep respirations that can lead to critical complications and is a priority intervention. Deep, rapid respirations and stupor are symptoms of hyperchloremia. Serum chloride levels are decreased and the restriction of salt will normally cause further chloride losses to occur. Diuretics will normally cause further chloride losses to occur, which could further compromise the client's status. **Cognitive Level:** Analyzing **Client Need:** Reduction of Risk Potential **Integrated Process:** Nursing Process: Planning **Content Area:** Adult Health **Strategy:** Recall first that metabolic alkalosis leads to hypochloremia. Eliminate two options because they would cause further hypochloremia. Recall signs of hypochloremia to choose correctly. **Reference:** LeMone, P., & Burke, K. (2008). *Medical surgical nursing: Critical thinking in client care* (4th ed.). Upper Saddle River, NJ: Pearson/Prentice Hall, pp. 213–217.

3 **Answer: 3** **Rationale:** The client presents with hypochloremia and most likely is experiencing other electrolyte deficiencies as well, most notably sodium and potassium. A solution with 0.45% saline with added potassium would correct expected fluid and electrolyte imbalances. 5% dextrose and water is a hypotonic solution once dextrose is metabolized and can further dilute the plasma and the serum chloride level. 0.9% sodium chloride would not be the most appropriate solution because it does not address the issue of additional electrolyte deficiencies, which are most likely occurring in addition to the chloride deficiency. Hypertonic saline is usually administered in cases of severe hyponatremia. **Cognitive Level:** Analyzing **Client Need:** Pharmacological and Parenteral Therapies **Integrated Process:** Nursing Process: Planning **Content Area:** Adult Health **Strategy:** First recognize the level is

dangerously low and recall sodium and potassium occur with low chloride and will need to be replaced. Only one option provides both of these electrolytes. **Reference:** LeMone, P., & Burke, K. (2008). *Medical surgical nursing: Critical thinking in client care* (4th ed.). Upper Saddle River, NJ: Pearson/Prentice Hall, pp. 203–215.

4 **Answer: 4** **Rationale:** Dates and bananas are high in chloride and therefore can be included in a dietary pattern to increase chloride levels. Foods containing rye should be included in the diet because they are high in chloride. Diuretics can increase the excretion of chloride and thereby reduce serum chloride levels. Although increasing the amount of citrus fruit in the diet provides nutritional benefit, it does not increase chloride levels. Citrus is high in potassium. **Cognitive Level:** Applying **Client Need:** Reduction of Risk Potential **Integrated Process:** Communication and Documentation **Content Area:** Adult Health **Strategy:** The core issue of the question is knowledge of foods that are naturally high in chloride. A critical word in the question is *dietary*, which helps to eliminate one option. Recall foods high in chloride to choose correctly. **Reference:** Kee, J. (2009). *Laboratory and diagnostic tests with nursing implications* (8th ed.). Upper Saddle River, NJ: Pearson/Prentice Hall, p. 384.

5 **Answer: 2, 5** **Rationale:** A serum value of 110 mEq/L reflects an elevated serum chloride level. Cushing's syndrome causes retention of excess sodium and chloride. In the presence of decreased renal function, the kidneys are unable to excrete hydrogen ions and reabsorb bicarbonate ions, which leads to metabolic acidosis and hyperchloremia. Addison's disease is associated with decreased levels of sodium and chloride. Elevated chloride levels are usually associated with metabolic acidosis. SIADH is associated with chloride deficit. **Cognitive Level:** Analyzing **Client Need:** Physiological Adaptation **Integrated Process:** Nursing Process: Assessment **Content Area:** Adult Health **Strategy:** First recognize the level is elevated. Recall hyperchloremia is seen with elevated sodium to direct you to the correct option. **Reference:** LeMone, P., & Burke, K. (2008). *Medical surgical nursing: Critical thinking in client care* (4th ed.). Upper Saddle River, NJ: Pearson/Prentice Hall, pp. 203–215.

6 **Answer: 3** **Rationale:** The stated value represents an elevated chloride level. Increased use of table salt will cause increase in both sodium and chloride levels. The use of NG suctioning would cause hydrochloric acid to be lost, thereby decreasing the chloride level. A level of 112 mEq/L is elevated. Muscle spasms would be expected with hypochloremia; but a level of 112 mEq/L reflects hyperchloremia. Neuromuscular stimulation is decreased with hyperchloremia. **Cognitive Level:** Analyzing **Client Need:** Physiological Adaptation **Integrated Process:** Nursing Process: Diagnosis **Content Area:** Adult Health **Strategy:** First determine the level is elevated. Eliminate incorrect options as they are associated with low chloride levels. **Reference:** LeMone, P., & Burke, K. (2008). *Medical surgical nursing: Critical thinking in client care* (4th ed.). Upper Saddle River, NJ: Pearson/ Prentice Hall, pp. 203–212.

7 **Answer: 1** **Rationale:** Chloride levels are typically drawn as part of general serum electrolytes and do not require special preparation. Caffeine and hormones will not interfere with test results. The client does not need to be NPO prior to the test because this will not alter the values. The client should continue to take the medications as prescribed by the physician. **Cognitive Level:** Applying **Client Need:** Reduction of Risk Potential **Integrated Process:** Nursing Process: Implementation **Content Area:** Adult Health **Strategy:** Recognize that caffeine and hormones do not affect chloride levels. Recall that chloride is drawn with other electrolytes to choose correctly. **Reference:** Kee, J. (2009). *Laboratory and diagnostic tests with nursing implications* (8th ed.). Upper Saddle River, NJ: Pearson/Prentice Hall, p. 120.

8 **Answer: 4** **Rationale:** It would be prudent to check serum chloride levels in order to determine the client's baseline in the presence of multiple electrolyte deficiencies. Ammonia does not reflect serum electrolytes and therefore will not change in proportion to the electrolyte changes. Uric acid should be unaffected as this is a product of purine metabolism. Creatinine is an indicator of kidney function. **Cognitive Level:** Applying **Client Need:** Reduction of Risk Potential **Integrated Process:** Nursing Process: Assessment **Content Area:** Adult Health **Strategy:** Recall that chloride goes in the same direction as sodium to help make the correct selection of which test to focus on. **Reference:** LeMone, P., & Burke, K. (2008). *Medical surgical nursing: Critical thinking in client care*

(4th ed.). Upper Saddle River, NJ: Pearson/Prentice Hall, pp. 203–210.

9 **Answer: 1** **Rationale:** The use of acetazolamide (Diamox) can lead to the development of hyperchloremic acidosis because it increases chloride levels. Antacids would lead to an alkalotic state. Thiazide diuretics would excrete sodium and chloride. Chronic laxative use would lead to chloride deficiencies that would result in an alkalotic state. **Cognitive Level:** Analyzing **Client Need:** Physiological Adaptation **Integrated Process:** Nursing Process: Assessment **Content Area:** Adult Health **Strategy:** Recognize that the incorrect options would contribute to loss of chloride and eliminate them. **Reference:** LeMone, P., & Burke, K. (2008). *Medical surgical nursing: Critical thinking in client care* (4th ed.). Upper Saddle River, NJ: Pearson/Prentice Hall, pp. 213–217.

10 **Answer: 1, 2** **Rationale:** A low urine sodium indicates retention in the body, especially with fluid excess, which would be seen with pitting edema. A low urine chloride indicates retention and is expected with fluid excess. Increased magnesium would indicate a fluid deficit. Calcium is not altered by fluid retention due to cardiac disorders. Phosphorus levels would not be affected. **Cognitive Level:** Applying **Client Need:** Physiological Adaptation **Integrated Process:** Nursing Process: Assessment **Content Area:** Adult Health **Strategy:** Critical words are *cardiac* and *pitting edema*. Recognize that sodium and chloride would be retained with edema and as result renal losses of chloride and sodium would decrease to choose correctly. **Reference:** LeMone, P., & Burke, K. (2008). *Medical surgical nursing: Critical thinking in client care* (4th ed.). Upper Saddle River, NJ: Pearson/Prentice Hall, pp. 195–236.

References

Adams, M. P., Josephson, D. L., & Holland, L. N. (2011). *Pharmacology for nurses: A pathophysiologic approach* (3rd ed.). Upper Saddle River, NJ: Pearson Education.

Berman, A., & Snyder, S. (2012). *Kozier & Erb's fundamentals of nursing: Concepts, process, and practice* (9th ed.). Upper Saddle River, NJ: Pearson Education.

Dudek, S. (2009). *Nutrition essentials for nursing practice* (6th ed.). Philadelphia: Lippincott Williams & Wilkins.

Hockenberry, M. J., & Wilson, D. (2008). *Wong's essentials of pediatric nursing* (8th ed.). St. Louis, MO: Mosby, Elsevier.

Ignatavicius, D., & Workman, M. (2009). *Medical-surgical nursing: Critical thinking in collaborative care* (6th ed.). St. Louis, MO: Elsevier Saunders.

Kee, J. L. (2009). *Handbook of laboratory and diagnostic tests with nursing implications* (6th ed.). Upper Saddle River, NJ: Pearson Education.

LeMone, P., & Burke, K. (2011). *Medical-surgical nursing: Critical thinking*

in client care (5th ed.). Upper Saddle River: NJ: Pearson Education.

London, M. L., Ladewig, P. W., Ball, J. W., Bindler, R. C., & Cowen, K. J. (2011). *Maternal & child nursing care* (3rd ed.). Upper Saddle River, NJ: Pearson Education.

Osborne, K. S., Wraa, C. E., & Watson, A. B. (2010). *Medical-surgical nursing: Preparation for practice.* Upper Saddle River, NJ: Pearson Education.

ANSWERS & RATIONALES

7 Phosphorus Balance and Imbalances

Chapter Outline

Overview of Phosphorus
  Regulation

Hypophosphatemia

Hyperphosphatemia

NCLEX-RN® Test Prep

Use the accompanying online resource,
NursingReviewsandRationales, to test
yourself with hundreds of NCLEX®-style
practice questions.

Objectives

➤ Review the basic functions of phosphorus in the body.
➤ Explain the pathophysiology and etiology of phosphorus imbalances.
➤ Identify specific assessment findings and diagnostic tests as they
  relate to phosphorus imbalances.
➤ Identify priority nursing diagnoses for phosphorus imbalances.
➤ Describe the therapeutic management of phosphorus imbalances.
➤ Describe the nursing management of a client who is experiencing
  a phosphorus imbalance.

Review at a Glance

**2,3-diphosphoglycerate
(2,3-DPG)** a substance found in red
blood cells that facilitates delivery of
oxygen to tissues

**adenosine triphosphate
(ATP)** a compound stored in muscle
containing three phosphorus groups that
produces energy when split

hyperphosphatemia serum
phosphate level greater than 4.5 mg/dL

hypophosphatemia serum
phosphate level less than 2.5 mg/dL

metastatic calcification
precipitate of calcium phosphate in soft
tissues, joints, and arteries as a
complication of hyperphosphatemia

**parathyroid hormone (PTH or
parathormone)** secreted by
parathyroid gland to regulate calcium
and phosphorus metabolism

phospholipids a lipid substance
containing phosphorus and fatty acids

phosphorus/phosphate a
nonmetallic element usually found in
combination with other elements; terms
are often used interchangeably

refeeding syndrome a state of
hypophosphatemia that can occur when
infusing high levels of calories into
clients who have alcoholism, anorexia, or
are otherwise malnourished

tetany a nervous system disorder
marked by intermittent tonic spasms that
are usually paroxysmal and involve the
extremities

**total parenteral nutrition
(TPN)** intravenous provision of total
nutritional needs for a client unable to
take appropriate amounts of food by
enteral route; administered via a central
venous access

vitamin D a fat-soluble vitamin essential for calcium and phosphorus absorption
from small intestine and metabolism

PRETEST

1 A six-month-old infant has a phosphorus level of 5.0 mEq/L. To help determine the cause of this level, the nurse should ask the infant's parent which question?

1. "Has the baby had a lot of diarrhea lately?"
2. "What kind of milk do you feed the baby?"
3. "Is the baby eating a lot of solid foods?"
4. "Has the baby been vomiting a lot lately?"

2 When checking serum phosphorus levels on a pediatric client with hypophosphatemia, the nurse anticipates finding which information?

1. Levels will be highest in the early morning.
2. Normal levels are slightly higher secondary to rapid skeletal growth.
3. A decrease will be seen initially after starting replacement therapy.
4. An arterial sample must be used to provide the most accurate level.

3 When checking laboratory values on a client, the nurse notes the phosphate level is 1.7 mg/dL. The nurse should also check laboratory values for evidence of which of the following?

1. An elevated platelet count
2. A decrease in hemoglobin level
3. A decrease in calcium level
4. An elevated magnesium level

4 The nurse would assess for manifestations of hypophosphatemia in the client who had which of the following predisposing clinical conditions? Select all that apply.

1. First-degree burns
2. Diabetic ketoacidosis
3. Hypermagnesemia
4. Oliguria
5. History of alcoholism

5 The nurse would plan to include the need for which foods in the diet when providing discharge teaching for a client with a phosphorus level of 1.5 mg/dL? Select all that apply.

1. Green leafy vegetables
2. White breads
3. Citrus fruits
4. Eggs
5. Liver

6 A client has just been started on total parenteral nutrition (TPN) for severe malnutrition. The nurse determines refeeding syndrome has occurred after noting which of the following laboratory test results?

1. Magnesium 2.5 mg/dL
2. Calcium 9.8 mg/dL
3. Phosphorus 1.2 mg/dL
4. Potassium 4.2 mEq/L

7 Which of the following findings in a client's history would alert the nurse to assess for signs and symptoms of hypophosphatemia?

1. Withdrawal from alcohol
2. The oliguric phase of acute tubular necrosis
3. Short-term gastric suction
4. Occasional use of aluminum-containing antacids

8 Which of the following concurrent electrolyte imbalances should the nurse anticipate while caring for a client with a phosphate level of 4.9 mg/dL?

1. Hyperkalemia
2. Hyponatremia
3. Hypocalcemia
4. Hypermagnesemia

9 A client has developed a serum phosphorus level of 5.0 mg/dL secondary to cytotoxic drug therapy. Because of the hyperuricemia that also occurs with this therapy, the nurse anticipates administration of which medication?

1. Aluminum hydroxide (Amphogel)
2. Allopurinol (Zyloprim)
3. Acetazolamide (Diamox)
4. Hydralazine (Apresoline)

10 When providing discharge teaching for a client who requires a diet high in phosphates, the nurse would include which statement?

1. "High levels of phosphates are found in food additives."
2. "Increase your vitamin A intake to enhance phosphorus absorption."
3. "Aluminum-based antacids increase phosphorus absorption."
4. "Soy and soy products are excellent sources of phosphorus."

➤ *See pages 145–147 for Answers and Rationales.*

I. OVERVIEW OF PHOSPHORUS REGULATION

A. Phosphorus balance
1. Serum levels
   a. Normal serum **phosphate** levels range from 2.5 to 4.5 mg/dL (1.7 to 2.6 mEq/L) in adults, 4.5 to 5.5 mg/dL in children, and 3.5 to 8.6 mg/dL in newborns
   b. Levels are greater in children because of their higher rate of skeletal growth
   c. Newborns have almost twice the adult level of **phosphorus**
   d. Serum levels may vary throughout the day
   e. Most phosphorus (P^+) exists in the body as the phosphate ion (PO_4^2)
   f. Phosphorus is the second most abundant mineral in the body
      1) 85% is combined with calcium in the teeth and bones, also in skeletal muscle
      2) 14% is found in intracellular fluid
      3) 1% is found in extracellular fluid and viscera
   g. Phosphorus is the primary anion of intracellular fluid
   h. Ionized calcium and phosphorus exist in a reciprocal balance in the blood
2. Functions in the body
   a. Essential for muscle function, red blood cells, and nervous system function, and plays a part in the metabolism of carbohydrates, fats, and proteins
   b. Plays a crucial role in the formation of teeth and bones
   c. Plays a part in the cellular metabolism of DNA and **adenosine triphosphate (ATP)**, a compound stored in muscle that contains three phosphorus groups and produces energy when split
   d. Assists in regulating calcium levels
   e. Aids renal regulation of acids and bases through its role in the phosphate buffer system
   f. Found in cell membranes as **phospholipids** that help maintain cell membrane integrity
   g. Required for the release of oxygen from hemoglobin in the form of **2,3-diphosphoglycerate (2,3-DPG)**
3. System interactions
   a. Serum levels vary throughout the day related to glucose intake, insulin administration, and hyperventilation, which increases cellular uptake of phosphorus
   b. Phosphorus assists in maintaining acid–base balance

Table 7-1	Lifespan Considerations for Health Maintenance: Phosphorus Balance	
Lifespan Considerations	**Common Risk Factors for Imbalances**	**Nursing Implications**
Infants	*Hyperphosphatemia* Use of cows' milk instead of formula or human milk.	Assess infant for signs of hyperphosphatemia.
Pediatrics	*Hypophosphatemia or hyperphosphatemia* Phosphorus is not a common imbalance in children, but imbalances may be seen in relation to calcium imbalances.	Check for low phosphorus levels when child has hypercalcemia. Check for high phosphorus levels when hypocalcemia is present.
Adults	*Hyperphosphatemia* Renal failure. Excessive use of phosphorus-containing enemas or laxatives. *Hypophosphatemia* Excessive use of phosphate-binding antacids.	Assess for signs of hyperphosphatemia. Assess client for signs of renal osteodystrophy. Instruct client to restrict intake of foods high in phosphorus and processed foods. Instruct clients on dangers of excessive use of phosphorus-containing enemas, such as Fleet's Phospho-soda. Instruct clients to avoid excessive use of aluminium containing antacids, such as Amphogel and Riopan

Practice to Pass

The school nurse is putting together a bulletin board that highlights foods high in various nutrients to use as a teaching tool for children and school visitors, including parents. What types of foods would the nurse identify on the display as being rich in phosphorus?

   c. An inverse relationship exists between phosphorus and calcium
     1) When calcium levels increase, phosphorus levels decrease; thus, calcium influences phosphorus regulation
     2) When phosphorus levels increase, calcium levels decrease; thus, calcium levels are influenced by phosphorus
   d. Phosphorus imbalances are often related to therapeutic interventions for other disorders
  4. See Table 7-1 for lifespan factors affecting phosphorus balance

B. Sources of phosphorus
  1. Cellular level
   a. Major anion of intracellular fluid; also found in extracellular fluid
   b. Kidneys are responsible for 90% of phosphate excretion
   c. Normal phosphate balance requires an efficient renal conservation mechanism
   d. During times of low phosphate intake, kidneys retain more phosphorus
  2. Dietary level
   a. Adequate intake is ensured by consumption of a balanced diet
   b. Average dietary intake ranges from 800 to 1600 mg/dL and is consistent with the recommended daily intake
   c. Found in high amounts in red and organ (brain, liver, kidney) meats, fish, poultry, eggs, milk and milk products, legumes, whole grains, and nuts
   d. Absorption via active and passive transport in the duodenum and jejunum
   e. Absorption influenced by **vitamin D**, a fat-soluble vitamin, and **parathyroid hormone (PTH)**, a hormone secreted by the parathyroid gland that regulates calcium and phosphorus levels
   f. Absorption inhibited by glucocorticoids, high magnesium diet, hypothyroidism, and aluminum-containing antacids
   g. Increased consumption of foods that contain food additives will result in increased ingestion of phosphates (see Box 7-1 for a list of examples of phosphorus-containing additives found in many processed foods)

Box 7-1	• Sodium phosphate: a texturizer
	• Aluminum phosphate: used in bread to improve texture
Phosphorus-Containing Additives Found in Many Processed Foods	• Calcium phosphate: a conditioner for bread dough
	• Potassium phosphate dibasic: an emulsifier and gelling agent
	• Ammonium phosphate: adjusts pH
	• Phosphate oxychloride liquid: a starch-modifying agent
	• Phosphoric acid: a pH adjuster used in beer and cheese
	• Potassium phosphate monobasic: a sequestering agent used in ice cream mixes
	• Sodium phosphate dibasic and monobasic: an emulsifier

II. *HYPOPHOSPHATEMIA*: A SERUM PHOSPHORUS LEVEL BELOW 2.5 MG/DL

A. Etiology and pathophysiology

1. Cellular level
   a. Defined as a serum phosphorus level of less than 2.5 mg/dL (1.7 mEq/L)
   b. Can result from transient shifts of phosphorus into the cells, as in respiratory or metabolic acidosis
   c. Increased releases of PTH decrease serum phosphorus levels
   d. The mobilization of calcium from other sources may reduce phosphorus levels
   e. Renal excretion of phosphorus may be increased
   f. Administration of highly concentrated glucose solutions may cause the release of insulin, which promotes the movement of glucose and phosphorus into the cell, known as **refeeding syndrome**; this secondarily causes hypophosphatemia
2. See Table 7-2 for a list of predisposing clinical conditions

B. Assessment

1. Clinical manifestations
   a. Signs begin to appear when serum phosphorus levels drop below 2.0 mg/dL
   b. Hematologic effects
      1) Anemia from the increased fragility of red blood cells from low ATP levels
      2) Altered granulocyte functioning
      3) Bruising and bleeding from platelet dysfunction and destruction
   c. Central nervous system effects
      1) Slurred speech
      2) Confusion, apprehension
      3) Seizures
      4) Coma
   d. Neuromuscular effects
      1) Reports of circumoral and fingertip/extremity numbness and tingling
      2) Muscle weakness, paresthesias
      3) Tremors, spasms, tetany
   e. Cardiovascular effects
      1) Reports of chest pain
      2) Dysrhythmias related to decreased oxygenation
      3) Heart failure and shock from decreased myocardial contractility
   f. Respiratory effects
      1) Alkalosis from an increased rate/depth of breathing in response to hypoxemia
      2) Respiratory muscle fatigue leading to respiratory failure

Table 7-2	Predisposing Clinical Conditions for Hypophosphatemia
Mechanism of Hypophosphatemia	**Associated Clinical Conditions**
Loss of Phosphorus	Increased intestinal losses from prolonged use of aluminum- and magnesium-containing antacids, which bind to phosphorus Severe vomiting and diarrhea; phosphorus is absorbed in the small intestine in the presence of vitamin D Prolonged gastric suction Increased renal excretion from hyperparathyroidism, hypomagnesemia, hypokalemia, thiazide diuretic therapy, diuretic phase of acute tubular necrosis, renal tubular disorders, polyuria, and glycosuria from uncontrolled diabetic ketoacidosis Hypercalcemia (may cause phosphaturia through stimulation of parathyroid hormone release) Medications: corticosteroids; androgens; aluminum component of some antacids combines with phosphorus, which lowers phosphorus levels; drugs containing large amounts of calcium can also lower phosphorus levels
Phosphorus Utilization	A depletion of ATP, which impairs a cell's energy supply, and a decrease in 2,3-DPG level in RBCs; this in turn reduces release of oxygen from hemoglobin, keeping it bound and less available to tissues Refeeding syndrome, which may carry a high mortality rate Diabetic ketoacidosis Administering TPN without adequate amounts of phosphorus Extracellular fluid volume expansion (a side effect of this) Respiratory alkalosis (may stimulate glycolysis—the breakdown of glucose—which stimulates movement of phosphorus into cells) Severe burns, possibly from hyperventilation and acceleration of glycolysis
Inadequate Phosphorus Intake or Absorption	Decreased intestinal absorption from vitamin D deficiency, malabsorption disorders, and starvation Alcoholism and severe alcohol abuse (especially during withdrawal) related to poor nutritional intake, vomiting, diarrhea, and use of antacids Poor dietary intake, malnutrition, and hypomagnesemia May be found more frequently in clients in critical care units because of nutritional deficiencies

    g. Gastrointestinal effects
       1) Hypoactive bowel sounds
       2) Anorexia, dysphagia, vomiting
       3) Gastric atony and ileus related to reduced gastric motility
2. Diagnostic and laboratory findings
    a. Plasma levels
       1) Mild hypophosphatemia: serum values of 1.0–2.5 mg/dL
       2) Severe hypophosphatemia: <1.0 mg/dL
    b. Associated electrolyte levels
       1) Serum magnesium: may be decreased because of increased renal excretion of magnesium
       2) Serum calcium: may be elevated because of the inverse relationship of calcium and phosphorus
       3) Arterial blood gases: may show respiratory or metabolic acidosis
    c. Trending of results
       1) Monitor laboratory values over time to determine effectiveness of therapy
       2) In prolonged hypophosphatemia, osteomalacia and pseudofractures may occur
    d. X-rays may show skeletal changes of osteomalacia

3. Identification of risk factors
   a. Alcohol withdrawal
   b. Malnourished clients
   c. Altered ability to eat normally
   d. **Total parenteral nutrition (TPN)** administration, in which total nutritional needs are provided intravenously through a central venous access catheter for a client unable to take appropriate amounts of food by enteral route
   e. Diabetic and uremic clients

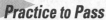

Practice to Pass

What neuromuscular manifestations should be assessed for in a client at risk for developing hypophosphatemia?

C. **Priority nursing diagnoses**
   1. Impaired Physical Mobility related to bone pain and fractures
   2. Risk for Injury (fractures) related to shifting of phosphorus out of bone tissue
   3. Impaired Gas Exchange related to weakened muscles of respiration
   4. Decreased Cardiac Output related to effects of hypophosphatemia on myocardial functioning
   5. Risk for Falls related to sensory or neuromuscular dysfunction

D. **Therapeutic management**
   1. Replacement therapies
      a. Administer phosphorus via oral supplements or intravenous replacement

      b. Avoid the use of phosphorus-binding antacids (those that contain aluminum)
      c. Adjust subsequent doses of replacement medication based on clinical presentation and serum phosphate levels
   2. Continued monitoring of the client
      a. Check serum levels periodically in clients at risk
      b. Assess diabetic clients for ketoacidosis
      c. Anticipate problems in clients who have a long history of antacid use; determine which products the client uses

      d. Be alert to clients who have difficulty speaking
      e. Note weakening respiratory efforts
      f. Monitor the ventilated client for increased incidence of hypophosphatemia from respiratory alkalosis
      g. Monitor for chest pain and cardiac dysrhythmias
      h. Assess serial hand grasps for increasing weakness
      i. Monitor for client reports of joint stiffness and arthralgia
      j. Investigate episodes of bleeding and/or bruising

      k. Watch for hypophosphatemia with the start of anabolism after prolonged periods of catabolism
      l. Monitor for other associated fluid and electrolyte imbalances, especially in those with nausea, vomiting, and/or diarrhea

E. **Restoration of balance**
   1. Achieved through oral, enteral, or parenteral replacement
   2. Normal phosphate levels should be achieved in 7–10 days

F. **Planning and implementation**

   1. Identify client populations at risk, especially those who are malnourished, receiving TPN, or receiving calories via enteral (tube) feedings
   2. Identify and eliminate the causes of hypophosphatemia
   3. Consult physician for orders to give appropriate supplementation
   4. Assess and document level of consciousness
   5. Assess orientation and neurologic status with each set of vital signs
   6. Inform the client/significant other that altered sensorium is temporary and will improve as phosphorus levels improve
   7. Use reality therapy by encouraging presence of family members and use of clock and calendar at the bedside

8. Incorporate seizure precautions into care
9. Have an appropriate size airway readily available
10. Assist the client in activities of daily living and ambulating
11. Monitor breath sounds for crackles, rhonchi, and shortness of breath
12. Monitor for elevated blood pressure and increased heart rate
13. Check temperature every four hours
14. If a wound infection is suspected, culture the wound(s) and drain
15. Use meticulous aseptic technique when giving care
16. Promote oral hygiene and skin care
17. Monitor for paresthesias, muscle weakness, pain, and mental changes
18. Medicate for pain
19. Assess serum phosphate levels and trends; watch for concurrent development of hypercalcemia in the presence of hypophosphatemia
20. Monitor for possible hyperphosphatemia after the initiation of therapy
21. Assess dietary I&O (intake and output)
    a. Carefully monitor fluid I&O
    b. Complete a diet history
    c. Log dietary intake
    d. Determine the client's food preferences

G. Medication therapy
1. Oral replacement therapy
   a. Monobasic potassium and sodium phosphates (K-Phos Neutral); potassium and sodium phosphates (Neutra-Phos)
      1) Usual dose is 250 mg four times a day
      2) Well absorbed following oral administration; vitamin D may enhance absorption
      3) Enters extracellular fluids and is then transported to sites of action
      4) Excreted mainly by the kidneys; acidifies the urine
      5) Contraindicated in hyperkalemia, hyperphosphatemia, hypocalcemia, severe renal impairment, and untreated Addison's disease
      6) Diarrhea is most frequent side effect
      7) Oxalates (in spinach and rhubarb) and phytates (in bran and whole grains) may decrease the absorption of phosphates by binding them in the GI tract
      8) Monitor serum phosphate, potassium, sodium, and calcium levels prior to and periodically throughout therapy
      9) Monitor renal function studies
   b. Phosphate/biphosphate (Fleet Phospho-Soda)
      1) Osmotically active bowel preparation and oral preparation used for its laxative effect
      2) Enema contains 7 grams sodium phosphate, and 19 grams sodium biphosphate; oral preparation contains 18 grams sodium phosphate and 48 grams sodium biphosphate
      3) Up to 20% of rectally administered sodium and phosphate may be absorbed
      4) Excreted by the kidneys
      5) Side effects include cramping, nausea
      6) May cause increased serum sodium and phosphorus levels, decreased serum calcium levels, and acidosis
      7) Oral preparations should be thoroughly dissolved in a full glass of water and administered after meals to minimize gastric irritation and the laxative effect and to enhance palatability
      8) Do not administer simultaneously with antacids containing aluminum, magnesium, or calcium

        9) Advise clients to maintain a high fluid intake to decrease the risk of developing kidney stones

        10) Instruct the client to promptly report diarrhea, weakness, fatigue, muscle cramps, unexplained weight gain, swelling of lower extremities, shortness of breath, and unusual thirst or tremors

  2. Parenteral replacement therapy

    a. Usually reserved for severe hypophosphatemia (<1 mg/dL)

    b. Potassium phosphate (KPO_4) or sodium phosphate ($NaPO_4$) used

    c. May be added to TPN solutions

    d. When giving potassium phosphate, do not exceed 10 mEq/hr; give slowly over two to six hours

    e. Complications of IV therapy may include:

      1) Tetany from hypocalcemia

      2) Calcium and phosphorus in the tissues may combine and form deposits

      3) Hypotension from too rapid an infusion rate

    f. Monitor infusion site for signs of infiltration, which may lead to tissue necrosis or sloughing

  3. Dietary therapy

    a. Daily requirements are 0.15 mM/kg/day or 10 mM/day; if under stress, requirements increase to 30–45 mM/day

    b. Phosphorus is plentiful in a normal diet

    c. Milk and milk products are excellent sources, as well as red meats, eggs, poultry, organ meats, legumes, and whole grains

H. Client education

  1. Teach the client and family to recognize signs and symptoms of hypophosphatemia

  2. Discuss the importance of avoiding phosphorus-binding antacids, such as aluminum hydroxide (Amphogel)

  3. Discuss with the client the pertinent conditions that cause hypophosphatemia

  4. Carry out dietary education and provide a list of foods high in phosphorus

I. Evaluation

  1. The client will regain a serum phosphorus value within the normal range

  2. The client can identify signs and symptoms of hypophosphatemia

  3. The client exhibits no evidence of injury caused by neurosensory changes

  4. The client exhibits adequate gas exchange as evidenced by a respiratory rate of 12 to 20 breaths/minute with normal depth and pattern and oxygen saturation (SaO_2) level of at least 92%

  5. Within 24 hours of the initiation of therapy, the client exhibits purposeful movement and has full range of motion and muscle strength

  6. The client has no signs or symptoms of heart failure and vital signs are within normal limits

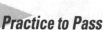

Practice to Pass

What are the important elements of care during administration of potassium phosphate in intravenous fluids for a client who has hypophosphatemia?

III. *HYPERPHOSPHATEMIA*: A SERUM PHOSPHORUS LEVEL ABOVE 4.5 MG/DL

  A. Etiology and pathophysiology (see Table 7-3)

  B. Assessment

    1. Clinical manifestations

      a. Common signs

        1) Most signs relate to the development of hypocalcemia or soft tissue calcification

        2) **Metastatic calcification** includes oliguria, corneal haziness, conjunctivitis, irregular heart rate

Table 7-3	Etiology and Pathophysiology of Hyperphosphatemia
Mechanism of Hyperphosphatemia	**Associated Clinical Conditions**
Cellular release of phosphorus (phosphate shifts from cells into extracellular fluid)	Respiratory or lactic acidosis or diabetic ketoacidosis because of movement of phosphorus out of cells Tumor lysis syndrome, which occurs with neoplastic diseases (leukemia, lymphoma) when treated with cytotoxic agents Rhabdomyolysis (breakdown of striated muscle), which releases phosphorus from cells because of tissue trauma, viral infections, heat stroke, increased metabolism, and catabolic states Chemotherapy for malignant tumors Massive transfusions because phosphorus can leak from cells during storage of blood
Phosphorus retention	Decreasing glomerular filtration rates (renal insufficiency, acute and chronic renal failure, chronic glomerulonephritis), which prevent adequate excretion of phosphates Decreased urinary losses unrelated to decreased renal function such as in hypoparathyroidism or volume depletion Hypocalcemia from antacids, diuretic agents, or steroids Hypoparathyroidism (primary or secondary), which causes a decrease in calcium and increased renal absorption of phosphorus Can occur with other conditions that cause cellular destruction and release of phosphorus into extracellular fluid Excess human growth hormone Hyperthyroidism, hypoparathyroidism Prolonged or excessive administration of heparin, tetracycline, pituitary extract, and salicylates
Excessive intake	Excessive intake of phosphorus or its supplements Infants fed cows' milk instead of human milk (940 mg of phosphorus in cows' milk compared to 150 mg in an equal amount of human milk) Vitamin D excess or increased GI absorption Large milk intake for the treatment of peptic ulcers Overzealous administration of oral or IV phosphorus supplements

      3) ECG changes and conduction disturbance, tachycardia

      4) The deposition of calcium phosphate in the cardiac tissues

      5) Tetany, which may increase in severity and spread to the limbs and face and be followed by numbness, muscle spasms, and pain

      6) The precipitation of calcium phosphate in nonosseous sites such as the kidney or heart

    b. Common symptoms

      1) Numbness and tingling around the mouth and in the fingertips, muscle spasms, and tetany from the increased phosphorus and corresponding decreased calcium

      2) Anorexia, nausea, vomiting

      3) Muscle weakness, hyperreflexia, tetany, flaccid paralysis

  2. Diagnostic and laboratory findings

    a. Serum phosphorus plasma levels are greater than 4.5 mg/dL (2.6 mEq/L)

    b. In clients with chronic renal failure, phosphorus values may be kept slightly higher (4–6 mg/dL) to ensure adequate levels of 2,3-DPG and thereby minimize effects of chronic anemia on oxygen delivery to tissues

    c. With increased phosphorus levels, serum calcium levels drop and hypocalcemia develops

      1) Hypocalcemia is more likely to occur in sudden, severe hyperphosphatemia (such as after intravenous administration of phosphates)

      2) Hypocalcemia may also occur in a client with chronic renal failure

  d. Chronic hyperphosphatemia in the client with chronic renal failure may contribute to the development of **renal osteodystrophy**, which may be assessed by skeletal x-rays

  1) A primary complication of hyperphosphatemia is metastatic calcification, the precipitation of calcium phosphate in the soft tissues, joints, and arteries

  2) Calcification formation and precipitation in the soft tissues may be anticipated if the product of the serum calcium level multiplied by the serum phosphorus level is greater than 70 mg/dL (normal product is about 30–40 mg/dL)

3. Identification of clients at risk

  a. Infants being fed cows' milk

  b. Clients using Phospho-Soda as an enema solution or regular laxative

  c. Clients in end-stage renal failure

C. Priority nursing diagnoses

1. Deficient Knowledge related to the purpose of phosphate-binding medications and the importance of reducing GI absorption of phosphorus to control hyperphosphatemia and prevent long-term complications

2. Risk for Injury related to internal factors associated with calcium phosphate precipitation in the soft tissues (corneas, lungs, kidneys, gastric mucosa, heart, blood vessels) and periarticular regions of the large joints (hips, shoulders, elbows) and development of hypocalcemic tetany

D. Therapeutic management

1. Decrease phosphorus intake

  a. Restrict or eliminate phosphorus intake in the diet

  b. Eliminate medications containing phosphorus, particularly over-the-counter preparations

2. Promote phosphorus excretion

  a. Increase gastrointestinal and renal excretion of phosphorus

  b. Perform renal dialysis in clients with renal failure

  c. Maintain fluid volume to ensure adequate blood pressure to enhance the excretion of phosphorus, particularly in clients receiving cytotoxic medications

3. Continue to monitor the client for increasing hypocalcemia

  a. Monitor for numbness and tingling of the fingers and circumoral region, and for hyperactive reflexes and muscle cramps

  b. Consult physician promptly if symptoms of hypocalcemia develop to avoid tetany

  c. Consult physician if client develops positive Trousseau or Chvostek sign

  d. Monitor renal function carefully, particularly urine output, BUN, and creatinine

  e. Monitor vital signs

  f. Calcium supplements and products containing vitamin D may be limited until phosphorus levels approach normal

  g. In clients with renal failure, serum phosphate values may be kept higher to ensure adequate levels of 2,3-DPG to improve tissue oxygenation

E. Planning and implementation

1. Monitor serum phosphorus and calcium levels

2. Calculate the calcium-phosphorus product and consult physician for abnormally high results

3. Identify clients at risk; treat the underlying cause

4. Monitor I&O; keep clients well hydrated; pay particular attention to the types of fluids being ingested (avoid carbonated beverages, which are high in phosphates); monitor urine output to be sure that it is adequate for phosphate excretion

Practice to Pass

What clinical manifestations may be seen in a client diagnosed with hyperphosphatemia?

5. Consult physician if client develops indications of soft tissue (metastatic) calcification (oliguria, corneal haziness, conjunctivitis, irregular heart rate, papular eruptions)

6. Monitor for signs and symptoms of tetany, such as positive Trousseau and Chvostek signs

7. Administer IV and oral phosphorus supplements cautiously in clients with normal phosphorus levels to avoid hyperphosphatemia; monitor serum phosphate levels periodically throughout administration

8. Avoid use of phosphate-containing enemas, especially in children and those with slowed bowel-emptying times

9. Encourage client to avoid intake of foods that are high in phosphorus content (previously described)

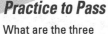

Practice to Pass

What are the three main types of phosphate binders that may be used to treat hyperphosphatemia?

F. **Medication therapy**

1. Specific drug therapies
   a. Avoid phosphate-containing laxatives and enemas, such as Fleet's Phospho-soda
   b. Use phosphate binders, such as Sevelamer (RenaGel), that are available in liquid, tablet, and capsule forms; administer these with meals to enhance binding of phosphate contained in the food

   c. Use aluminum-containing antacids to bind phosphates in the GI tract; be aware that aluminum-based products may lead to dementia if used over prolonged periods of time (such as those with renal failure) and cause constipation; examples include aluminum carbonate (Basojel) and aluminum hydroxide (Amphojel)

   d. Calcium carbonate (Tums) is useful as a supplement for clients with renal failure because this will help to counteract hypocalcemia, the imbalance that tends to accompany hyperphosphatemia

   e. In clients with hyperphosphatemia from use of cytotoxic drugs, use allopurinol (Zyloprim) as ordered to decrease uric acid production, which prevents the formation of uric acid calculi in the kidney and uric acid nephropathy

G. **Client education**

1. Awareness of precipitating factors

   a. Teach the client the purpose of phosphate binders and to take them as prescribed with or after meals to maximize their effectiveness
   b. Symptoms of hyperphosphatemia may be minimal; therefore, the client needs to be aware of preventing long-term complications through education

   c. Teach to avoid over-the-counter phosphorus medications such as laxatives, enemas, and vitamin-mineral supplements
   d. Instruct the client to identify signs and symptoms of hyperphosphatemia
   e. Teach to read labels to identify phosphorus and phosphate inclusions

2. Dietary education
   a. Use bulk-building supplements or stool softeners to combat the constipating effects of some phosphate binders, especially those with an aluminum base
   b. Avoid or limit foods high in phosphorus, as previously described, and avoid carbonated beverages, which have low nutrient value and are also high in phosphates

H. **Evaluation**

1. The client describes the symptoms of hyperphosphatemia and the ways in which it can be prevented

2. The client creates a three-day meal plan using foods low in or without phosphorus

3. The client verbalizes how to take medication therapy properly

Case Study

Mr. G. is a 56-year-old client with newly diagnosed chronic renal failure as a complication of diabetes mellitus. He will be beginning therapy with hemodialysis. He is married and lives at home with his wife; he has three grown children who do not live in the area. You have been assigned as his case manager and need to coordinate plans for his treatment and for client and family education.

1. Do you expect Mr. G. to have hypophosphatemia or hyperphosphatemia? What is the rationale for your choice?

2. How will you explain the etiology of this electrolyte imbalance to Mr. G?

3. What dietary modifications need to be made in order to keep serum phosphorus levels under control?

4. What role will dialysis play in managing phosphorus levels?

5. What medication therapy teaching do you anticipate will be needed?

For suggested responses, see pages 204–205.

POSTTEST

1. The nurse utilizes which of the following concepts about phosphate levels in the newborn when implementing client care?
   1. Phosphate levels are consistent throughout the day.
   2. Phosphate levels in newborns are nearly twice the adult level.
   3. Normal serum phosphate levels range from 1.5 to 2.0 mg/dL.
   4. Phosphorus is the most abundant mineral in the body.

2. When caring for a client with a phosphorus level of 1.8 mg/dL, the nurse plans interventions to promote which of the following?
   1. Conservation of energy
   2. Increased renal perfusion
   3. A decrease in peristalsis
   4. Deep and rapid breathing

3. A client experiencing hypophosphatemia has been started on sodium phosphate (Neutra-Phos). The nurse instructs the client that it is acceptable to take the medication with which of the following foods? Select all that apply.
   1. Whole grains
   2. Milk
   3. Orange juice
   4. Chicken
   5. Spinach

4. The nurse would assess for manifestations of hypophosphatemia in the client who has which predisposing clinical condition?
   1. Severe vomiting and diarrhea
   2. Occasional use of magnesium-containing antacids
   3. Infusion of balanced total parenteral nutrition (TPN) solutions
   4. Vitamin D excess

5. When caring for a client with a serum phosphorus level of 1.9 mg/dL, the nurse should be alert to which of the following signs?
   1. Hyperactive bowel sounds
   2. Dysrhythmias related to decreased oxygenation
   3. Increased muscle tone
   4. Polycythemia

6 When caring for a client with a phosphorus level of 5.2 mg/dL, the nurse should anticipate reports of which of the following?

1. Circumoral numbness
2. Hunger
3. Chest pain
4. Thirst

7 A client with chronic renal failure (CRF) has been started on a sevelamer (Renagel) for treatment of hyperphosphatemia. To enhance effectiveness of the medication, the nurse plans to administer it in which way?

1. On an empty stomach
2. Thirty minutes before the meal
3. With meals
4. Two hours after a meal

8 When administering an infusion of potassium phosphate, the nurse administers the infusion carefully, using an infusion pump so that phosphorus replacement does not exceed _____ mEq per hour.

Fill in your answer below:
_____ mEq/hr

9 The nurse determines that a client with a phosphorus level of 4.9 mg/dL indicates an understanding of dietary instructions when the client limits intake of which food item?

1. Pork chops
2. White rice
3. Sirloin steak
4. Green peas

10 The nurse identifies that a client who chronically uses which type of over-the-counter products is at greatest risk for developing hyperphosphatemia?

1. Enemas
2. Cough preparations
3. Cold preparations
4. Bedtime sleeping aids

➤ *See pages 147–148 for Answers and Rationales.*

POSTTEST

ANSWERS & RATIONALES

Pretest

1 **Answer: 2** **Rationale:** Infant levels of phosphorus are higher than an adult's levels due to the rapid turnover of bone, but a level of 5.0 mEq/L is elevated for an infant. The nurse needs to determine what is contributing to the elevated level. Infant formulas and breast milk would not cause elevated levels, whereas cows' milk is naturally high in phosphorus. **Cognitive Level:** Applying **Client Need:** Physiological Adaptation **Integrated Process:** Nursing Process: Evaluation **Content Area:** Child Health **Strategy:** First recognize that the phosphorus level is elevated. Recall causes of elevated phosphorus to delete the options for vomiting and diarrhea. Recall sources of phosphorus to choose the correct option. **Reference:** London, M.L., Ladewig, P.W., et al. (2011). *Maternal and child nursing care* (3rd ed.). Upper Saddle River, NJ: Pearson/ Prentice Hall, pp. 1232–1260.

2 **Answer: 2** **Rationale:** Children have higher phosphate levels than adults because of their more rapid bone development rate. Serum phosphate levels vary throughout the day. Replacement therapy would result in an increase in phosphorus level. A venous sample, not arterial, is taken. **Cognitive Level:** Applying **Client Need:** Physiological Adaptation **Integrated Process:** Nursing Process: Diagnosis **Content Area:** Child Health **Strategy:** First recognize that this is a pediatric client, and pediatric phosphorus levels would normally be higher. Eliminate arterial sampling as arterial blood gases are the only common lab drawn arterially. After starting phosphorus replacement, the levels should rise. **Reference:** Kee, J., Paulanka, B., & Polek, C. (2010). *Handbook of fluids and electrolytes and acid-base imbalance* (3rd ed.). Clifton, NY: Delmar, pp. 118–120.

3 **Answer: 2** **Rationale:** A phosphate level of 1.7 mg/dL reflects hypophosphatemia. Phosphorus is needed for formation of the red blood cell enzyme 2,3-DPG, and so a deficiency of phosphorus can lead to anemia, reflected by a decrease in hemoglobin level. Because phosphorus is needed for many cellular enzyme reactions necessary

ANSWERS & RATIONALES

for red blood cell and platelet synthesis, the platelet count may be decreased, not increased. Calcium and phosphorus levels have a reciprocal relationship and so an elevation of calcium would be expected. Low magnesium levels, not elevated, are associated with a low phosphorus level. **Cognitive Level:** Analyzing **Client Need:** Reduction of Risk Potential **Integrated Process:** Nursing Process: Assessment **Content Area:** Adult Health **Strategy:** First recognize the level reflects hypophosphatemia. Recall the role of phosphorus in red blood cell production to direct you to the correct option. **Reference:** LeMone, P., & Burke, K. (2008). *Medical surgical nursing: Critical thinking in client care* (4th ed.). Upper Saddle River, NJ: Pearson/Prentice Hall, pp. 236–237.

4 Answer: 2, 5 Rationale: Because of the elevated glucose levels seen with diabetic ketoacidosis, osmotic diuresis causes a loss of phosphorus. Clients with a history of alcoholism often have poor dietary intake of foods high in phosphorus, contributing to hypophosphatemia. There is not a shift of fluids or significant cellular damage occurring with first-degree burns that would affect phosphorus levels. Hypomagnesemia would be seen with hypophosphatemia due to renal excretion of phosphorus. A decrease in urine output would contribute to less renal excretion of phosphorus, and the level would increase, not decrease. **Cognitive Level:** Applying **Client Need:** Physiological Adaptation **Integrated Process:** Nursing Process: Assessment **Content Area:** Adult Health **Strategy:** Critical words are *hypophosphatemia* and *predisposing clinical conditions*. Analyze each option recalling phosphorus is lost in the urine. Recognize that polyuria seen with acidosis will contribute to phosphorus loss to choose diabetic ketoacidosis, and poor intake of phosphorus causes decreased serum levels to choose the option for history of alcoholism. **Reference:** LeMone, P., & Burke, K. (2008). *Medical surgical nursing: Critical thinking in client care* (4th ed.). Upper Saddle River, NJ: Pearson/Prentice Hall, pp. 236–237.

5 Answer: 4, 5 Rationale: Although phosphorus is found in a large number of food items, it is found in the greatest quantities in red and organ meats, fish, poultry, eggs, milk and milk products, legumes, whole grains, and nuts. The other options identify foods that have lesser amounts of phosphorus. **Cognitive Level:** Applying **Client Need:** Physiological Adaptation **Integrated Process:** Teaching and Learning **Content Area:** Adult Health **Strategy:** Recall foods high in phosphorus to choose correctly. **Reference:** Kee, J., Paulanka, B., & Polek, C.L. (2010). *Handbook of fluids and electrolytes and acid base imbalance* (3rd ed.). Clifton, NY: Delmar, pp. 118–122.

6 Answer: 3 Rationale: Phosphorus is utilized in the metabolism of TPN, causing a shift of phosphorus into the cells and lowering serum phosphorus levels, reflected by the low level of 1.2 mg/dL. Because of the many enzyme reactions needed for the metabolism of TPN, magnesium is utilized and levels drop with refeeding syndrome. A magnesium level of 2.5 mg is at the upper

end of normal. Calcium levels sometimes drop with refeeding syndrome secondary to cellular shifts. A calcium level of 9.8 mg/dL is normal. This is a normal potassium level. Potassium levels may decrease as cellular shifts occur with the metabolism of TPN. **Cognitive Level:** Analyzing **Client Need:** Physiological Adaptation **Integrated Process:** Nursing Process: Evaluation **Content Area:** Adult Health **Strategy:** First recall the purpose and content of TPN. Recall that electrolytes are utilized for enzyme reactions and metabolism and recognize which value is low to choose the correct option. **Reference:** LeMone, P., & Burke, K. (2008). *Medical surgical nursing: Critical thinking in client care* (4th ed.). Upper Saddle River, NJ: Pearson/Prentice Hall, pp. 236–237.

7 Answer: 1 Rationale: Poor nutritional intake, vomiting, diarrhea, and overuse of antacids are related to alcoholism and alcohol abuse, and can lead to hypophosphatemia. During the oliguric phase, renal excretion of phosphorus would be diminished, contributing to elevated serum levels of phosphorus. Clients with prolonged (not short-term) gastric suction are more likely to experience hypophosphatemia. Prolonged or continuous use of aluminum-containing antacids (not occasional use) leads to hypophosphatemia. **Cognitive Level:** Analyzing **Client Need:** Physiological Adaptation **Integrated Process:** Nursing Process: Assessment **Content Area:** Adult Health **Strategy:** Recognize that some of the options have conditions that would contribute to a low phosphorus level, but identify withdrawal from alcohol as having the greatest risk. **Reference:** LeMone, P. & Burke, K. (2008). *Medical surgical nursing: Critical thinking in client care* (4th ed.). Upper Saddle River, NJ: Pearson/Prentice Hall, pp. 236–237.

8 Answer: 3 Rationale: A phosphate level of 4.9 mg/dL reflects an elevated phosphorus level. Because a reciprocal relationship occurs with calcium, hypocalcemia is expected. Hypocalcemia would be expected, not hyperkalemia. Because a reciprocal relationship occurs with calcium, hypocalcemia would be expected rather than hyponatremia. Magnesium would not be affected. **Cognitive Level:** Analyzing **Client Need:** Physiological Adaptation **Integrated Process:** Nursing Process: Assessment **Content Area:** Adult Health **Strategy:** Recall the relationship between calcium and phosphorus to direct you to the correct option. **Reference:** LeMone, P., & Burke, K. (2008). *Medical surgical nursing: Critical thinking in client care* (4th ed.). Upper Saddle River, NJ: Pearson/Prentice Hall, pp. 237–238.

9 Answer: 2 Rationale: In clients with hyperphosphatemia (normal 2.5–4.5 mg/dL) from use of cytotoxic drugs, allopurinol (Zyloprim) may be ordered to decrease uric acid production, which prevents the formation of uric acid calculi in the kidney and uric acid nephropathy. Although Amphogel might be given to treat the elevated phosphorus level, the question asks which drug will be given to treat the elevated uric acid. Diamox is a carbonic anhydrase inhibitor, which is a type of diuretic used to treat glaucoma. Apresoline is a vasodilator used in the treatment of hypertension. **Cognitive Level:** Applying **Client Need:** Pharmacological and Parenteral Therapies **Integrated Process:** Nursing Process: Diagnosis **Content Area:** Adult Health **Strategy:** Note that there are two conditions in the question—hyperphosphatemia and hyperuricemia—but the question addresses treatment of the latter only. Use knowledge of pharmacology and the process of elimination to make a selection. **Reference:** Adams, M. P., Josephson, D. C., & Holland, C.N. (2011). *Pharmacology for nurses: A pathophysiologic approach* (3rd ed.).Upper Saddle River, NJ: Pearson/Prentice Hall, pp. 424, 744.

10 Answer: 1 Rationale: Many types of food additives and preservatives contain phosphorus and would be acceptable for the client who needs to increase dietary phosphorus. Vitamin A does not have an effect on phosphorus absorption. Aluminum binds to phosphorus and would be contraindicated for the client needing to increase phosphorus levels. Soy-based foods are not a good source of phosphorus. Phosphorus is found in dairy products, meats, whole grains, and nuts. **Cognitive Level:** Applying **Client Need:** Health Promotion and Maintenance **Integrated Process:** Teaching and Learning **Content Area:** Adult Health **Strategy:** Key words are *discharge teaching* and *diet high in phosphates*. Recall knowledge of phosphorus sources to direct you to the correct option. **Reference:** Dudek, S. (2010). *Nutrition essentials for nursing practice* (6th ed.). Philadelphia: Lippincott Williams & Wilkins, pp. 128, 130–131.

Posttest

1 Answer: 2 Rationale: Newborn levels of phosphate can range from 4.0 to 7.0 mg/dL. Phosphate levels differ throughout the day. Normal serum phosphate levels range from 2.5 to 4.5 mg/dL. Phosphate is the second most abundant mineral in the body. **Cognitive Level:** Applying **Client Need:** Reduction of Risk Potential **Integrated Process:** Nursing Process: Diagnosis **Content Area:** Child Health **Strategy:** The critical word is *newborn*. Recognize the three incorrect statements to eliminate them. **Reference:** Corbett, J. (2008). *Laboratory tests and diagnostic procedures with nursing diagnoses* (7th ed.). Upper Saddle River, NJ: Pearson/Prentice Hall, p. 177.

2 Answer: 1 Rationale: Phosphorus is needed for adenosine triphosphate (ATP) production, which in turn is utilized for cellular energy. A level of 1.8 mg/dL reflects a low level of phosphorus, indicating a deficit will present for energy production in the body. Increased renal perfusion would contribute to increased secretion of phosphorus. Peristalsis is already decreased in hypophosphatemia; measures should be taken to prevent constipation. Hypophosphatemia can lead to hypoxemia and increased deep and rapid breathing. Measures should be taken to reduce energy expenditure and prevent respiratory distress. **Cognitive**

Level: Analyzing **Client Need:** Reduction of Risk Potential **Integrated Process:** Nursing Process: Planning **Content Area:** Adult Health **Strategy:** Recall that the normal phosphorus level is 2.5–4.5 mg/dL and then choose an intervention that will help with hypophosphatemia. **Reference:** LeMone, P., & Burke, K. (2008). *Medical surgical nursing: Critical thinking in client care* (4th ed.). Upper Saddle River, NJ: Pearson/Prentice Hall, pp. 236–237.

3 Answer: 2, 3, 4 Rationale: Oxalate (in spinach and rhubarb) and phytates (found in bran and whole grains) can interfere with the absorption of phosphate by binding with them in the intestines. Milk, orange juice, and chicken do not pose this problem for absorption of phosphate. **Cognitive Level:** Applying **Client Need:** Pharmacological and Parenteral Therapies **Integrated Process:** Nursing Process: Implementation **Content Area:** Adult Health **Strategy:** Recall that calcium and phosphorus have an inverse relationship, and phytates and oxalates inhibit phosphorus absorption. **Reference:** Adams, M. P., Josephson, D. C., & Holland, C.N. (2011). *Pharmacology for nurses: A pathophysiologic approach.* (3rd ed.). Upper Saddle River, NJ: Pearson/Prentice Hall, pp. 644–648.

4 Answer: 1 Rationale: Phosphorus can be lost via the gastrointestinal tract through vomiting and diarrhea. Prolonged or excessive use of aluminum- or magnesium-containing antacids can contribute to hypophosphatemia, but the occasional use should not pose a problem. A balanced infusion of TPN should contain appropriate amounts of phosphorus to prevent hypophosphatemia. When TPN is first initiated, refeeding syndrome may contribute to phosphorus utilization and low levels may be seen. A deficiency of vitamin D can lead to decreased intestinal absorption of phosphorus. **Cognitive Level:** Analyzing **Client Need:** Physiological Adaptation **Integrated Process:** Nursing Process: Assessment **Content Area:** Adult Health **Strategy:** Critical words are *predisposing clinical condition*. Note the word *severe* in the correct option and recognize phosphorus will be lost with vomiting and diarrhea. **Reference:** LeMone, P., & Burke, K. (2008). *Medical surgical nursing: Critical thinking in client care* (4th ed.). Upper Saddle River, NJ: Pearson/Prentice Hall, pp. 236–237.

5 Answer: 2 Rationale: Hypophosphatemia results in decreased adenosine triphosphate (ATP) production, decreasing enzyme levels of 2,3-DPG, which in turn keeps oxygen bound to hemoglobin and less available to the tissues. Clients with hypophosphatemia will experience hypoactive bowel sounds, muscle weakness, paresthesias, and anemia due to red blood cell (RBC) fragility from low ATP levels. **Cognitive Level:** Analyzing **Client Need:** Reduction of Risk Potential **Integrated Process:** Nursing Process: Assessment **Content Area:** Adult Health **Strategy:** Recall that phosphorus is needed for ATP production and oxygenation. Recognize that these deficiencies can contribute to irregular heart rhythms to direct you to the correct option. **Reference:** LeMone, P., & Burke, K. (2008). *Medical surgical nursing: Critical* *thinking in client care* (4th ed.). Upper Saddle River, NJ: Pearson/Prentice Hall, pp. 236–137.

6 **Answer: 1** **Rationale:** A phosphorus level of 5.2 mg/dL reflects hyperphosphatemia, which is usually accompanied by hypocalcemia. Numbness and tingling around the mouth in the fingertips is associated with hypocalcemia. Anorexia, nausea, and vomiting are associated with hyperphosphatemia. Chest pain may be seen with hypophosphatemia associated with a decline in 2,3-DPG levels, reducing the release of oxygen to the tissues. Thirst is not a sign of this imbalance. **Cognitive Level:** Applying **Client Need:** Physiological Adaptation **Integrated Process:** Nursing Process: Assessment **Content Area:** Adult Health **Strategy:** First recognize the level reflects hyperphosphatemia. Recall that hypocalcemia is associated with hyperphosphatemia to choose correctly. **Reference:** LeMone, P., & Burke, K. (2008). *Medical surgical nursing: Critical thinking in client care* (4th ed.). Upper Saddle River, NJ: Pearson/Prentice Hall, pp. 237–238.

7 **Answer: 3** **Rationale:** Sevelamer is a phosphate binder frequently used in patients with renal failure. In order to maximize binding of the phosphate, phosphate binders should be given with a meal or shortly after in order for the medication to have contact with the phosphate in the food. **Cognitive Level:** Applying **Client Need:** Pharmacological and Parenteral Therapies **Integrated Process:** Nursing Process: Planning **Content Area:** Adult Health **Strategy:** Note the similarities between taking sevelamer on an empty stomach and two hours after a meal to eliminate them. Recognize the purpose and action of the medication to direct you to the correct option. **Reference:** Adams, M. P., Josephson, D. C., & Holland C.N. (2011). *Pharmacology for nurses: A pathophysiologic approach.* (3rd ed.). Upper Saddle River, NJ: Pearson/Prentice Hall, pp. 644–648.

8 **Answer: 10** **Rationale:** Intravenous phosphorus replacement should not exceed 10 mEq/hr in order to prevent phlebitis or potassium overload and to allow gradual return of phosphorus levels. **Cognitive Level:** Applying **Client Need:** Pharmacological and Parenteral Therapies **Integrated Process:** Nursing Process: Implementation **Content Area:** Adult Health **Strategy:** Recall safety measures related to administration of electrolytes. **Reference:** LeMone, P., & Burke, K. (2008.). *Medical surgical nursing: Critical thinking in client care* (4th ed.). Upper Saddle River, NJ: Pearson/Prentice Hall, pp. 236–237.

9 **Answer: 3** **Rationale:** A phosphorus level of 4.9 mg/dL is elevated, indicating a need to restrict foods high in phosphorus, which include red meats, dairy products, eggs, poultry, organ meats, legumes, and whole grains. Sirloin steak is a red meat and high in phosphorus. Pork chops are not as high in phosphorus as the choice of sirloin steak. White rice is lower in phosphorus because it is not a whole grain. Green peas would not be excessively high in phosphorus. **Cognitive Level:** Applying **Client Need:** Physiological Adaptation **Integrated Process:** Nursing Process: Evaluation **Content Area:** Adult Health **Strategy:** Recall foods high in phosphorus to direct you to the correct option. **Reference:** Dudek, S. (2010). *Nutrition essentials for nursing practice* (6th ed.). Philadelphia: Lippincott Williams & Wilkins, pp. 128–131.

10 **Answer: 1** **Rationale:** Enemas can be high in phosphorus, thus making the client at risk for hyperphosphatemia if they are frequently used. The other products listed do not necessarily have large amounts of phosphorus in them. **Cognitive Level:** Analyzing **Client Need:** Pharmacological and Parenteral Therapies **Integrated Process:** Nursing Process: Assessment **Content Area:** Adult Health **Strategy:** Analyze each option for phosphorus content, eliminating cough and cold preparations and bedtime sleeping aids because they are not high in phosphorus. **Reference:** LeMone, P., & Burke, K. (2008). *Medical surgical nursing: Critical thinking in client care* (4th ed.). Upper Saddle River, NJ: Pearson/Prentice Hall, pp. 237–238.

References

Adams, M. P., Josephson, D. L., & Holland, L. N. (2011). *Pharmacology for nurses: A pathophysiologic approach* (3rd ed.). Upper Saddle River, NJ: Pearson Education.

Berman, A., & Snyder, S. (2012). *Kozier & Erb's fundamentals of nursing: Concepts, process, and practice* (9th ed.). Upper Saddle River, NJ: Pearson Education.

Dudek, S. (2009). *Nutrition essentials for nursing practice* (6th ed.). Philadelphia: Lippincott Williams & Wilkins.

Hockenberry, M. J., & Wilson, D. (2008). *Wong's Essentials of pediatric nursing* (8th ed.). St. Louis, MO: Mosby, Elsevier.

Ignatavicius, D., & Workman, M. (2009). *Medical-surgical nursing: Critical thinking in collaborative care* (6th ed.). St. Louis, MO: Elsevier Saunders.

Kee, J. L. (2009). *Handbook of laboratory and diagnostic tests with nursing implications* (6th ed.). Upper Saddle River, NJ: Pearson Education.

LeMone, P., & Burke, K. (2011). *Medical-surgical nursing: Critical thinking in client care* (5th ed.). Upper Saddle River: NJ: Pearson Education.

London, M. L., Ladewig, P. W., Ball, J. W., Bindler, R. C., & Cowen, K. J. (2011). *Maternal & child nursing care* (3rd ed.). Upper Saddle River, NJ: Pearson Education.

Osborne, K. S., Wraa, C. E., & Watson, A. B., (2010). *Medical-surgical nursing: Preparation for practice.* Upper Saddle River, NJ: Pearson Education.

ANSWERS & RATIONALES

Acid–Base Balance and Imbalances

8

Chapter Outline

Overview of Acid–Base
    Physiology
Respiratory Acidosis

Respiratory Alkalosis
Metabolic Acidosis
Metabolic Alkalosis

Mixed Acid–Base
    Disturbances

Objectives

➤ Review the basic physiology of acid–base balance.
➤ Identify potential acid–base imbalances.
➤ Identify priority nursing diagnoses for acid–base imbalances.
➤ Describe the therapeutic management of acid–base imbalances.
➤ Describe the nursing management of a client who is experiencing
    an acid–base imbalance.

NCLEX-RN® Test Prep

Use the accompanying online resource,
NursingReviewsandRationales, to test
yourself with hundreds of NCLEX®-style
practice questions.

Review at a Glance

acid a substance that releases a hydrogen (H^+) ion when dissolved in water

base a substance that binds to a hydrogen (H^+) ion when dissolved in water

buffer prevents major changes in extracellular fluid (ECF) by releasing or accepting hydrogen (H^+) ions

compensation body process of using its regulatory mechanisms to return pH to normal level

HCO_3^- bicarbonate, an alkalotic substance; a direct reflection of renal system's ability to compensate for pH changes

metabolic acidosis a gain of hydrogen (H^+) ions or a loss of HCO_3^-; pH decreases and HCO_3^- decreases

metabolic alkalosis a loss of hydrogen (H^+) ion or a gain in HCO_3^-; pH increases and HCO_3^- increases

mixed acid–base disorder occurs when two or more independent acid–base disorders occur at same time

$PaCO_2$ measurement of CO_2 pressure that is being exerted on the plasma and is directly related to the amount of CO_2 being produced

PaO_2 measures amount of pressure exerted by oxygen on plasma

pH negative logarithm of H^+ ion concentration in mEq per liter

respiratory acidosis a condition that occurs in response to hypoventilation; CO_2 is retained and pH is decreased

respiratory alkalosis a decreased level of CO_2; sometimes called a H_2CO_3 deficit; pH is elevated and $PaCO_2$ is decreased

SaO_2 amount of oxygen attached to a hemoglobin molecule

PRETEST

1 Arterial blood gases on a client with pneumonia indicate the client is in respiratory acidosis. In order to best improve this acid–base imbalance, the nurse implements which of the following nursing interventions? Select all that apply.

1. Restrict oral fluid intake to water only.
2. Ambulate client in hallways twice each shift.
3. Encourage frequent cough and deep breathing exercises.
4. Medicate with a nonopiate pain medication frequently for intercostal muscle pain.
5. Give magnesium.

2 A client receiving intravenous (IV) sodium bicarbonate for treatment of metabolic acidosis develops muscle twitching and an irregular pulse. Which action should be taken by the nurse initially?

1. Stop the infusion and notify the physician.
2. Reduce the infusion by one-half of the ordered rate and observe client closely.
3. Monitor heart rate, blood pressure, and mentation every 15 minutes.
4. Check pulse oximetry and place client on bedrest.

3 Which of the following arterial blood gases (ABGs) would the nurse expect to see when a client has apnea and develops acidosis?

1. pH 7.42, $PaCO_2$ 48 mm Hg, HCO_3^- 25 mEq/L
2. pH 7.29, $PaCO_2$ 62 mm Hg, HCO_3^- 23 mEq/L
3. pH 7.36, $PaCO_2$ 42 mm Hg, HCO_3^- 26 mEq/L
4. pH 7.49, $PaCO_2$ 30 mm Hg, HCO_3^- 35 mEq/L

4 The nurse concludes that which statement by a student nurse reflects correct understanding about the client's physiological attempt to restore homeostasis during acidosis?

1. "The kidneys start to work within seconds after an imbalance occurs and are very effective in restoring the body to a correct acid–base balance."
2. "The kidneys may not start to function immediately but are very effective as a buffer system to restore the acid–base balance."
3. "The kidneys are not as effective as the lungs in restoring the acid–base balance because the bicarbonate ion is not a good buffer."
4. "The kidneys are very slow to respond to any acid–base imbalance but are very effective in ridding the body of carbonic acid."

5 Which of the following ABG results would the nurse expect to see when a client is admitted with diarrhea that has lasted for four days?

1. pH 7.50, $PaCO_2$ 60 mm Hg, HCO_3^- 28 mEq/L
2. pH 7.30, $PaCO_2$ 40 mm Hg, HCO_3^- 18 mEq/L
3. pH 7.40, $PaCO_2$ 38 mm Hg, HCO_3^- 28 mEq/L
4. pH 7.50, $PaCO_2$ 38 mm Hg, HCO_3^- 32 mEq/L

6 The nurse has been caring for a client who has become extremely anxious and agitated. When assessing the client, the nurse would expect to find which of the following that could ultimately lead to an acid–base imbalance?

1. Rapid, deep respiratory pattern
2. Rapid, shallow respiratory pattern
3. Rapid, irregular heart rate
4. Slow, irregular heart rate

7 Which of the following pH values would the nurse expect to see in an anxious client?

1. 7.45
2. 7.38
3. 7.50
4. 7.20

8 The nurse anticipates which of the following responses in a client who develops metabolic acidosis?

1. Heart rate will increase.
2. Urinary output will increase.
3. Respiratory rate will increase.
4. Temperature will increase.

9 The nurse assesses a client with uncontrolled type 1 diabetes mellitus (DM) for which primary acid–base imbalance?

1. Metabolic alkalosis
2. Respiratory alkalosis
3. Respiratory acidosis
4. Metabolic acidosis

10 The client with respiratory acidosis from COPD asks the nurse why a continuous pulse oximeter is ordered. Which response by the nurse is best?

1. "The pulse oximeter measures your CO_2 level so ABGs need to be drawn once a day only."
2. "The pulse oximeter measures the oxygen saturation in your blood at any given time."
3. "The pulse oximeter is being used so we do not have to draw ABGs on you while you are in the hospital."
4. "The machine is used to adequately assess your ventilatory effort while you are in bed."

➤ *See pages 167–169 for Answers and Rationales.*

I. OVERVIEW OF ACID–BASE PHYSIOLOGY

A. Nature of acids and bases
1. An **acid** is a substance that releases a hydrogen (H^+) ion when dissolved in water
2. A **base** is a substance that will bind to an H^+ ion when dissolved in water
3. Weak acids do not completely separate in water; they only release some of the H^+ ions
4. A weak base accepts the H^+ ion less easily but it is extremely valuable in preventing major alterations in the pH of the extracellular fluid (ECF)

B. Chemical buffer systems in the body
1. A **buffer** prevents major changes in the ECF by releasing or accepting hydrogen (H^+) ions
2. The major chemical buffers are found in the blood and include the carbonic acid–bicarbonate buffer system, the phosphate buffer system, and the protein buffer system
3. Chemical buffers are present in both intracellular fluid (ICF) and ECF
4. Buffers are found in all tissues of the body, including bone
5. Chemical buffers act within seconds to neutralize acids and bases and keep the pH within the narrow normal range of 7.35 to 7.45
6. Bicarbonate buffer system
   a. This system consists of a water solution that contains a weak acid, carbonic acid (H_2CO_3), and a bicarbonate salt, usually sodium bicarbonate ($NaHCO_3$)
   b. Normally the body maintains the pH by keeping the ratio of bicarbonate (HCO_3^-) to H_2CO_3 at a proportion of 20:1
      1) This ratio is changed if the pH goes up or down depending on the alteration
      2) Once compensation occurs, the ratio becomes stable again
   c. The bicarbonate/carbonic acid buffer system is linked to both the respiratory and renal systems to protect the body from changes in pH
      1) H_2CO_3 is the respiratory compensatory component because it can dissociate into carbon dioxide (CO_2) and water, with CO_2 being exhaled by the lungs
      2) HCO_3^- is the primary renal compensatory component because it can be excreted by the kidneys

[handwritten margin note: So excess CO₂ = ↓ pH. (give pt. Bicarb)]

    3) This function is illustrated by the following equation:

$$CO_2 + H_2O \leftrightarrow H_2CO_3 \leftrightarrow HCO_3^- + H^+$$

  7. The phosphate buffer system buffers both ICF and ECF to maintain a normal pH

  8. The protein buffer system acts in a similar manner to the bicarbonate-carbonic acid buffer system because it releases or accepts H^+ readily and can exist as either an acid or a base; it is a major intracellular buffer

  9. The hemoglobin–oxyhemoglobin buffer system helps to maintain pH within normal range in both arterial and venous blood, which have different amounts of CO_2

C. Physiologic buffers in the body

  1. Pulmonary regulation

    a. Lungs control the respiratory carbonic acid buffer system

    b. Lungs compensate for acid–base disturbances that are primarily metabolic in nature (lactic acidosis that occurs with exercise, for example)

    c. Under control of the medulla oblongata, the lungs increase or decrease the respiratory rate and depth in response to the amount of CO_2 in the ECF

    d. In an acid environment, respirations increase to blow off CO_2; in an alkaline environment, respirations slow to retain CO_2

    e. The respiratory system is extremely sensitive to changes in the pH and begins compensatory efforts within seconds to minutes

      1) These mechanisms can become quickly exhausted

      2) This system is not as efficient as renal compensatory efforts

    f. The elderly have a reduced amount of gas exchange during breathing and also have less alveolar membrane so CO_2 retention and increased H^+ ions are a problem

  2. Renal regulation

    a. The kidneys control the metabolic buffer $NaHCO_3^-$ by excreting an acidic urine or an alkaline urine

    b. This system works within several hours to days, but is powerfully effective in that it can eliminate either acids or bases as needed

    c. The kidneys control the HCO_3^- in ECF by either reabsorbing or excreting the H^+ ion

      1) They can reabsorb HCO_3^- as needed

      2) They can secrete free H^+ ions into the renal tubules from the peritubular capillaries

      3) They can combine ammonia (NaH_3) with hydrochloric acid (HCl) to form ammonium (NH_4Cl), which is excreted by the kidneys; approximately 50% of excess H^+ can be excreted by this mechanism

    d. The kidneys can actually excrete weak acids into the urine

    e. The body depends on the kidneys to excrete acids from cellular metabolism; thus the urine is normally acidic (average pH is 6)

    f. Renal function decreases with age so elderly clients do not excrete H^+ ions or synthesize HCO_3^- as efficiently; therefore, their acid–base imbalances are more difficult to correct, especially if other conditions, such as pneumonia, fever, or infection, occur

  3. Compensation for an acid–base imbalance occurs when the body uses regulatory mechanisms to return pH to normal by transforming acids and bases within the body; the body will either fully compensate, partially compensate, or progress to an uncompensated state

    a. A primary metabolic disturbance will cause a respiratory compensation

    b. A primary respiratory disturbance will cause an acute metabolic response due to buffering system and a more chronic compensation due to renal function

    c. Fully compensated means that the pH remains within normal range, although other values (CO_2 and bicarbonate) may still be abnormal

       d. Partial compensation means that the buffers are in the process of working to restore homeostasis; however, the pH remains abnormal

       e. Decompensation refers to a worsening state of acid–base imbalance and the pH remains abnormal

   4. Correction of the acid–base imbalance occurs when lungs and/or kidneys eliminate the offending substance(s) from the body; the CO_2 and HCO_3^- levels are returned to normal, not just the pH

  D. Measurement of acid–base status: assessed by using arterial blood gases (ABGs) (see Table 8-1)

   1. pH: the negative logarithm of H^+ ion concentration in mEq per liter

       a. The actual concentration of the H^+ ions is very small (< 0.0001 mEq/liter); therefore, it has a negative logarithm

       b. Because the pH is calculated as a negative value, there is an inverse relationship between the pH and the H^+ ion concentration; therefore, as the H^+ ion concentration increases, pH decreases

       c. The normal value for the pH in arterial blood is 7.35 to 7.45; in venous blood, the pH is 7.32 to 7.42

       d. A pH less than 7.35 is termed *acidotic*

       e. Conversely, a pH greater than 7.45 is called *alkalotic*

   2. $PaCO_2$ (partial pressure of carbon dioxide): the measurement of the CO_2 pressure that is being exerted on the plasma and is directly related to the amount of CO_2 being produced

       a. The normal value of $PaCO_2$ is 35–45 mm Hg

       b. The $PaCO_2$ is regulated by the lungs and indicates the amount of H_2CO_3 that is available to act as a buffer

       c. The $PaCO_2$ is the respiratory component of the ABG

       d. Values less than 35 mm Hg are indicative of alkalosis (consistent with hyperventilation)

       e. Acidosis occurs when the value rises above 45 mm Hg (consistent with hypoventilation)

   3. PaO_2 (partial pressure of oxygen): measures the amount of pressure exerted by oxygen on the plasma

       a. The range of normal values for PaO_2 is 80–100 mm Hg for adults under 60 years of age

       b. For every year above 60, there is an expected decrease in PaO_2 of 1 mm Hg

       c. If the PaO_2 drops dramatically, it indicates hypoxemia, which leads to tissue hypoxia; oxygen saturation will also decrease greatly

Table 8-1   **Arterial Blood Gas Interpretation**

Blood Gas Values	Acidosis	Normal	Alkalosis
pH	<7.35	7.35–7.45	>7.45
$PaCO_2$ Abnormal $PaCO_2$ with a normal HCO_3^- indicates a respiratory basis for imbalance	>45 mm Hg respiratory	35–45 mm Hg	<35 mm Hg respiratory
HCO_3^- Abnormal with a normal $PaCO_2$ indicates a metabolic basis for imbalance	<22 mEq/L metabolic	22–26 mEq/L	>26 mEq/L metabolic

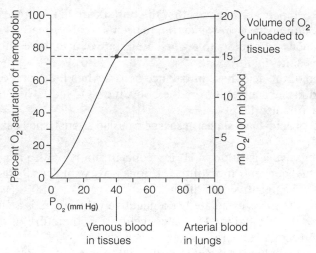

Figure 8-1

Oxygen-hemoglobin dissociation curve. The lower the PaO$_2$ level, the more readily hemoglobin will onload or offload oxygen.

4. **SaO$_2$**: refers to the percent of hemoglobin bound with oxygen; normal range is 95–100%
   a. Because most oxygen is carried on hemoglobin, the total oxygen concentration is measured using the hemoglobin saturation (SaO$_2$)
   b. There is a relationship between the PaO$_2$ and SaO$_2$ that influences binding affinity and dissociation of oxygen and hemoglobin (see Figure 8-1)
   c. Acidosis causes a shift to the right on the oxyhemoglobin dissociation curve that results in a decreased affinity; oxygen is more easily released to the tissues
   d. Alkalosis causes a shift to the left on the oxyhemoglobin dissociation curve that results in an increased affinity; oxygen is held more tightly and is less available to tissues
   e. There are other factors that affect oxygen affinity, such as body temperature and transfusion of banked blood
5. Electrolyte interactions

   a. HCO$_3^-$ (normal 22–26 mEq/L) is a direct reflection of the renal system's ability to compensate for pH changes
      1) A decreased HCO$_3^-$ level indicates acidosis
      2) Alkalosis occurs when the HCO$_3^-$ level rises above normal
   b. The base excess (BE) is an indication of the amount of HCO$_3^-$ available in the ECF
      1) Either a negative or positive amount of HCO$_3^-$ is available for use
      2) Normal base excess ranges from a −3.0 to a +3.0 in adults
      3) Values above +3.0 indicate metabolic alkalosis
      4) Metabolic acidosis exists when the value is below −3.0
   c. Serum anion gap (AG) represents an attempt to calculate concentrations of anions (HCO$_3$, chloride [Cl], proteins, phosphates, and sulfates) and cations (sodium [Na$^+$], potassium [K$^+$], magnesium [Mg^{++}], calcium [Ca^{++}])
      1) Normal range is 10–12 mEq/L
      2) Calculated value is Na$^+$ − [CL$^-$ + HCO$_3^-$]
      3) Increased AG of >16 mEq/L indicates metabolic acidosis (anion gap acidosis); always check anion gap if client has acidosis
      4) Normal AG can exist with a metabolic acidosis (non-anion-gap acidosis) when there is a decrease in HCO$_3^-$ balanced by an increase in Cl$^-$
      5) Serum K$^+$ levels are also evaluated in connection with normal AG levels

      6) Decreased AG can be seen in clients with low albumin levels or in conditions where there is an increase in unmeasured cations (multiple myeloma, lithium toxicity, or nephrotic syndrome)

    d. Chloride levels are used to evaluate clients who are at risk for metabolic alkalosis

      1) Urinary levels <10 mEq/L are associated with chloride-responsive metabolic alkalosis (the more commonly occurring type that is usually seen with ECF volume depletion and renal and GI losses; bicarbonate retention occurs)

      2) Urinary levels >10 mEq/L are associated with chloride-resistant metabolic alkalosis (less common and is seen in clients with adrenal problems, hypertension, and Mg^{++} or K^+ depletion)

E. Identification of simple acid–base disturbances (refer again to Table 8-1)

  1. Interpret the pH

    a. Is the pH less than 7.35? This indicates acidosis

    b. Is the pH greater than 7.45? This indicates alkalosis

  2. Identify primary cause—respiratory or metabolic

    a. Examine the $PaCO_2$ and the HCO_3^- values

    b. If the $PaCO_2$ is abnormal, then the problem is respiratory

    c. If the HCO_3^- is abnormal, a metabolic problem exists

  3. Determine presence of compensation

    a. Determine if the $PaCO_2$ and HCO_3^- are decreased or increased as the body attempts to maintain the ratio of HCO_3^- to H_2CO_3 at 20:1

    b. Partial compensation exists when the pH remains abnormal but changes start to occur in the opposite system (example: the pH indicates an acidotic state but the HCO_3^- is increasing, indicating that the body is utilizing the buffer system to bring the pH back into line)

    c. Full or complete compensation occurs when the buffer system is working effectively and brings the pH back to a value of 7.35 to 7.45, although both the CO_2 and HCO_3^- values are abnormal

      1) If the ABG is fully compensated, in order to determine if it is acidotic or alkalotic, if the pH is normal but less than 7.40, it is considered acidotic

      2) Conversely, if the pH is normal but is greater than 7.40, it is considered alkalotic

II. RESPIRATORY ACIDOSIS

A. Overview

  1. Respiratory acidosis: a condition in which carbon dioxide is retained and the pH is decreased (see Table 8-2)

  2. It occurs in response to hypoventilation, which occurs with respiratory depression, inadequate chest expansion, airway obstruction, or interference with alveolar-capillary exchange

B. Clinical presentation

  1. Cardiovascular

    a. Hypotension

    b. Delayed cardiac conduction that can lead to heart block, peaked T waves, prolonged PR intervals, and widened QRS complexes

    c. Peripheral vasodilation with thready, weak pulse

    d. Tachycardia

    e. Warm, flushed skin related to the peripheral vasodilation as well as to impaired gas exchange

  2. Respiratory

    a. Dyspnea

    b. May have hypoventilation with hypoxia

Practice to Pass

How would the nurse determine if a client was in uncompensated respiratory acidosis?

Table 8-2 Respiratory Alterations in Acid–Base Balance

Clinical Picture	Acidosis	Alkalosis
pH	<7.35	>7.45
PaCO$_2$	>45	<35
HCO$_3^-$	Elevated with compensation	Decreased with compensation
Signs and Symptoms		
Cardiovascular	Hypotension, heart block, peaked T waves, prolonged PR interval, weak and thready pulse, tachycardia, warm and flushed skin	Increased myocardial irritability, increased heart rate, increased sensitivity to digitalis preparations
Respiratory	Rapid and shallow respiratory pattern	Dyspnea, chest tightness
CNS	Headache, seizures, altered mental status, papilledema, decreased LOC, drowsiness, coma	Dizziness, anxiety, panic, tetany, seizures, blurred vision
Causes	Chronic obstructive pulmonary disease, sedative or barbiturate overdose, chest wall abnormalities, pneumonia, atelectasis, respiratory muscle weakness, underventilation	Hyperventilation caused by hypoxia, fear, fever, pain, exercise, anxiety, pulmonary embolus Mechanical overventilation Stimulated respiratory centers caused by septicemia, encephalitis, brain injury, salicylate poisoning, hypokalemia
Compensation	Kidneys eliminate H$^+$ ions and retain HCO$_3^-$	Kidneys conserve H$^+$ ions and excrete HCO$_3^-$

Practice to Pass

Why is the nurse concerned about hyperkalemia in the client who has respiratory acidosis?

   3. Central nervous system (CNS)
      a. Headache
      b. Seizures
      c. Altered mental status, confusion
      d. Papilledema
      e. Muscle twitching
      f. Decreased level of consciousness
      g. Drowsiness that can progress to a coma
C. Diagnostic findings
   1. pH decreased below 7.35
   2. PaCO$_2$ elevated above 45 mm Hg
   3. Hyperkalemia
D. Compensation
   1. Increased rate and depth of respirations to blow off CO$_2$
   2. Kidneys eliminate H$^+$ ions and retain HCO$_3^-$ (urine pH less than 6)
   3. HCO$_3^-$ levels rise when the body is compensating for the acidosis
E. Priority nursing diagnoses
   1. Ineffective Breathing Pattern related to hypoventilation
   2. Impaired Gas Exchange related to alveolar hypoventilation
   3. Impaired Sensory Perception related to acid–base alterations
   4. Anxiety related to breathlessness
   5. Risk for Injury related to decreased level of consciousness
   6. Risk for Decreased Cardiac Output related to dysrhythmias
F. Therapeutic management
   1. Treatment is directed toward correcting the underlying cause and improving ventilation
   2. It is important to implement pulmonary hygiene measures to clear the respiratory tract of mucus and purulent drainage

3. Provide adequate fluid intake to liquefy secretions
4. If indicated, administer supplemental oxygen cautiously to a client with chronic respiratory acidosis; O_2 rather than CO_2 may stimulate respirations
   a. It is important to note that clients with chronic acidosis have compensated and are adjusted to living with higher $PaCO_2$ levels
   b. Remember the CO_2 level is the usual mechanism stimulating the respiratory drive
   c. Oxygen administration at higher levels can lead to a decreased ventilatory drive and can cause further hypoxia in a client with COPD
   d. Low flow oxygen is the expected treatment for clients with COPD
   e. Collaborate with physician and respiratory therapist in the management of clients with chronic respiratory disease
5. Mechanical ventilation may be required to improve respiratory status and to decrease the CO_2 gradually to prevent alkalosis and seizures from occurring

G. Planning and implementation
1. Assess respiratory rate, depth, and breath sounds; encourage coughing and deep breathing
2. Monitor the client for complications and response to therapy
3. Take apical pulse and assess for tachycardia and irregularities
4. Assess level of consciousness
5. Monitor ECG for dysrhythmias
6. Draw serum electrolytes, especially potassium and ABGs
7. Administer oxygen as indicated and ordered; suction as needed to clear respiratory tract of secretions that interfere with oxygenation
8. Administer medications as ordered
9. Provide good oral hygiene frequently
10. Keep side rails up, the bed at the lowest level, and the call bell within reach of the client
11. Maintain a calm, quiet environment
12. Assess color of skin, nail beds, and mucous membranes
13. If client is confused, orient frequently to person, place, and time
14. Place in semi-Fowler's to Fowler's position to facilitate maximum lung expansion
15. Provide adequate fluid intake
16. Encourage pursed-lip breathing to promote CO_2 elimination as appropriate
17. Encourage frequent position changes; out of bed as tolerated

H. Medication therapy
1. The type of drug and route of administration depend on the client's baseline condition and whether the disease is either acute or chronic with an acute exacerbation
2. Medications that could be used include the following:
   a. Bronchodilators to decrease bronchospasm
   b. Antibiotics to treat infections in the respiratory tract
   c. Respiratory agents to decrease viscosity of pulmonary secretions, such as acetylcysteine (Mucomyst)
   d. Anticoagulants and thrombolytics to prevent or treat pulmonary emboli
3. Medications are usually administered via IV in acute situations and then changed to PO as client's condition stabilizes
4. Respiratory therapists often administer medications as part of a treatment plan; they are often called on a PRN basis to assist client during acute episodes

I. Client education
1. Teach preventive measures to clients at risk
2. Teach deep breathing techniques
3. Teach signs and symptoms of infection to report to the health care provider
4. Report signs of infections, shortness of breath, fatigue, and increased pulse rate to the health care provider

J. Evaluation

1. ABGs return to as near normal as possible for the client
2. Anxiety level diminishes, leading to improved work of breathing with less effort
3. Client is oriented to person, place, and time
4. Client remains free of injury
5. No cardiac dysrhythmias occur
6. Level of consciousness improves
7. Respiratory pattern becomes deeper and rate decreases

III. RESPIRATORY ALKALOSIS

A. Overview

1. **Respiratory alkalosis**: a condition in which pH is elevated and $PaCO_2$ is decreased
2. Occurs with hyperventilation and leads to a decreased level of CO_2; sometimes called an H_2CO_3 deficit
3. Other causes can include:
   a. Respiratory center stimulation from fever, salicylate intoxication, and trauma to the CNS
   b. Infection
   c. Excessive mechanical ventilation
   d. Refer back to Table 8-2

B. Clinical presentation

1. Cardiovascular
   a. Increased myocardial irritability; palpitations
   b. Increased heart rate
   c. Increased sensitivity to digoxin
2. Respiratory
   a. Rapid, shallow breathing
   b. Chest tightness and palpitations
3. CNS
   a. Dizziness
   b. Lightheadedness
   c. Anxiety, panic
   d. Tetany
   e. Seizures
   f. Difficulty concentrating
   g. Blurred vision
   h. Numbness and tingling in extremities
   i. Hyperactive reflexes

C. Diagnostic findings

1. High pH (>7.45)
2. Low $PaCO_2$ (<35 mm Hg)
3. Hypokalemia
4. Hypocalcemia (as pH increases, calcium binding occurs in the serum and calcium level decreases; accounts for numbness and tingling)

D. Compensation

1. Kidneys conserve H^+ and excrete HCO_3^- (urine pH greater than 6)
2. Low HCO_3^- indicates the body is attempting to compensate

E. Priority nursing diagnoses

1. Impaired Sensory/Perception related to neurological deficits
2. Impaired Thought Processes related to altered cerebral functioning

Practice to Pass

Why would a client with uncontrolled type 1 diabetes develop metabolic acidosis, and how can this be prevented?

3. Ineffective Breathing Pattern related to hyperventilation
4. Risk for Injury related to weakness or seizures
5. Risk for Injury related to tetany
F. **Therapeutic management**
1. Treat the underlying cause
2. Have client rebreathe CO_2 by using a rebreather mask or a paper bag
3. Give oxygen therapy if the client is hypoxemic
4. Medicate as needed with anti-anxiety drugs
G. **Planning and implementation**
1. Assess respiratory rate, depth, breath sounds
2. Ensure a calm, quiet environment; provide support and reassurance
3. Treat fever if this is a possible cause
4. Monitor vital signs and ABGs
5. Assist client to breathe more slowly
6. If needed, provide client with rebreather mask or paper bag to breathe into
7. Protect from injury
8. Administer anti-anxiety, sedative, or analgesic medications as prescribed
9. Monitor response to therapy
H. **Medication therapy**
1. Sedatives or anti-anxiety agents may be used to control hyperventilation due to anxiety
2. Pain medications may be used to control pain as a contributing factor
I. **Client education**
1. Teach client relaxation techniques
2. Encourage client to attend stress management classes
3. Teach parents to keep aspirin and other salicylates out of reach of children and in an inaccessible area
J. **Evaluation**
1. Respiratory rate decreases
2. Numbness and tingling in extremities dissipates
3. ABGs return to normal
4. Anxiety diminishes
5. Client remains free from injury

IV. METABOLIC ACIDOSIS

A. **Overview**
1. **Metabolic acidosis**: an imbalance in which pH decreases and HCO_3 decreases
2. Occurs when acids other than carbonic acid accumulate in the ECF or when there is a loss of HCO_3^-
3. This condition rarely occurs spontaneously but rather is accompanied by other problems, such as GI conditions (starvation, malnutrition, and chronic diarrhea), renal (kidney failure), DKA, hyperthyroidism, trauma, shock, increased exercise, severe infection, and fever
B. **Clinical presentation**
1. Cardiovascular
   a. Hypotension
   b. Dysrhythmias and cardiac arrest
   c. Peripheral vasodilation
   d. Cold, clammy skin
2. Respiratory
   a. Deep, rapid pattern
   b. Kussmaul's respirations

3. CNS
   a. Drowsiness
   b. Coma
   c. Headache
    d. Confusion
   e. Lethargy
   f. Weakness
4. Gastrointestinal
   a. Nausea and vomiting
   b. Diarrhea
   c. Abdominal pain

C. Diagnostic findings
1. pH less than 7.35
2. HCO_3^- less than 22 mEq/L
3. Hyperkalemia frequently seen
4. ECG may show changes related to increased potassium levels
5. Anion gap calculation increases; base excess decreases
6. Increased lactate levels in sepsis/septic shock
7. Elevated ionized (free) calcium
8. Decreased magnesium levels

D. Compensation
1. Lungs eliminate CO_2; kidneys conserve HCO_3^-
2. Urine pH less than 6
3. $PaCO_2$ decreases when compensation is occurring

E. Priority nursing diagnoses
1. Decreased Cardiac Output secondary to dysrhythmias and/or fluid volume deficits
2. Risk for Impaired Sensory/Perception related to changes in neurological functioning secondary to acidosis
3. Risk for Injury related to confusion, weakness, and drowsiness
4. Risk for Deficient Fluid Volume related to excessive loss from the kidneys or gastro-intestinal system

F. Therapeutic management
1. Treatment is aimed at correcting the underlying problem
2. Provide hydration to restore water, nutrients, and electrolytes
3. Administration of alkalotic IV solution (sodium bicarbonate or sodium lactate) may be indicated to correct acidosis
4. Mechanical ventilation is used only if other treatment modalities are ineffective

G. Planning and implementation
1. Monitor ABGs
2. Monitor intake and output (I&O), assess for edema
3. Measure daily weights
4. Assess vital signs, especially respiration for rate and depth
5. Assess level of consciousness
6. Assess gastrointestinal function
7. Monitor ECG for conduction problems
8. Monitor serum electrolytes
9. Protect from injury
10. Administer medications and IV fluids as prescribed

H. Medication therapy: based on underlying cause
1. If cause is secondary to diabetic ketoacidosis, implement hydration with normal saline, regular insulin, and potassium

2. If diarrhea is the cause, treat with hydration and antidiarrheal agents
3. Administer $NaHCO_3$ cautiously and only when HCO_3^- levels are very low (below 16–18 mEq/L)
   a. Can cause metabolic alkalosis and hypokalemia
   b. The medication must be titrated closely so as to avoid further acid–base imbalances

I. Client education
1. Teach clients to seek health care if they have prolonged diarrhea
2. Teach diabetic clients the importance of preventing occurrences of DKA and how to manage DKA should it occur

J. Evaluation
1. Client remains free from injury
2. No dysrhythmias occur
3. ABGs return to normal
4. Fluid volume deficits are corrected
5. Level of consciousness returns to normal
6. Gastrointestinal upset is corrected

Practice to Pass

How would the nurse prevent the client from losing H^+ ions when nasogastric suctioning is being used?

V. METABOLIC ALKALOSIS

A. Overview
1. **Metabolic alkalosis**: a condition in which there is an increased pH and increased HCO_3^-
2. Occurs when there is a loss of H^+ ion (such as in vomiting or nasogastric suctioning) or an increase in the HCO_3^- level (such as with ingestion of bicarbonate-based antacids)
3. See Table 8-3

Table 8-3 Metabolic Alterations in Acid–Base Balance

Clinical Picture	Acidosis	Alkalosis
pH	<7.35	>7.45
$PaCO_2$	<35 with compensation	>45 with compensation
HCO_3^-	<22	>26
Signs and Symptoms		
Cardiovascular	Hypotension, dysrhythmias, peripheral vasodilation, cold, clammy skin	Tachycardia, dysrhythmias secondary to hypokalemia, hypotension, premature ventricular contractions, atrial tachycardia
Respiratory	Deep, rapid respiratory pattern (Kussmaul's respirations)	Hypoventilation, respiratory failure
CNS	Drowsiness, coma, headache, confusion, lethargy, weakness, nausea and vomiting, diarrhea, abdominal pain	Dizziness, irritability, nervousness, confusion, tremors, muscle cramps, tetany, hyperreflexia, paresthesias in fingers and toes, seizures
Causes	Diabetic ketoacidosis, lactic acidosis, starvation, severe diarrhea, renal tubule acidosis, renal failure, GI fistulas, shock	Severe vomiting, excessive NG suctioning, diuretic therapy, hypokalemia, licorice, excessive $NaHCO_3$ use, excessive mineralocorticoids
Compensation	Lungs eliminate CO_2; kidneys conserve HCO_3^-	Lungs retain CO_2; kidneys excrete HCO_3^-

B. Clinical presentation
  1. Cardiovascular
      a. Tachycardia
      b. Dysrhythmias
      c. Hypertension
      d. Atrial tachycardia
      e. Premature ventricular contractions
  2. Respiratory

      a. Hypoventilation
      b. Respiratory failure
  3. CNS
      a. Dizziness
      b. Irritability
      c. Nervousness
      d. Confusion
      e. Tremors
      f. Muscle cramps
      g. Hyperreflexia
      h. Tetany
      i. Paresthesias in fingers and toes
      j. Seizures
  4. Gastrointestinal
      a. Anorexia
      b. Nausea and vomiting
      c. Paralytic ileus if hypokalemia occurs

C. Diagnostic findings
  1. pH greater than 7.45
  2. HCO_3^- above 26 mEq/L
  3. Hypokalemia
  4. Hypocalcemia (as pH increases, calcium binding occurs and serum calcium levels decrease)
  5. Hyponatremia and hypochloremia
  6. Urine chloride levels reveal whether client is chloride responsive (<10 mEq/L) or chloride resistant (>10 mEq/L)
  7. Base excess increases

D. Compensation
  1. Lungs retain CO_2; kidneys conserve H^+ and excrete HCO_3^-
  2. $PaCO_2$ increases with compensation
  3. Urine pH greater than 6

E. Priority nursing diagnoses
  1. Deficient Fluid Volume related to excess gastrointestinal fluid loss
  2. Decreased Cardiac Output related to fluid volume deficit and altered cardiac conduction secondary to hypokalemia and alkalosis
  3. Deficient Knowledge related to appropriate use of potassium-wasting diuretics and antacids
  4. Risk for Impaired Gas Exchange related to hypoventilation
  5. Risk for Injury related to hypotension secondary to fluid volume deficit

F. Therapeutic management
  1. Treatment aimed at correcting underlying problem
  2. Provide sufficient chloride to enhance renal absorption of sodium and excretion of HCO_3^-
  3. Restore normal fluid balance

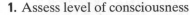

G. Planning and implementation
   1. Assess level of consciousness
   2. Assess vital signs, especially respiratory rate and depth, and oxygen saturation
   3. Administer medication and IV fluids as ordered
   4. Monitor I&O
   5. Monitor response to therapy
   6. Protect from injury
   7. Monitor ECG for conduction abnormalities
   8. Monitor ABGs and serum electrolytes
   9. Monitor skin color
   10. Position to allow for maximum lung expansion; semi-Fowler's to Fowler's position
   11. Plan to allow for rest periods between activities
   12. Administer oxygen as prescribed
   13. Obtain daily weight

Practice to Pass

Why does the client with metabolic alkalosis have cardiac conduction problems that must be monitored?

H. Medication therapy
   1. Normal saline-based IV fluid replacement
   2. Potassium supplementation if hypokalemic
   3. Histamine-2 receptor antagonists such as cimetidine (Tagamet) or ranitidine (Zantac) to reduce production of H^+ ions and loss of H^+ ions from gastrointestinal drainage
   4. If client is chloride responsive, then administer acetazolamide (Diamox) to increase renal bicarbonate excretion
   5. If client is chloride resistant, then correct K^+ and Mg^{++} deficits with appropriate supplementation

I. Client education
   1. Teach clients to take antacids correctly
   2. Teach signs and symptoms to report to health care provider for those at risk, especially the elderly
   3. Teach signs and symptoms of hypokalemia to report to health care provider

J. Evaluation
   1. Client remains free from injury
   2. ABGs return to normal
   3. Hypertension is corrected
   4. Electrolytes restored to normal
   5. Cardiac conduction abnormalities do not occur
   6. Client states ways to prevent problem from recurring

VI. MIXED ACID–BASE DISTURBANCES

A. Identification and treatment of primary disorder
   1. A **mixed acid–base disorder** occurs when two or more independent acid–base disorders occur at the same time
   2. The pH is dependent on the type and severity of each simple disorder
   3. Respiratory acidosis and alkalosis cannot occur concurrently; it is impossible to have hyperventilation and hypoventilation at the same time
   4. Treatment is aimed at correcting the underlying cause of each disorder
   5. When identifying acid–base imbalances, mathematical formulas can be used to assess degree of expected compensation
      a. The use of these equations is usually done on an intermediate level of acid–base balance
      b. However, it is important for the nurse to know that there are calculations that will identify the degree of compensatory changes
   6. Anion gap and urine pH values will also assist in determining which imbalance is occurring

B. Chronic and superimposed acid–base disturbances
  1. Mixed metabolic acidosis and respiratory acidosis
      a. Clients with acute pulmonary edema
      b. Clients with cardiac arrest as a result of buildup of lactic acidosis and CO_2 retention due to inadequate ventilation
      c. pH values decrease and are more pronounced because of decreasing HCO_3^- level coupled with increasing CO_2 level
  2. Mixed metabolic alkalosis and respiratory acidosis
      a. Seen in clients with chronic obstructive pulmonary disease (COPD) secondary to treatment with potassium-wasting diuretics, severe vomiting, or development of diarrhea
      b. Seen in clients with COPD who have a quick improvement in ventilation
      c. pH values tend to become balanced because of an increase in both HCO_3^- and PCO_2 values
  3. Mixed metabolic acidosis with respiratory alkalosis
      a. Seen in clients with a rapid correction of metabolic acidosis
      b. Seen in clients with salicylate intoxication
      c. Seen in clients with gram-negative septicemia
      d. pH values tend to become balanced because of decreases in both HCO_3^- and pCO_2
  4. Mixed metabolic alkalosis and respiratory alkalosis
      a. Seen in clients postoperatively with severe hemorrhage
      b. Seen in clients who have massive transfusions
      c. Seen in clients with excessive NG drainage
      d. pH values increase and are more pronounced because of an increase in HCO_3^- coupled with a decrease in CO_2 levels
  5. Mixed metabolic acidosis and metabolic alkalosis
      a. Seen in clients with gastroenteritis, vomiting, and diarrhea
      b. If imbalance is present in the same proportion, there is usually no change in values (pH, HCO_3^-, and pCO_2) even though there is hypovolemia
  6. Chronic and acute respiratory acidosis
      a. Clients with chronic respiratory conditions with an acute condition superimposed can lead to increased pCO_2 levels, causing further pulmonary dysfunction and leading to serious consequences that can compromise both treatment and expected response to treatment
      b. Clients who have both a chronic and a superimposed acute respiratory acid–base imbalance should be closely monitored by a pulmonologist
      c. Respiratory therapy should be part of the collaborative health care team during the management of this client

C. Diagnostic and laboratory findings
  1. For ABG interpretations when pH is abnormal pH, see Table 8-4
  2. Normal pH values
      a. Increased pCO_2 leads to respiratory acidosis with compensated metabolic alkalosis
      b. Decreased pCO_2 leads to respiratory alkalosis with compensated metabolic acidosis
  3. Changes in anion gap levels and bicarbonate levels
  4. Abnormal serum electrolyte levels can reflect changes in acid–base balance
  5. ECG results may show electrolyte disturbances
  6. CXR may show underlying cardiac or pulmonary disease
  7. Hemoglobin and hematocrit levels can indicate oxygen-carrying potential

D. Priority nursing diagnoses
  1. Decreased Cardiac Output related to dysrhythmias secondary to fluid volume or potassium alterations
  2. Impaired Sensory/Perception related to acid–base imbalance
  3. Risk for Injury related to neurological changes secondary to acid–base imbalances

Table 8-4		Abnormalities in Arterial Blood Gases
pH	**CO$_2$**	**Associated Acid–Base Imbalances**
↓	↑	Respiratory acidosis with incompletely compensating metabolic alkalosis Respiratory acidosis with coexisting metabolic acidosis
↓	↓	Metabolic acidosis with incompletely compensating respiratory alkalosis Metabolic acidosis with coexisting respiratory alkalosis
↑	↓	Respiratory alkalosis with incompletely compensating metabolic acidosis Respiratory alkalosis with coexisting metabolic alkalosis
↑	↑	Metabolic alkalosis with incompletely compensating respiratory acidosis Metabolic alkalosis with coexisting respiratory acidosis

E. Therapeutic management
1. Treatment focuses on correcting the underlying causes of the disorder
2. The mixed disorders must be treated before acid–base balance can be restored
3. A collaborative team approach (including a pulmonologist, respiratory therapist, nurses, and dietitian) is needed to assist client in restoring acid–base balance, increasing activity tolerance, and improving physiological function

F. Planning and implementation
1. Monitor vital signs
2. Monitor ABGs, pulmonary function tests, pulse oximetry, and CXR
3. Protect from injury
4. Monitor level of consciousness
5. Monitor ECG, H&H, and serum electrolytes
6. Ensure adequate fluid intake
7. Implement therapeutic measures as ordered

G. Medication therapy
1. Therapy is aimed at resolving the underlying causes of disorders
2. Administer oxygen per physician order and respiratory therapy guidelines
3. The presence of chronic disease will influence selection of medications

H. Client education
1. Clients with chronic respiratory conditions should report exacerbations to the health care provider
2. Clients who experience fluid losses through emesis or diarrhea are at increased risk for acid–base imbalance and should notify the health care provider if the condition is not self-limiting
3. Clients who are diabetic are at risk for acid–base imbalance due to alterations in glucose levels and should closely monitor serum glucose levels and use appropriate interventions to maintain normal levels
4. Clients who have renal problems are prone to develop acid–base imbalance due to alterations in electrolyte levels; closely monitor renal status to identify potential disturbances and allow for intervention

I. Evaluation
1. Client remains free from injury
2. Mixed disorder is treated quickly and effectively
3. ABGs return to normal
4. ECG conduction problems do not occur
5. Fluid volume is maintained
6. Electrolytes return to normal
7. Level of consciousness improves
8. Client reports ways to prevent problem from reoccurring

Case Study

A 69-year-old client with chronic obstructive pulmonary disease (COPD) is admitted with an acute respiratory infection. You are the nurse assigned to the care of this client.

1. What would this client's ABGs look like?

2. What will you do to help improve the client's respiratory status?

3. Why is a client with COPD given oxygen at a low flow rate?

4. Why is this client's $PaCO_2$ different than a client who does not have COPD?

5. What teaching does this client require in order to prevent development of metabolic alkalosis?

For suggested responses, see page 205.

POSTTEST

1 A client with COPD is admitted to the hospital with an exacerbation of the disease. Arterial blood gas (ABG) results are pH 7.30, $PaCO_2$ 51, and HCO_3^- 25. How would the nurse interpret these results?

1. Respiratory acidosis, uncompensated
2. Respiratory alkalosis partially compensated
3. Respiratory acidosis, compensated
4. Metabolic acidosis, compensated

2 A client admitted to the emergency department (ED) with chest injuries following a motor vehicle accident complains that it hurts to breathe. The client's respiratory rate is 12 and very shallow. The nurse would anticipate which results on arterial blood gases (ABGs)?

1. pH 7.42, $PaCO_2$ 41 mm Hg, HCO_3^- 23 mEq/L, SaO_2 96%
2. pH 7.31, $PaCO_2$ 49 mm Hg, HCO_3^- 24 mEq/L, SaO_2 87%
3. pH 7.49, $PaCO_2$ 34 mm Hg, HCO_3^- 30 mEq/L, SaO_2 89%
4. pH 7.38, $PaCO_2$ 38 mm Hg, HCO_3^- 22 mEq/L, SaO_2 90%

3 What action should the nurse take initially to avoid acid–base imbalance when a client becomes anxious and starts to hyperventilate?

1. Tell the client to stop breathing so fast because he may pass out.
2. Give the client a sedative to decrease anxiety and stop hyperventilation.
3. Give the client a paper bag to breathe into.
4. Notify the physician.

4 The nurse would closely monitor a client with renal failure for which of following primary acid–base imbalances?

1. Metabolic acidosis
2. Metabolic alkalosis
3. Respiratory acidosis
4. Respiratory alkalosis

5 A 36-year-old female is admitted with vomiting and dehydration after having the flu for three days. Arterial blood gas (ABG) results are pH 7.46, $PaCO_2$ 50, HCO_3^- 33, SaO_2 95%. What do these values indicate to the nurse?

1. Metabolic acidosis, uncompensated
2. Respiratory acidosis, compensated
3. Metabolic alkalosis, partially compensated
4. Metabolic alkalosis, uncompensated

6 A client in a full cardiac arrest is admitted to the emergency department (ED). Arterial blood gases (ABGs) indicate a respiratory acidosis. How does the nurse respond to correct this condition?

1. Administer $NaHCO_3$ to correct the acidosis.
2. Administer epinephrine to get a heart rate so the acidosis can be corrected.
3. Ventilate client to "blow off" excess CO_2.
4. Defibrillate the client.

7 The nurse identifies which of the following clients to be at risk for developing metabolic alkalosis? Select all that apply.

1. A client who has a nasogastric tube (NGT) to continuous suction
2. A client who has had diarrhea for two days
3. A client who is admitted with salicylate toxicity
4. A client who takes antacids frequently for heartburn
5. A client who is admitted with asthmatic bronchitis

8 The arterial blood gas (ABG) results of a 68-year-old client admitted with pneumonia are pH 7.46, $PaCO_2$ 30, HCO_3^- 19, SaO_2 72. How should the nurse interpret these results?

1. Respiratory acidosis, uncompensated
2. Respiratory alkalosis, partially compensated
3. Respiratory alkalosis, uncompensated
4. Metabolic alkalosis, partially compensated

9 A 71-year-old client develops hypertension, tachycardia, and increased respirations two days after surgery. Arterial blood gas (ABG) results are pH 7.29, $PaCO_2$ 52, HCO_3^- 24, SaO_2 95%. The nurse interprets that these results indicate which of the following?

1. Respiratory acidosis, uncompensated
2. Respiratory acidosis, partially compensated
3. Metabolic acidosis, uncompensated
4. Metabolic acidosis, partially compensated

10 A 57-year-old client is admitted with a diagnosis of acute myocardial infarction. Arterial blood gas (ABG) results are pH 7.36, $PaCO_2$ 29, HCO_3^- 20, SaO_2 100%. The nurse draws which conclusion about this client's status?

1. Well oxygenated with uncompensated respiratory alkalosis
2. Hypoxemic with compensated respiratory acidosis
3. Well oxygenated with compensated metabolic acidosis
4. Hypoxemic with compensated metabolic acidosis

➤ *See pages 169–170 for Answers and Rationales.*

ANSWERS & RATIONALES

Pretest

1 **Answer: 3, 4** **Rationale:** The respiratory acidosis in this client is secondary to retention of carbon dioxide. Cough and deep breathing exercises will stimulate expectoration of secretions, allowing for improved gas exchange. Fluids will help to liquefy secretions and do not need to be restricted to water. It would be helpful to ambulate the client, which will promote lung expansion and improve gas exchange. Medicating the client frequently with narcotics may decrease respiratory drive, but a nonnarcotic medication may enable the client to breathe deeply. Magnesium has no effect on acid–base. **Cognitive Level:** Applying **Client Need:** Reduction of Risk Potential **Integrated Process:** Nursing Process: Implementation **Content Area:** Adult Health **Strategy:** Recall causes of respiratory acidosis are related to retention of carbon

dioxide. Determine that coughing and deep breathing, ambulating, and fluids provide measures to best promote improved gas exchange in the lungs. **Reference:** LeMone, P., & Burke, K. (2008.). *Medical surgical nursing: Critical thinking in client care* (4th ed.). Upper Saddle River, NJ: Pearson/Prentice Hall, pp. 238–246.

2 **Answer: 1** **Rationale:** Symptoms of alkalosis include irritability, confusion, cyanosis, irregular pulse, slow respirations, and muscle twitching. These symptoms warrant discontinuing the medication and notifying the primary health care provider because the client may have received excessive sodium bicarbonate. After this action is initiated, the nurse should closely monitor the client. **Cognitive Level:** Analyzing **Client Need:** Pharmacological and Parenteral Therapies **Integrated Process:** Nursing Process: Implementation **Content Area:** Adult Health **Strategy:** The critical word is *initially*, indicating all or some of the options are correct, but one takes first priority. Recognize the client is experiencing metabolic alkalosis and the severity of this to choose the correct option. **Reference:** Adams, M., Josephson, D., & Holland, L. (2011). *Pharmacology for nurses: A pathophysiologic approach*. (3rd ed.). Upper Saddle River, NJ: Pearson/Prentice Hall, p. 663.

3 Answer: 2 Rationale: Apnea and hypoventilation result in rising carbon dioxide levels, which leads to acidosis. The ABG would likely reflect respiratory acidosis without compensation, as reflected by a pH of less than 7.35, an elevated $PaCO_2$, and an HCO_3^- that is within normal limits. **Cognitive Level:** Analyzing **Client Need:** Physiological Adaptation **Integrated Process:** Nursing Process: Assessment **Content Area:** Adult Health **Strategy:** Critical words are *apnea* and *acidosis*, indicating the cause will be respiratory in nature. Look for the ABG with a pH indicating acidosis to direct you to the correct option. **Reference:** LeMone, P., & Burke, K. (2008). *Medical surgical nursing: Critical thinking in client care* (4th ed.). Upper Saddle River, NJ: Pearson/Prentice Hall, pp. 237–242.

4 Answer: 2 Rationale: The kidneys respond more slowly to acid–base imbalances but are more effective than the lungs in restoring acid–base balance to the extracellular fluid. The primary response to acidosis is with lung compensation. **Cognitive Level:** Understanding **Client Need:** Physiological Adaptation **Integrated Process:** Communication and Documentation **Content Area:** Adult Health **Strategy:** Note some of the options are only partially correct. Recall the role of the kidney in maintaining acid–base balance to choose the correct option. **Reference:** LeMone, P., & Burke, K. (2008). *Medical surgical nursing: Critical thinking in client care* (4th ed.). Upper Saddle River, NJ: Pearson/Prentice Hall, pp. 237–240.

5 Answer: 2 Rationale: Diarrhea leads to loss of bicarbonate from the intestinal tract. This can cause metabolic acidosis. With metabolic acidosis, the pH is low and the HCO_3^- is also decreased. **Cognitive Level:** Analyzing **Client Need:** Physiological Adaptation **Integrated Process:** Nursing Process: Assessment **Content Area:** Adult Health **Strategy:** The critical word is *diarrhea*. Recall this leads to a loss of alkaline fluids, which will cause acidosis to direct you to the choice with a pH of greater than 7.45 and a low $PaCO_2$ level. **Reference:** LeMone, P., & Burke, K. (2008). *Medical surgical nursing: Critical thinking in client care* (4th ed.). Upper Saddle River, NJ: Pearson/Prentice Hall, pp. 238–240.

6 Answer: 2 Rationale: Clients who are extremely anxious tend to hyperventilate and have a rapid, shallow respiratory pattern. Cardiac rhythm and regulation are independent of respiratory function, and the rate may vary depending on the client's medical condition and/or treatment. A rapid, deep respiratory pattern is associated with further respiratory compromise. **Cognitive Level:** Applying **Client Need:** Physiological Adaptation **Integrated Process:** Nursing Process: Assessment

Content Area: Adult Health **Strategy:** Critical words are *anxious* and *agitated*. Visualize this client when considering options. Eliminate the options that are related to pulse and not breathing. Recall breathing patterns seen in anxious clients to choose the correct option. **Reference:** LeMone, P. & Burke, K. (2008). *Medical surgical nursing: Critical thinking in client care* (4th ed.). Upper Saddle River, NJ: Pearson/Prentice Hall, pp. 238–242.

7 Answer: 3 Rationale: An anxious client often hyperventilates, leading to loss of carbon dioxide and alkalosis. A pH of 7.50 indicates an alkalotic state. 7.45 is at the high end of the normal range for pH. A pH of 7.38 is normal. A pH of 7.20 is extremely acidotic and would be unexpected in a client who is anxious. **Cognitive Level:** Applying **Client Need:** Physiological Adaptation **Integrated Process:** Nursing Process: Assessment **Content Area:** Adult Health **Strategy:** The critical word is *anxious*. Recall anxiety will cause an increase in respiratory rate with loss of carbon dioxide, resulting in alkalosis. **Reference:** LeMone, P., & Burke, K. (2008). *Medical surgical nursing: Critical thinking in client care* (4th ed.). Upper Saddle River, NJ: Pearson/Prentice Hall, pp. 238–242.

8 Answer: 3 Rationale: A client with metabolic acidosis will have an increase in respiratory rate and depth in an attempt to compensate for the acidosis. Increases in heart rate, temperature, and urinary output are all metabolic responses that are not directly associated with maintaining acid–base balance. Initial compensation with metabolic acidosis will be via the lungs. **Cognitive Level:** Applying **Client Need:** Physiological Adaptation **Integrated Process:** Nursing Process: Assessment **Content Area:** Adult Health **Strategy:** Recall the respiratory system will try to compensate for acidosis by blowing off carbon dioxide and water to direct you to the correct option. **Reference:** LeMone, P., & Burke, K. (2008). *Medical surgical nursing: Critical thinking in client care* (4th ed.). Upper Saddle River, NJ: Pearson/Prentice Hall, pp. 125, 238–240.

9 Answer: 4 Rationale: Diabetic clients are more likely to develop metabolic acidosis, secondary to accumulation of ketones when fatty acids are broken down for energy. Metabolic alkalosis would not be expected. Respiratory alkalosis could occur in response to the client's metabolic acidosis, but the respiratory alkalosis is not the primary disturbance. The cause is metabolic in nature, not respiratory. **Cognitive Level:** Applying **Client Need:** Physiological Adaptation **Integrated Process:** Nursing Process: Assessment **Content Area:** Adult Health **Strategy:** Recognize this condition leads to ketoacidosis with retention of metabolic acids to direct you to the correct option. **Reference:** LeMone, P., & Burke, K. (2008). *Medical surgical nursing: Critical thinking in client care* (4th ed.). Upper Saddle River, NJ: Pearson/Prentice Hall, pp. 240, 1081.

10 Answer: 2 Rationale: The pulse oximeter does measure oxygen saturation. The pulse oximeter measures the amount of oxygen, not carbon dioxide, in the blood. The pulse oximeter does not replace the need to do ABGs, although it provides a good indication of the client's oxygenation status. The pulse oximeter does not measure the ventilator effort of the client. **Cognitive Level:** Applying **Client Need:** Physiological Adaptation **Integrated Process:** Nursing Process: Implementation **Content Area:** Adult Health **Strategy:** Critical words are *COPD* and *pulse oximeter*. Recall the function and purpose of the latter to choose the correct option. **Reference:** Kozier, B., Erb, G., Berman, A., & Snyder, S. (2008). *Fundamentals of nursing: Concepts, process, and practice* (8th ed.). Upper Saddle River, NJ: Pearson/Prentice Hall, p. 517.

Posttest

1 **Answer: 1** **Rationale:** A pH of 7.30 indicates acidosis. A $PaCO_2$ of 51 indicates a respiratory acidosis is occurring. Because the $PaCO_2$ is elevated with a normal HCO_3^-, an uncompensated respiratory acidosis is occurring. **Cognitive Level:** Analyzing **Client Need:** Reduction of Risk Potential **Integrated Process:** Nursing Process: Assessment **Content Area:** Adult Health **Strategy:** First determine that the pH indicates acidosis and then examine CO_2 to determine that the cause is respiratory. Because bicarbonate is normal with uncompensated acidosis, choose that option. **Reference:** LeMone, P., & Burke, K. (2008). *Medical surgical nursing: Critical thinking in client care* (4th ed.). Upper Saddle River, NJ: Pearson/Prentice Hall, pp. 237–239.

2 **Answer: 2** **Rationale:** A client with a chest injury is likely to hypoventilate (have a shallow respiratory pattern) as a result of pain due to associated trauma. It is unknown at this time whether there are any internal injuries that could affect the client's oxygen saturation. This type of respiratory pattern is associated with respiratory acidosis. The incorrect options represent normal values or metabolic alkalosis. **Cognitive Level:** Analyzing **Client Need:** Reduction of Risk Potential **Integrated Process:** Nursing Process: Assessment **Content Area:** Adult Health **Strategy:** Before looking at the options, recognize the client is at greatest risk for respiratory acidosis. Eliminate the options where the pH is normal or it reflects alkalosis. **Reference:** LeMone, P., & Burke, K. (2008). *Medical surgical nursing: Critical thinking in client care* (4th ed.). Upper Saddle River, NJ: Pearson/Prentice Hall, pp. 237–239.

3 **Answer: 3** **Rationale:** Giving the client a paper bag to breathe into helps to prevent the CO_2 from dropping lower as the client rebreathes the gas that has been exhaled into the bag. Just telling the client to stop breathing fast does nothing to assist the client and could make the client become more anxious and breathe even faster. A sedative may be indicated to help the client relax and slow down respirations, but this is not the best initial action. The physician may need to be notified if the client needs further assistance, but this is not the

best initial action for the nurse to take. **Cognitive Level:** Applying **Client Need:** Reduction of Risk Potential **Integrated Process:** Nursing Process: Implementation **Content Area:** Adult Health **Strategy:** Critical words are *initially* and *hyperventilate*. Recognize some of the options are partially correct, but choose the option that offers a readily available solution that can be tried before the other options may be needed. **Reference:** LeMone, P., & Burke, K. (2008). *Medical surgical nursing: Critical thinking in client care* (4th ed.). Upper Saddle River, NJ: Pearson/Prentice Hall, p. 239.

4 **Answer: 1** **Rationale:** Because the diseased kidneys are unable to reabsorb bicarbonate and excrete excess hydrogen ions, the client with renal failure develops metabolic acidosis. Metabolic alkalosis is the opposite problem of the one the client is experiencing. The client does have acidosis but it is not respiratory in nature. The client does not have respiratory alkalosis. **Cognitive Level:** Applying **Client Need:** Physiological Adaptation **Integrated Process:** Nursing Process: Assessment **Content Area:** Adult Health **Strategy:** Recall the kidneys' role in maintaining acid–base balance and recall the major imbalance that occurs as a result of renal failure. **Reference:** LeMone, P., & Burke, K. (2008). *Medical surgical nursing: Critical thinking in client care* (4th ed.). Upper Saddle River, NJ: Pearson/Prentice Hall, p. 238.

5 **Answer: 3** **Rationale:** The pH indicates alkalosis, and the HCO_3^- is elevated, indicating a metabolic basis. The $PaCO_2$ is slightly elevated, indicating that compensation is occurring. **Cognitive Level:** Analyzing **Client Need:** Physiological Adaptation **Integrated Process:** Nursing Process: Assessment **Content Area:** Adult Health **Strategy:** First determine that the pH reflects slight alkalosis. Note the increased bicarbonate level reflects that the cause is metabolic, and because the CO_2 is elevated, the pH is partially compensated. **Reference:** LeMone, P., & Burke, K. (2008). *Medical surgical nursing: Critical thinking in client care* (4th ed.). Upper Saddle River, NJ: Pearson/Prentice Hall, pp. 237–239.

6 **Answer: 3** **Rationale:** Because the cause of the acidosis is respiratory, the client needs to be ventilated in order to oxygenate the client and facilitate removal of the retained carbon dioxide. $NaHCO_3$ may need to be administered, but this is more helpful to correct metabolic acidosis, and the cause of the client's acidosis is respiratory. Epinephrine may need to be administered but the respiratory acidosis will need to be corrected through ventilation. Defibrillation may be needed depending on the client's cardiac rhythm, but this does not address the respiratory acidosis. **Cognitive Level:** Applying **Client Need:** Reduction of Risk Potential **Integrated Process:** Nursing Process: Implementation **Content Area:** Adult Health **Strategy:** The focus of the question is respiratory acidosis, so choose the option that directly assists in reversing this problem. **Reference:** LeMone, P., & Burke, K. (2008). *Medical surgical* *nursing: Critical thinking in client care* (4th ed.). Upper Saddle River, NJ: Pearson/Prentice Hall, pp. 238–240.

7 **Answer: 1, 4** **Rationale:** Loss of acidic contents via NG drainage can lead to alkalosis and intake of antacids, which are frequently alkaline substances. Diarrhea leads to a loss of alkalotic fluids, predisposing the client to acidosis. Salicylate toxicity results in acidosis. The client with asthmatic bronchitis retains carbon dioxide, leading to respiratory acidosis. **Cognitive Level:** Applying **Client Need:** Physiological Adaptation **Integrated Process:** Nursing Process: Diagnosis **Content Area:** Adult Health **Strategy:** Recall conditions that contribute to a loss of acidic body fluids and a gain of alkaline substances to direct you to the correct options. **Reference:** LeMone, P., & Burke, K. (2008). *Medical surgical nursing: Critical thinking in client care* (4th ed.). Upper Saddle River, NJ: Pearson/Prentice Hall, pp. 237–240.

8 **Answer: 2** **Rationale:** The slightly elevated pH (alkalosis), the low $PaCO_2$ (respiratory origin), and the low HCO_3^- indicate compensation is starting but is not yet fully complete, because the pH is still abnormal. In addition, SaO_2 level is decreased significantly, which is not consistent with aging alone. **Cognitive Level:** Analyzing **Client Need:** Physiological Adaptation **Integrated Process:** Nursing Process: Assessment **Content Area:** Adult Health **Strategy:** First determine that the pH is alkalotic. Then recognize the CO_2 is low to determine the cause is respiratory. Choose the option in which bicarbonate reflects some compensation. **Reference:** LeMone, P., & Burke, K. (2008). *Medical surgical nursing: Critical thinking in client care* (4th ed.). Upper Saddle River, NJ: Pearson/Prentice Hall, pp. 238–242.

9 **Answer: 1** **Rationale:** The pH is low (acidosis) and the $PaCO_2$ is high (respiratory origin). The HCO_3^- is normal, indicating that compensation has not occurred. The client is experiencing hyperventilation, but blood gases reveal a respiratory acidosis, probably because of prior hypoventilation. **Cognitive Level:** Analyzing **Client Need:** Physiological Adaptation **Integrated Process:** Nursing Process: Assessment **Content Area:** Adult Health **Strategy:** First determine that the pH indicates acidosis. Next analyze the CO_2 to determine that the cause is respiratory. **Reference:** LeMone, P., & Burke, K. (2008). *Medical surgical nursing: Critical thinking in client care* (4th ed.). Upper Saddle River, NJ: Pearson/Prentice Hall, pp. 238–242.

10 **Answer: 3** **Rationale:** The pH is normal (but is nearer to the acidotic end), while the $PaCO_2$ is low (compensation has occurred) and the HCO_3^- is low (indicating metabolic origin). The oxygen saturation of 100% indicates the blood is well oxygenated. Because the pH is within normal limits, it is more likely that there are mixed acid–base disorders occurring that are compensating each other. Because the $PaCO_2$ and HCO_3^- are low, metabolic acidosis is occurring with a respiratory alkalosis. **Cognitive Level:** Analyzing **Client Need:** Physiological Adaptation **Integrated Process:** Nursing Process: Assessment **Content Area:** Adult Health **Strategy:** This question requires you to identify ABG results and the quality of oxygenation. Because the oxygen level is 100%, eliminate options that are hypoxemic. Recognize the pH is within normal limits to choose a compensated condition. **Reference:** LeMone, P., & Burke, K. (2008). *Medical surgical nursing: Critical thinking in client care* (4th ed.). Upper Saddle River, NJ: Pearson/Prentice Hall, pp. 237–240.

References

Adams, M. P., Josephson, D. L., & Holland, L. N. (2011). *Pharmacology for nurses: A pathophysiologic approach* (3rd ed.). Upper Saddle River, NJ: Pearson Education.

Berman, A., & Snyder, S. (2012). *Kozier & Erb's fundamentals of nursing: Concepts, process, and practice* (9th ed.). Upper Saddle River, NJ: Pearson Education.

Dudek, S. (2009). *Nutrition essentials for nursing practice* (6th ed.). Philadelphia: Lippincott Williams & Wilkins.

Hockenberry, M. J., & Wilson, D. (2008). *Wong's essentials of pediatric nursing* (8th ed.). St. Louis, MO: Mosby, Elsevier.

Ignatavicius, D., & Workman, M. (2009). *Medical-surgical nursing: Critical thinking in collaborative care* (6th ed.). St. Louis, MO: Elsevier Saunders.

Kee, J. L. (2009). *Handbook of laboratory and diagnostic tests with nursing implications* (6th ed.). Upper Saddle River, NJ: Pearson Education.

LeMone, P., & Burke, K. (2011). *Medical-surgical nursing: Critical thinking in client care* (5th ed.). Upper Saddle River: NJ: Pearson Education.

London, M. L., Ladewig, P. W., Ball, J. W., Bindler, R. C., & Cowen, K. J. (2011). *Maternal & child nursing care* (3rd ed.). Upper Saddle River, NJ: Pearson Education.

Osborne, K. S., Wraa, C. E., & Watson, A. B., (2010). *Medical-surgical nursing. Preparation for practice.* Upper Saddle River, NJ: Pearson Education.

ANSWERS & RATIONALES

Replacement Therapies for Fluid and Electrolyte Imbalances

9

Chapter Outline

Fluid Therapies

Diagnostic and Laboratory Findings

Selection of Fluid and Electrolyte Therapies

Objectives

➤ Review concepts related to hydration therapy.
➤ Review assessment data and diagnostic testing used to evaluate fluid balance.
➤ Identify specific solutions used for the treatment of fluid imbalance.
➤ Identify priority nursing diagnoses for clients receiving fluid and electrolyte replacement therapy.
➤ Describe the therapeutic management of a client receiving fluid replacement therapy.
➤ Describe the nursing management of a client receiving fluid replacement therapy.

NCLEX-RN® Test Prep

Use the accompanying online resource, NursingReviewsandRationales, to test yourself with hundreds of NCLEX®-style practice questions.

Review at a Glance

ABO blood typing blood-typing system that identifies naturally occurring antigens and antibodies located on the membrane of red blood cells (RBCs); helps to identify the correct recipient and donor for administration of blood products

anaphylaxis a severe, potentially life-threatening allergic reaction accompanied by itching, urticaria, bronchospasm, laryngeal edema, hypotension, and vascular collapse

autologous transfusion represents donation of blood by an individual for use during perioperative period or for use as a salvage method during perioperative phase

colloid a high molecular weight substance that pulls fluids out of intracellular and interstitial spaces and expands intravascular volume

crystalloid a solution containing small molecules that can pass through a semipermeable membrane; may be hypotonic, isotonic, or hypertonic

fresh frozen plasma (FFP) a blood product removed from whole blood that contains all the coagulation factors and liquid plasma portion

granulocytes consist of basophils, eosinophils, and neutrophils (with platelets or platelet-poor) used to treat acquired neutropenia or severe infections unresponsive to conventional antibiotic therapy; infusion of these is currently not approved by the FDA but is undergoing clinical investigation

hemolytic transfusion reaction most serious and potentially life-threatening reaction usually stemming from administration of ABO or Rh-incompatible blood and resulting in chills, low back pain, hemoglobinuria, renal failure, and shock

homologous transfusion donation of blood for other clients or for own use (designated homologous transfusion); also called *allogenic transfusion*

human leukocyte antigen (HLA) alloimmunization process

by which an individual exposed to HLA antigens via nonleukocyte-depleted blood develops antibodies to those antigens that limit the effectiveness of future platelet transfusions

irradiated blood blood that is exposed to radiation to kill cells that might initiate transfusion graft vs. host disease (TGVHD) in an immunocompromised individual

leukocyte-depleted blood packed red blood cells and platelets that have been filtered to remove leukocytes to decrease incidence of transfusion-related febrile reactions, CMV transmission, and HLA alloimmunization

leukopheresis process by which leukocytes are extracted from withdrawn blood, which is then retransfused into donor

packed red blood cells (PRBCs) a blood product that provides the same number of RBCs as whole blood but with most plasma removed, leading to a solution with an increased hematocrit

transfusion graft vs. host disease (TGVHD) condition in which donor lymphocytes attack an immunocompromised individual, resulting in an erythematous (sunburn) rash, liver dysfunction, and pancytopenia

type and cross-match process by which recipient's blood is typed to determine ABO blood group and Rh factor and recipient's serum is mixed with donor RBCs to check for antibodies to donor's minor antigens

type and screen process whereby blood antigens and antibodies are determined but no blood product is physically held for client

PRETEST

1 A trauma victim admitted to the emergency department (ED) is hemorrhaging, in shock, and has lost a significant percentage of blood volume. Because there is no time to perform a cross-match, which actions should the nurse take immediately? Select all that apply.

1. Transfuse type AB, Rh-positive blood.
2. Transfuse albumin to expand the remaining plasma volume.
3. Transfuse type O, Rh-negative blood.
4. Transfuse platelets to restore adequate clotting ability.
5. Establish an intravenous line.

2 A client with gastrointestinal (GI) bleeding suddenly develops diaphoresis with a rapid and thready pulse, and the nurse finds it difficult to hear a blood pressure. Which intravenous (IV) fluid does the nurse anticipate the health care provider will order STAT?

1. Dextrose in water (D_5W)
2. 0.9% sodium chloride (normal saline)
3. 0.45% sodium chloride (½ normal saline)
4. Dextrose 5% in 0.45% sodium chloride ($D_5$1/2NS)

3 A client with pretransfusion hemoglobin and hematocrit values of 9 grams and 27%, respectively, received two units of packed red blood cells (PRBCs) on the evening shift. The nurse determines the transfusions were effective when repeat laboratory tests indicate which results?

1. 11 grams, 33%
2. 12 grams, 36%
3. 13 grams, 30%
4. 15 grams, 39%

4 In addition to monitoring for bleeding, which interventions should the nurse anticipate being ordered for a client who has accidentally taken too much warfarin (Coumadin)? Select all that apply.

1. Check prothrombin time (PT) or International Normalized Ratio (INR).
2. Check partial thromboplastin time (PTT) or activated PTT (aPTT).
3. Prepare to administer albumin.
4. Prepare to administer platelets.
5. Prepare to administer fresh frozen plasma.

5 The nurse is caring for a client experiencing severe abdominal ascites secondary to cirrhosis. The nurse determines an infusion of albumin has been effective when assessment findings indicate which of the following?

1. A decrease in abdominal girth
2. A decrease in blood pressure
3. An increase in pulse
4. An increase in weight

6 Which of the following changes in laboratory values would the nurse anticipate after administering isotonic intravenous fluids to a client experiencing hypertonic dehydration?

1. Increased serum osmolality, increased blood urea nitrogen (BUN), and decreased hematocrit (HCT)
2. Decreased serum osmolality, decreased BUN, and decreased HCT
3. Increased serum osmolality, increased BUN, and increased HCT
4. Decreased serum osmolality, decreased BUN, and increased HCT

7 A client with a history of congestive heart failure (CHF) has been carefully rehydrated with normal saline (0.9% sodium chloride) for isotonic dehydration related to overzealous diuresis. Which statement by the client indicates that the nurse's discharge teaching has been effective?

1. "I will increase my salt intake and double up on my fluid intake."
2. "I will take my diuretic pill every other day."
3. "I will weigh myself daily and notify the physician if I develop a fever or diarrhea."
4. "I will drink only one glass of water a day so I can eventually stop taking my pill."

8 A female client with type B, Rh-negative blood has been exposed to Rh-positive blood in the past. The nurse will evaluate that instruction regarding blood compatibility has been effective when the client verbalizes it is safe to receive which types of blood?

1. Type B positive and type O positive blood
2. Type B negative and type O negative blood
3. Type AB negative and type O negative blood
4. Type A positive and type O positive blood

9 A client in need of a blood transfusion is concerned about the possibility of disease transmission. Which of the following statements by the nurse may help to alleviate some anxiety for the client?

1. "All blood products are absolutely safe after testing, and there is no need to worry."
2. "If you do not want the transfusion, do not sign the consent. Perhaps the physician can give you some iron pills."
3. "More sophisticated screening tests have made the blood supply safer and the risk of infection, while it exists, is very low."
4. "Have a family member or friend donate blood for you because this will guarantee its safety."

10 Which of the following blood products does the nurse anticipate the physician will prescribe for a client diagnosed with hemophilia?

1. Whole blood
2. Packed red blood cells (PRBCs)
3. Fresh frozen plasma (FFP)
4. Albumin

➤ *See pages 193–194 for Answers and Rationales.*

I. FLUID THERAPIES

A. Crystalloids: solutions that contain small molecules and are able to pass through semipermeable membranes (flowing readily from the vascular to interstitial space and cells)

1. Isotonic solutions
   a. Have approximately the same concentration (osmolality) as that of the extracellular fluid (ECF), thereby remaining within the ECF space
   b. Are given to expand the ECF volume
   c. Have no net effect on cellular dynamics because of their osmolarity

   d. Examples: normal saline (NS or 0.9% NaCl), Lactated Ringer's (LR)
2. Hypotonic solutions
   a. Osmolality is lower than that of serum plasma
   b. Are given to reverse dehydration; provides hydration to cells
   c. With regard to cellular dynamics, cause cells to swell and possibly burst
   d. Fluid shifting occurs with administration as fluids shift out of blood vessels and into interstitial spaces, causing intravascular volume depletion
   e. Due to fluid-shifting effects, hypotonic fluids should be administered cautiously

   f. Examples: ½ NS (0.45% NaCl), dextrose 2.5% in water ($D_{2.5}W$), and dextrose 5% in water (D_5W); note that D_5W is considered hypotonic to the RBC after metabolism of dextrose occurs (is isotonic in IV bag)

3. Hypertonic solutions
   a. Osmolality is higher than that of serum plasma
   b. Are given to increase the ECF volume and decrease cellular swelling
   c. With regard to cellular dynamics, cause cells to shrink and contribute to ECF volume overload
   d. Should be administered cautiously due to fluid shifting and potential for vein irritation due to high osmolar concentration
   e. Examples: 5% dextrose in 0.9% NaCl (D_5NS), 10% dextrose in water ($D_{10}W$), and 3% NaCl; 5% dextrose in lactated Ringers (D_5LR)

B. **Colloids**: solutions containing high molecular weight proteins or starch that do not cross capillary semipermeable membrane and remain in intravascular space (pulling fluid out of intracellular and interstitial spaces) for several days, assuming client has an intact capillary membrane; although colloids contain no clotting factors, they can affect coagulation process—this fact must be considered in reference to certain treatment therapies

1. Albumin
   a. Major plasma protein available in two forms: 5% (isotonic—equivalent to 12.5 grams or 250 mL) and 25% (hypertonic—equivalent to 25 grams or 50 mL)
   b. Normal human serum albumin is derived from donor plasma and is heat treated for viral inactivation (free from hepatitis; no known risk for acquired immunodeficiency syndrome [AIDS])
   c. Changes in albumin concentration affect cellular dynamics
      1) Increased albumin concentration results in fluid moving back into the capillaries from the interstitial space
      2) Decreased albumin concentration results in fluid leaking through the capillary walls into the interstitial space (edema)
      3) Clients suffering from underlying medical/nutritional problems (malnutrition, cirrhosis, or nephritic syndrome) can have chronically low albumin levels
   d. Comparison with crystalloid solutions
      1) Remain in the vascular space longer than crystalloids
      2) More expensive than crystalloids
      3) May cause febrile reactions
      4) Because they remain in the intravascular space for a longer period of time, they are more likely to cause circulatory overload than crystalloid solutions
   e. Indications and contraindications
      1) Primary clinical use is as a volume expander when treating hypovolemic shock from trauma or surgery, which results in increased blood pressure and cardiac output
      2) Given as a volume expander in a client who needs whole blood while the cross-match is being done
      3) Used to support blood pressure during a hypotensive episode, create diuresis in fluid volume excess, and facilitate remobilization of fluid from third-space fluid shifts
      4) Also used to treat burns, trauma, acute liver failure, hypoproteinemia, and overzealous diuresis in clients with cirrhosis or nephrotic syndrome, and to prevent and treat cerebral edema
      5) Are contraindicated in severe anemia and avoided in clients who are dehydrated
      6) Are given cautiously to clients with cardiac and pulmonary problems or in clinical situations where there is increased capillary leakage (sepsis, trauma, or burns)
   f. Administration and nursing actions
      1) Use glass bottle with administration set and filter that requires vented tubing
      2) Should be used within a four-hour time frame, as there are no preservatives
      3) Requires dedicated line for infusion

Practice to Pass

The physician has prescribed 0.9% NaCl IV at 250 mL per hour for a newly admitted client in diabetic ketoacidosis. How will you evaluate the effectiveness of this IV therapy for this client?

Practice to Pass

The physician has just prescribed 25% albumin for a 75-year-old female client in hypovolemic shock. Detail your priority assessments, interventions, and expected outcomes for the client.

4) Dose and rate of infusion are based on client's blood volume and underlying condition; infuse as rapidly as tolerated in clients with hypovolemic shock to replace vascular volume; in a client with normal blood volume, infuse 5% albumin at 2–4 mL/minute and 25% albumin at 1 mL/minute

        5) Assess for urticaria, fever, and manifestations of fluid volume overload; monitor vital signs and breath sounds of all clients regardless of underlying condition and rate of administration

2. Dextran

    a. A glucose solution with colloidal activity similar to albumin that expands the plasma volume by pulling fluid from the interstitial to intravascular space, thereby promoting dehydration of tissues

    b. No risk of transfusion-related illnesses (not extracted from human plasma)

    c. Increased likelihood of hypersensitivity reactions during the first minutes of administration due to presence of polysaccharide-reacting antibody

    d. Available in two strengths

        1) Dextran 40—low molecular weight dextran (refer to Box 9-1 for specific drug information)

        2) Dextran 70—high molecular weight dextran (refer to Box 9-2 for specific drug information)

Box 9-1

Specific Information Related to Dextran 40

- Acts as a hypertonic colloidal solution that rapidly expands the plasma volume
- Stays in the vascular space for up to six hours, depending on renal clearance
- Appropriate for all types of shock states and acts as an adjunct to restore volume
- Parenteral infusion is given via dedicated line because it has a high incompatibility profile
- Will alter clotting factors because it has antiplatelet activity (decreases the adhesiveness of RBCs and improves peripheral blood flow)
- Can lead to false elevations in some laboratory tests and interfere with blood typing
- Used prophylactically during surgical procedures that present a high risk for clotting to prevent DVT and PE and can be used for pump priming in extracorporeal circulation
- Contraindicated in clients who have defined hypersensitivities, renal failure, cardiac failure, severe anemia, pregnancy, and clients receiving anticoagulant therapy
- Clients with chronic liver disease, severe dehydration, or at risk for developing renal or cardiac failure require cautious use and monitoring if therapy is indicated by the physician

---

Box 9-2

Specific Information Related to Dextran 70

- Has higher molecular weight that is broken down more slowly in the body
- Interferes with coagulation because it can prolong bleeding time, increase platelet adhesiveness, and increase blood viscosity
- Can lead to false elevations in some laboratory tests and interfere with blood typing
- Shows volume expansion within minutes with a duration of 20 hours
- Give parenteral infusion via a dedicated line because it has a high incompatibility profile
- Use in emergency situations to treat impending or existing hypovolemic or hemorrhagic shock as a result of burns, trauma, or surgery
- Contraindicated for clients who have severe coagulopathy, known sensitivity to dextran, and severe cardiac or renal failure

e. Alterations of diagnostic tests
   1) Can affect **type and cross-match** (process by which compatibility between donor and recipient blood is determined) due to presence of Rouleaux formation (RBCs stacked together in long chains)
   2) Can result in *false increases* in blood glucose, total protein, total bilirubin, and urine specific gravity
   3) Can increase liver enzymes, such as AST and ALT levels
   4) Can alter coagulation indices and increase bleeding times by inhibiting platelet aggregation

f. Administration and nursing actions
   1) Draw blood for type and cross-match (especially) and other labs as needed prior to beginning the dextran infusion if possible; at minimum, notify laboratory personnel that the client is receiving dextran
   2) Obtain baseline hematocrit prior to dextran infusion and maintain Hct >30% during course of therapy or notify physician of decreased volume
   3) Assess for signs and symptoms of **anaphylaxis** (tightness in chest, wheezing, bronchospasm, and urticaria)
   4) Dextran 1 (Promit) is usually given IV prior to infusion of dextran to prevent formation of immune complexes by site binding on the antibody
   5) Maintain hydration of client with supplemental IV fluids
   6) Observe for signs and symptoms of bleeding
   7) Monitor pertinent labs including Hct, serum chemistries, and serum protein levels on a frequent basis

3. Hetastarch (Hespan, Hextend)
   a. Synthetic colloid made from cornstarch and available in a 6% solution (approximates albumin and dextran in terms of colloidal activity) that is diluted in 500 mL of NS (Hespan), and a 6% solution that is diluted in 500 and 1,000 mL of an electrolyte-lactated solution (Hextend)
   b. Expands the plasma and is used in shock precipitated by hemorrhage, trauma, burns, and sepsis; will stay in the vascular space up to 36 hours, but the plasma volume expansion starts decreasing at about 24 hours; causes osmotic diuresis
   c. Hespan is also used in the process of **leukopheresis** (the process by which leukocytes are extracted from withdrawn blood) when **granulocytes** are being harvested from a donor in order to be transfused into a neutropenic client
   d. Alterations of diagnostic tests
      1) Will not interfere with blood typing or cross-matching but can dilute clotting factors; PT, PTT, and clotting times may be transiently prolonged
      2) Serum amylase will increase after Hespan administration (up to four times normal levels)
      3) Can increase serum bilirubin levels but total bilirubin levels usually remain normal
   e. Excretion is both renal and hepatic; do not administer to clients in renal failure with oliguria or anuria; use caution in clients with liver disease
   f. Use caution in clients with CHF or bleeding disorders; contraindicated in severe bleeding disorders
   g. Administration and nursing actions
      1) Use opened containers immediately; contains no preservatives
      2) Monitor every client receiving Hespan for signs of hypervolemia (increased blood pressure, dyspnea, and bounding pulse)
      3) Monitor for transient changes in PT and PTT; check serum amylase level prior to beginning the infusion

4) Assess for adequate tissue perfusion; expect an increased urine output as Hespan causes osmotic diuresis; the increased urine output is not an indicator of adequate blood volume

5) Be alert to signs and symptoms of anaphylaxis and intervene accordingly (stop infusion; provide oxygen; hydrate with NS; administer epinephrine, steroids; antihistamines as ordered; be prepared to intubate and maintain circulatory support)

6) Clients who are diabetic or who have acid–base imbalances due to increased lactate levels should not be given this medication because it can worsen the alkalosis (Hextend) or contribute to lactic acidosis

4. Plasma protein fraction (PPF)

   a. Major component is albumin with immunoglobulins and sodium; used to expand the intravascular volume

   b. Indicated for emergency treatment of hypovolemic shock, burns, and low protein states; functions as a blood-product volume expander

   c. Monitoring parameters include vital signs (hemodynamic—central venous pressure [CVP] if possible) and urine output during the first hour at a frequency of every 5 to 15 minutes

   d. Monitor clients closely for potential fluid volume overload, pulmonary edema, or heart failure

   e. Monitor serum protein, electrolytes, and hemoglobin and hematocrit during course of therapy

   f. Contraindicated in clients with CHF, history of bypass surgery, allergic reactions to albumin, and severe anemia

   g. Vial must be used within four hours of opening; incompatible with alcohol, amino acids, and protein hydrolysate

C. Blood and blood products

   1. **Packed red blood cells (PRBCs)**

      a. Prepared from whole blood with each unit approximately 250 mL (some plasma, leukocytes, and platelets from the whole blood are still present); usually takes six donors to make one unit of PRBCs

      b. Platelets and leukocytes are not viable but can cause problems for the recipient in that they contain human leukocyte antigens (HLAs); recipient can form antibodies against these antigens (HLA alloimmunization); this can create problems with future transfusions especially when receiving platelets

      c. Typically, PRBCs are **leukocyte depleted** (blood is filtered to remove leukocytes) to minimize the possibility that HLA alloimmunization will occur

      d. Contain the same red blood cell concentration as whole blood from which they are derived; advantage is the client receives the same increase in oxygen-carrying capacity without being exposed to risk of fluid volume overload as with whole blood

      e. Increase colloidal oncotic pressure; pull fluids from extravascular to intravascular space and increase plasma volume

      f. Identification methods used for transfusion therapy

         1) Recipient's blood must be typed to determine **ABO blood typing** and Rh factor to ensure that the client receives compatible blood

         2) Recipient must not have antibodies to donor's major antigens on the RBCs (refer to Table 9-1)

         3) Cross-matching: to detect presence of recipient antibodies to donor's minor antigens

            a) Recipient's serum is mixed with donor's RBCs; if antibodies to donor's antigens are present, agglutination will occur (no match)

Practice to Pass

A client receiving Hespan for hypovolemia related to hemorrhage becomes very pale and diaphoretic, complains of chest tightness, and begins wheezing. Physical examination reveals hives covering the client's chest. What nursing actions should be taken immediately?

Table 9-1	ABO Compatibility System and Safe Transfusion	
Client Blood Type (Recipient)	Donor Blood That Can Be Safely Administered	Rationale
Type A	Type A	Client has no anti-A antibodies.
	Type O	*Universal donor.* Donor has no antigens to which the recipient can react.
Type B	Type B	Client has no anti-B antibodies.
	Type O	*Universal donor.* Donor has no antigens to which the recipient can react.
Type AB	Type A, B, or AB	*Universal recipient.* Client has no anti-A or anti-B antibodies.
	Type O	*Universal donor.* Donor has no antigens to which the recipient can react.
Type O	Type O	*Universal donor.* Donor has no antigens to which the recipient can react.

Note: Rh status must also be determined as part of the blood-typing procedure. Rh-positive clients can receive Rh-positive and Rh-negative blood. Rh-negative clients can only receive Rh-negative blood.

  b) If no antibodies to the donor's RBCs are present, agglutination will not occur (desired)

  c) Takes approximately 20 minutes to perform; type and cross-match is good for 48 hours only; must be repeated if time expires and the client needs blood; blood is physically held for a specific client

 4) A **type and screen** can be used to identify blood type, surface antigens, and Rh factor but blood is not physically held; is useful in nonemergency situations when it is expected that blood will have to be administered

 5) In an emergency situation, type O negative blood (universal donor) can be administered to a client, foregoing the type and cross-matching procedure

 6) May transmit viruses; additional tests for donated blood: hepatitis A, B, C, HIV, syphilis, ALT level (increased may be suspicious for hepatitis)

g. Specific treatments related to blood processing

 1) Irradiated blood: blood is treated with radiation that kills donor cells that could attack an immunocompromised client (bone marrow transplant recipients, clients with Hodgkin's disease, leukemia, intrauterine neonatal transfusion, or in clients being aggressively treated with chemotherapy)

  a) Goal is to prevent the transmission of **transfusion graft vs. host disease (TGVHD)**—donor lymphocytes attack recipient, cause liver dysfunction and bone marrow suppression, and can be fatal

  b) Leukocyte-depleted blood (Leukopor) will not prevent TGVH disease

 2) Cytomegalovirus (CMV) negative blood: for immunocompromised clients including AIDS clients; CMV remains in a latent state in donor's leukocytes if previously infected with the virus; transfer of the leukocytes to immunocompromised recipients could cause severe illness; leukodepletion may eliminate CMV

h. One unit of PRBCs should raise hemoglobin one gram and hematocrit by 3% (assuming there is no ongoing blood loss if bleeding was either a cause or a contributing factor)

i. Are expensive as compared to other colloids and crystalloids (collecting, testing, and screening blood and all the special processing contribute heavily to the expense)

j. Indications

 1) To improve oxygen-carrying capacity in clients with symptomatic anemia

2) To restore blood loss caused by hemorrhage (gastrointestinal or trauma related) or surgical blood loss

k. Transfusion options

1) Autologous transfusion (to self) may be planned prior to surgical procedure (preoperative donation) or blood may also be collected and reinfused during or after surgery (perioperative, intraoperative, or postoperative blood salvage)

2) Homologous transfusion (or allogenic) represents blood collected from clients for use for other clients (volunteer), or for themselves (designated)

3) The blood collected for homologous transfusion undergoes testing for antibodies, pathologic organisms (HIV, CMV, hepatitis variants, HTLV, and syphilis)

4) Minimum standards are set by the American Association of Blood Banks (AABB) regarding criteria for donor requirements, citing age, baseline hemoglobin and hematocrit, vital signs, weight, no evidence of transmittable disease or drug use, and frequency of blood donation

l. Administration (refer to Box 9-3)

1) Pretransfusion: verify order and follow hospital policy and procedure with regard to all transfusion therapy; ensure that client has received informed consent and has signed consent form

2) Start an IV if one not already in place; use an 18- to 20-gauge angiocath, which is preferred

3) Note that if the client is elderly with small fragile veins, a 22- to 24-gauge angiocath may be used without an infusion pump (force created by pump through a small gauge catheter may cause cells to lyse); blood will infuse more slowly but RBCs will remain intact; blood bank may be able to split the unit into two bags (one bag can infuse while the other remains properly refrigerated in the blood bank); check hospital policy for managing elderly client with fragile veins

4) Administer blood with normal saline only to prevent cell lysis; obtain 500 mL of NS and Y tubing and prime Y tubing that contains blood filter; additional filters may be required, such as Pall filter, depending on blood product used and/or general health condition of client; may connect to client and run at KVO (to keep vein open) rate if blood will arrive soon

5) Once blood bank indicates that blood is ready, premedicate client if ordered; common premedications are diphenhydramine (Benadryl), acetaminophen (Tylenol), and occasionally a corticosteroid or H_2 receptor blocker; premedication may be indicated to minimize allergic potential and symptoms; furosemide (Lasix) can be given either as premedication or between units to minimize risk of potential fluid volume overload

Box 9-3 **Principles of Transfusion Therapy**	• Obtain informed consent for transfusion therapy. • Ensure patent IV access prior to retrieving blood from the blood bank using appropriate tubing with NS as the priming solution. • Follow hospital policy and procedure regarding blood typing, acquisition of unit from blood bank, and verification of orders with two registered nurses. • Identify client at the bedside confirming client name and identification (ID) number, blood bank identification band (if used), unit number, blood type, and expiration date. • Remain at client's bedside during the first 15 minutes of transfusion therapy and monitor vital signs per protocol. • Obtain follow-up blood work to determine response to transfusion therapy.

6) Obtain blood from blood bank following hospital procedure and record baseline vital signs

7) Two RNs must verify identification of pertinent blood unit information (type, Rh factor, unit number, expiration date, matching with client's blood identification bracelet and original physician order); RNs must also identify client using two unique identifiers (such as stating name and date of birth)

8) Prior to hanging any blood product, inspect for discoloration and/or bubbling that could indicate bacterial contamination; if there is any suspicion, then return blood unit to blood bank

9) In preparation for blood administration, don gloves and hang blood, keeping the spike and blood bag opening sterile, prime filter and tubing with blood; make sure that filter is completely filled with blood; may use pump for administration of blood if hospital policy permits

10) Remain with the client for the first 15 minutes of therapy and monitor vital signs as per policy (refer to Box 9-4)

11) If client will receive another unit of blood, check to see if physician has ordered a diuretic in between units if client is at risk for fluid volume overload

12) Lab work (hemoglobin and hematocrit) should be ordered two hours post-transfusion in order to assess client's response to therapy

m. Clients who undergo multiple transfusions are at risk for developing additional electrolyte problems; these may include hyperkalemia or increased ammonia levels (because of cellular release from stored blood products) and hypocalcemia (because of chelation of calcium with citrate anticoagulant used as a blood preservative)

n. Clients may still experience a transfusion reaction, regardless of all the precautions that are used to prevent such an occurrence (refer to Box 9-5)

2. Platelets

a. Require ABO typing only but Rh matching preferred; if no ABO-compatible platelets are available, mismatched platelets may be given, which can lead to

---

Box 9-4	
Timing Issues Relevant to Transfusion Therapy	• Transfusion should be started within 30 minutes of the time that the unit is checked out of the blood bank. • Remain with the client during the first 15 minutes of the transfusion and monitor accordingly for signs and symptoms of possible transfusion reaction. • Stop blood if any signs or symptoms of a transfusion reaction occur and notify the physician. • Run each unit over two hours unless otherwise ordered by the physician. • Blood cannot hang more than four hours at room temperature because this can lead to cellular breakdown of the blood product.

Box 9-5	
Transfusion Reaction Principles	• Stop blood immediately if you suspect client is exhibiting a significant reaction. • Monitor client's vital signs, keep IV access with NS (switch tubing), and insert indwelling urinary catheter if needed. • Give old tubing and remaining blood product to lab for investigation. • Notify physician and lab for follow-up blood draws and report client's condition. • Keep client warm and provide supplemental oxygen at low flow rates. • Medicate as ordered following hospital policy and procedure and emerging physician orders.

potential allergic reactions; HLA-matched platelets are recommended to decrease the likelihood of allergic reactions

b. Can be random donor (pooled platelets from 6 to 10 donors) or single donor

c. Are stored at room temperature for up to five days with frequent gentle agitation of bag to keep platelets viable; half-life of platelets is three to four days; platelet transfusion may be repeated every one to three days

d. If platelet count <20,000/mm^3 and client is experiencing major bleeding, platelets may be needed; 1 platelet concentrate (1 unit) should increase recipient platelet count by approximately 5000 to 10,000/mm^3; usual dose is 6 to 10 units of concentrate

e. Clients receiving platelets over a long period of time develop antibodies to the HLA antigens found on the surface of the circulating platelets (causing antigen–antibody reaction, febrile reaction, and platelet destruction); over time, the client's platelet count is less responsive to platelet transfusions because alloimmunization is occurring; in response to the platelet administration, the count would show little or no rise after transfusion; actions to decrease likelihood of reaction include the following:

1) Use single-donor platelet transfusions from the onset of therapy

2) Use WBC filters to minimize infusion of WBCs because this will help to decrease antibody production

3) Try to find HLA-matched donor platelets for the recipient

4) Premedicate with diphenhydramine (Benadryl), acetaminophen (Tylenol), or hydrocortisone (Cortef) to decrease possibility of a reaction

5) Fever, infection, and active bleeding can modify the effectiveness of the transfusion

f. Indications

1) Thrombocytopenia resulting from decreased platelet production (aplastic anemia, leukemia), increased platelet loss (bleeding), increased platelet destruction (hypersplenism in cirrhosis, transfusion reaction), and increased use or consumption as in disseminated intravascular coagulopathy (DIC)

2) Clients undergoing needed surgery with a platelet count less than 100,0000/mm^3 or experiencing platelet dysfunction and/or coexisting coagulation disorders

g. Contraindications

1) Not indicated for idiopathic thrombocytopenic purpura (ITP) unless client is actively bleeding because administered platelets will also be destroyed

2) Avoid administering platelets when client is febrile

h. Administration and nursing actions

1) Premedicate as ordered, especially if client has a history of platelet transfusion reaction

2) Obtain IV access with 20- to 22-gauge angiocath, Y tubing, and NS to prime tubing

3) Begin platelet transfusion slowly and observe for signs of a reaction; adjust rate to 1–2 mL/minute and infuse each unit over 5 to 10 minutes as tolerated (platelets tend to clump, which is why they should be infused quickly)

4) A poor 15-minute platelet count means HLA antibodies are present, indicating the need to use HLA-matched platelets; if there is a good 15-minute count but poor 24-hour count, this suggests consumption (fever, sepsis), but the client does not need HLA-matched platelets

5) Administer single-donor platelets if at all possible for all clients; if client will receive multiple transfusions, use single-donor platelets and use a leukodepletion filter (some platelets may be prepared as leukodepleted; check the bag label); if the client will receive aggressive chemotherapy or a transplant, check

Practice to Pass

A client being aggressively treated with chemotherapy for acute leukemia will receive two units of irradiated CMV-negative PRBCs. The client wants to know why the blood needs special treatment. What will you tell this client?

for anti-HLA antibodies first so that blood product administration can be carefully planned

3. Whole blood
   a. One unit of donated whole blood can be broken down into one unit of packed cells, one unit of platelets, and one unit of fresh frozen plasma to replace whichever component(s) the client may need
   b. Not routinely used; indicated for treatment of acute massive hemorrhage and loss of >25–30% of blood volume; may also be used with cardiac surgeries, trauma situations, or major burns
   c. Must be ABO and Rh compatible
   d. Increases colloidal oncotic pressure and plasma volume, increases red cell mass, and improves tissue oxygenation; however, it can result in fluid volume overload
   e. Should not be administered to clients with chronic anemia who only need RBCs and should have a normal blood volume
   f. Stored whole blood is high in potassium
   g. Administration and nursing actions
      1) One unit equals approximately 500 mL; use an 18- to 20-gauge angiocath and Y tubing; use only NS as primer; infuse over two to four hours
      2) Observe for signs and symptoms of a transfusion reaction, such as **hemolytic transfusion reaction** (refer to Table 9-2), fluid volume overload, hypothermia, electrolyte disturbances, citrate toxicity (citrate is a preservative used in blood), and infection
      3) Expect a one-gram increase in hemoglobin and a 3–4% rise in hematocrit for each unit of whole blood infused, assuming no further bleeding

4. **Fresh frozen plasma (FFP)**
   a. Derived from one unit of donated whole blood whereby plasma is separated from the RBCs and then frozen; contains clotting factors and fibrinogen, but no platelets; volume of each unit is approximately 225 mL
   b. Must know the client's ABO group to ensure client's RBCs are compatible with antibodies that may be present in the plasma; group AB FFP may be administered if client's blood type is unknown; Rh matching (although not required) is preferred
   c. Increases colloidal oncotic pressure and moves fluid into the vascular space
   d. May cause fluid volume overload, hypersensitivity reaction, or hemolytic reactions
   e. Indications
      1) Replaces plasma volume in hemorrhage and/or hypovolemic shock
      2) Replaces plasma proteins lost from burn injuries
      3) Replaces clotting factors for client with a known (specific clotting factor may not be available) or unknown deficiency
      4) Indicated for the following clinical conditions: liver disease with significantly impaired clotting factor synthesis, DIC with active bleeding, prolonged PT/INR with active bleeding or when immediate surgery is needed, and dilutional coagulopathy (substantial volume overload)

Table 9-2	**Transfusion Reactions**			
Type	**Etiology**	**Clinical Presentation**	**Nursing Actions**	**Prevention**
Hemolytic	ABO or Rh incompatibility. Most severe and potentially life-threatening, but accounts for a very small percentage. Severe antigen–antibody reaction due to clumping of cells.	Chills, low back pain, headache, chest pain, tachycardia, dyspnea, hypotension, nausea, vomiting, restlessness, anxiety, shock, flank pain, and oliguria. Symptoms occur during first 30 minutes of infusion or in response to 100–200 mL of incompatible blood.	*Stop transfusion immediately.* Keep IV line open with NS and new tubing. Follow ABCs. Notify appropriate personnel (blood bank, physician, and lab). Follow hospital protocol. Medicate per protocol.	Follow established protocol. Verify orders. Monitor client during therapy.
Blood Contamination (Bacterial)	Organisms that survive the cold such as *pseudomonas or staphylococcus.*	Sudden chills, fever, dry flushed skin, headache, abdominal pain, lumbar pain, nausea, vomiting, diarrhea, hypotension, and/or signs of renal failure.	*Stop transfusion immediately.* Keep IV line open with NS and new tubing. Follow ABCs. Notify appropriate personnel (blood bank, physician, and lab). Follow hospital protocol. Medicate per protocol.	Change administration set and filter per protocol (per unit). Infuse unit over prescribed time period. Do not run blood unit >4 hours. Maintain sterile technique.
Febrile (Nonhemolytic)	Most common transfusion reaction. Sensitizations to HLA antibodies or plasma occur.	Mild reaction-chills and fever. Severe reaction—high fever, chills, headache, tightness in chest, palpitations, tachycardia, facial flushing, or flank pain. Symptoms can occur within 30 minutes but may start as late as 1–2 hours post transfusion.	Physician may note parameters to run blood even if the client presents with slight temperature elevation. Validate order prior to hanging to be aware of parameters. With a severe reaction, *stop the transfusion* and proceed with hospital protocol for a hemolytic reaction.	Keep client warm. For clients with prior history of this reaction, premedicate with acetaminophen (Tylenol), or diphenhydramine (Benadryl), administer leukocyte-poor blood products, HLA-compatible products, or washed RBCs.
Allergic	Sensitivity reaction, antigen-antibody reaction to plasma proteins. IgE molecules on mast cells react to form histamine release.	Mild reaction involves urticaria and hives. Severe reaction involves chills, fever, facial and airway swelling, SOB, wheezing, loss of consciousness, shock, or possible cardiac arrest.	Mild reaction—follow hospital policy and procedure, slow down transfusion, notify the physician, medicate as ordered. Severe reaction—*stop transfusion.* Follow hospital policy and protocol. Medicate as ordered. With critical situations, client may need to be intubated and managed by in-house physician.	Premedication for clients who have history of allergic reactions or multiple transfusions. Washed RBCs, leukocyte-depleted products, and additional filters may be needed on a routine basis for transfusion therapy.

Note: It is critical to follow agency policy and procedure for ALL transfusion therapies. Many reactions can be prevented or minimized if correct administration techniques are used and client is promptly assessed and monitored. Remain at the client's bedside during the first 15 minutes of any transfusion therapy. Have all necessary equipment readily available should the client experience a reaction (additional tubing and oxygen setup).

f. Administration and nursing actions

      1) Use as soon as possible after it is thawed or within six hours (takes about 30 minutes to thaw)

      2) Use a 20- to 22-gauge angiocath, NS not required (no RBCs present)

      3) Administer as rapidly as possible, suggested rate is 4 to 10 mL/minute; most units are completed in one to two hours

      4) Observe for signs and symptoms of allergic or febrile reaction and fluid volume overload; there is also a risk for hepatitis transmission

      5) Clients receiving large amounts of FFP may become hypocalcemic due to citric acid binding with calcium in the plasma; observe for signs and symptoms of hypocalcemia; may need calcium gluconate intravenously

5. Cryoprecipitate

    a. Derived from one unit of FFP and contains Factor VIII (antihemophilia factor), Factor XIII (Von Willebrand factor), and Factor IX (fibrinogen)

    b. ABO compatibility testing is not required; however, may cause ABO incompatibility; donor plasma and recipient RBCs should be ABO compatible (because some donor plasma is present and plasma contains the antibodies); if client's (recipient) blood group is unknown, type AB cryoprecipitate is preferred; Rh matching is not required (Rh factor is on the RBC and RBCs are not being transfused)

    c. Used to treat hemophilia A, Von Willebrand disease, hypofibrinogenemia, DIC (will quickly raise fibrinogen level), and massive transfusion with hemodilution; used in uremic clients to control bleeding

    d. Possibility of hepatitis or HIV transmission exists

    e. Administration and nursing actions

      1) Use within six hours once thawed; usual dose is 6 to 10 units

      2) Use 20- to 22-gauge angiocath and standard blood filter

      3) Administer as rapidly as tolerated (10 mL/min)

6. Granulocytes

    a. Harvested by leukopheresis from a single donor; must be transfused within 24 hours after obtaining from donor

    b. Each unit consists of granulocytes, lymphocytes, platelets, and RBCs in plasma

    c. Donor must be ABO and Rh compatible (RBCs present in unit); it is preferable to be HLA compatible as well

    d. Granulocytes are not FDA approved at the current time and are being used in clinical research trials to support febrile neutropenic clients who are not responding to other methods (antibiotic therapy or neupogen injections) to improve white blood cell (WBC) count

    e. Infusion can cause fever, allergic reaction, severe chills, mild hypertension, disorientation, and hallucinations; premedicate with diphenhydramine (Benadryl), steroids, and antipyretics as prescribed

    f. Use an 18- to 20-gauge angiocath and Y tubing with standard inline filter; no microaggregate filter is used because it would trap the WBCs; administer slowly, generally 50 mL/hour within four hours

    g. Treat chills with antipyretics or blankets; treat hypertension if needed; only discontinue transfusion if client has severe respiratory distress

    h. Generally one unit per day is transfused for at least four to five days or until infection resolves

Practice to Pass

A client with disseminated intravascular coagulopathy (DIC) is receiving platelets, fresh frozen plasma, and packed red blood cells. What laboratory results will you review in evaluating the effectiveness of the transfusions? How does the disease process complicate the clinical picture?

Practice to Pass

A neutropenic client undergoing aggressive chemotherapy is febrile with positive blood cultures. The physician orders granulocytes for this client. How would you safely administer this product to the client?

II. DIAGNOSTIC AND LABORATORY FINDINGS

A. Serum or plasma osmolality (275–295 mOsm/kg)

1. Hydration status affects serum/plasma osmolality, and specific parenteral therapies can affect osmolality due to nature of solution (tonicity of fluid) and crystalloid or colloid status

2. Increases are seen in dehydration, hyperglycemia, and in conditions where BUN is also increased; decreases are seen in clinical states resulting in overhydration

3. Allows nurse to assess client's baseline hydration status and evaluate response to replacement therapy

B. Serum chemistries

1. Blood urea nitrogen (BUN) (8–22 mg/dL) and creatinine (0.8–1.6 mg/dL) are indicators of renal function; BUN is also affected by hydration status

    a. Increased levels seen in dehydration (BUN only), renal disease, and gastrointestinal bleeding, due to retention of urea; decreased levels are seen in clinical states that result in overhydration

    b. Creatinine is a more accurate indicator of renal function than BUN because it is a constant metabolic end product of muscle metabolism and reflects glomerular filtration rate; increased levels reflect renal dysfunction

    c. Creatinine is generally unaffected by fluid intake; however, marked fluid volume deficit can decrease glomerular filtration and slightly increase the creatinine level

    d. Adequate renal function needs to be determined before fluid and electrolyte replacement begins (except in the case of a fluid challenge to check the kidneys' responsiveness); abnormal renal function can put the client at risk for fluid volume overload and electrolyte disturbances

2. Electrolytes

    a. Sodium (Na^+) and chloride (Cl^-) concentration should be considered in replacement therapies because they are part of the content of many crystalloid fluids; specific parenteral solutions (hypotonic or hypertonic) can result in fluid shifting and impact serum and urinary levels; see Chapters 2 and 6

    b. Potassium (K^+) is usually considered in replacement therapies as an additive being used to restore normal serum levels; it is important to know the client's baseline, trend pertinent laboratory values, and administer replacement according to protocol; see Chapter 3

    c. Critical laboratory values exist for both hypokalemic and hyperkalemic states with resultant effects on the cardiac system

    d. Acid–base imbalances can arise from alterations in potassium and chloride levels, and the client should be properly monitored using serial arterial blood gases (ABGs); see Chapter 8

    e. Calcium levels can be affected by replacement therapies, such as multiple blood unit administration (citrate anticoagulant resulting in hypocalcemia), that require calcium administration; correlate calcium levels with serum albumin levels because binding occurs that could affect the results

    f. Specific therapies such as diuretic administration, prolonged infusion of hypotonic fluids, dehydration states (malnutrition), overhydration, and underlying disease states can further impact serum electrolyte levels and response to replacement therapies

3. Serum glucose (70–110 mg/dL)

    a. Regulation of serum glucose levels is necessary in order to maintain normal cognitive function and prevent adverse health conditions that result in coma

    b. Because many IV solutions contain dextrose, the client must be evaluated and monitored closely for possible effects on blood glucose; in addition, other medications (such as dextran, diuretics, and steroids) and parenteral therapies (such as TPN) can lead to increases in blood glucose

4. Serum albumin (3.5–5.0 mg/dL)
   a. Major protein in plasma that regulates colloidal oncotic pressure and maintains intravascular integrity
   b. Hydration status affects albumin level with dehydration leading to increased albumin levels; decreased albumin from volume excess leads to fluid shifting and third spacing of fluids
   c. It is important to know the albumin level when evaluating serum calcium level, because calcium exists in the body in both ionized and nonionized forms and the ionized form is bound to protein; a low albumin level can therefore be accompanied by hypocalcemia

C. **Blood counts and clotting studies**
   1. RBC count
      a. Normal range: male 4.5–5.3 million/mm^3, female 4.1–5.1 million/mm^3
      b. Hydration states can affect RBC count; dehydration falsely elevates the RBC count and overhydration decreases the RBC count
      c. CBC with differential and a peripheral smear will provide pertinent information relative to RBC indices and morphology
   2. Hematocrit
      a. Packed cell volume with normal range for males 37 to 49%; females 36 to 46%, which is usually three times the hemoglobin value
      b. Hydration status can affect serum values due to hemoconcentration (seen in dehydration causing falsely high values) and hemodilution (seen in overhydration causing decreased values)
      c. Serial hematocrit levels are drawn for a client with ongoing bleeding
      d. In a healthy client, transfusion is generally not needed if hemoglobin is >8 grams/dL and hematocrit is above 24% (variation depends on age and any underlying clinical condition)
      e. Each unit of PRBCs will increase hematocrit by 3%; a unit of whole blood will increase hematocrit by 3 to 4%
   3. Hemoglobin
      a. Normal range for males is 13 to 18 grams/dL and for females is 12 to 16 grams/dL
      b. Serial hemoglobin levels are drawn in client with ongoing blood loss
      c. Hydration can affect serum values (dehydration causes false high and overhydration decreases concentration, causing a lower value)
      d. Each unit of PRBCs or whole blood will increase hemoglobin by one gram
   4. Platelets
      a. Normal range is 150,000 to 400,000/mm^3
      b. Increased levels are seen with iron deficiency anemia (IDA) and decreased levels are seen with hemorrhage or coagulation disorders
      c. Each unit of platelets administered should increase the platelet count by approximately 5000 to 10,000/mm^3 unless alloimmunization has occurred
      d. Dextran has antiplatelet activity
   5. Prothrombin time (PT)
      a. Used to evaluate the competence of the extrinsic coagulation pathway and final common coagulation pathway
      b. If the clotting factors making up the pathway are inadequate, the PT is prolonged
      c. Normal range is 9.5 to 12.0 seconds
      d. Vitamin K is necessary to make prothrombin; drug interaction is seen with sodium warfarin (Coumadin) anticoagulant therapy because it interferes with production of vitamin K–dependent clotting factors, thus prolonging PT and

increasing risk for bleeding; assess client for signs and symptoms of bleeding; INR may be monitored instead of PT to determine effectiveness of warfarin therapy

  e. Inadequate clotting may require the transfusion of FFP, cryoprecipitate, or administration of vitamin K depending on cause and urgency of situation

  f. Hespan can transiently prolong the PT

 6. Partial thromboplastin time (PTT)

  a. Used to evaluate the intrinsic clotting system and final common pathway

  b. Normal range for PTT is 60 to 70 seconds, and for activated PTT (aPTT) 20 to 39 seconds

  c. Used to monitor heparin therapy; therapeutic range for heparin is 1.5 to 2.5 times the control in seconds; PTT >100 seconds or aPTT >70 seconds greatly increases risk of bleeding

  d. PTT may be abnormally prolonged due to hemophilia A or B, DIC, liver disease, or biliary obstruction

  e. Assess for signs and symptoms of bleeding

  f. FFP or cryoprecipitate may be indicated to restore missing clotting factors and vitamin K in the case of biliary obstruction

  g. Hespan can transiently prolong PTT

 7. Antibody and immunoglobulin testing

  a. Direct antiglobulin test (direct Coomb's) detects immunoglobulins on RBC surfaces and can be used to investigate hemolytic transfusion reactions, aid in differential diagnosis of hemolytic anemia, and test for hemolytic disease of newborn

  b. Antibody screening (indirect Coomb's) determines Rh-positive antibodies in maternal blood and assists with identification of ABO incompatibility in newborns

  c. HLA antigens are identified on surface of circulating platelets, WBCs, and most tissue cells; this can be used to match blood products to minimize reactions (such as **HLA alloimmunization**) and identify disease processes

D. Daily weights and body surface area (BSA)

 1. Clients receiving IV fluids should be weighed daily (before breakfast and after voiding; use same scale; have client wear similar clothing each time—i.e., hospital gown)

 2. One kg (2.2 lbs) of body weight is approximately equal to one liter of IV fluid; abrupt changes in weight are an important clue to changes in fluid status

 3. Despite a weight gain, a client may have a significant fluid volume deficit if there is third spacing of fluid; thorough client system assessment is critical; a weight loss is generally expected during diuretic therapy and a weight gain is expected when a client is being rehydrated for a fluid volume deficit

 4. Calculation of BSA provides a more accurate determination of fluid needs for a client with critical needs; a nomogram is used to assist in calculating BSA from height and weight data

III. SELECTION OF FLUID AND ELECTROLYTE THERAPIES

A. Replacement therapies

 1. Oral

  a. May be indicated if fluid loss is not excessive, client is not vomiting, client has intact gag and swallowing reflexes and adequate GI absorption, client has intact thirst mechanism and is able to drink

  b. Physician may prescribe to "push fluids" for clients with actual or potential fluid volume deficits (fever, mild diarrhea)

  c. In choosing oral fluid replacement, consider client preferences, offer fluids frequently, and assist clients who have impaired swallowing by proper positioning

Practice to Pass

An elderly client with a history of CVA was admitted with fluid volume deficit related to inadequate intake and fever. What instructions will you include in discharge teaching for the client and the home health aide assigned to the client's care?

(upright with head and neck flexed forward slightly) and providing thickened liquids or semisolid foods such as gelatin, pudding, or milk shakes

> **d.** It is critical to keep an accurate record of intake and output (I&O), trend results, and notify the physician accordingly if imbalances occur

2. Parenteral

    a. Indicated when client cannot take PO fluids because of clinical presentation, when client is NPO and requires maintenance to replace insensible losses, to provide nutrients and electrolytes when GI tract is not functional, or to replace abnormal losses (GI suction, vomiting, diarrhea, fever, hemorrhage)

> **b.** Infusion rate affected by maintenance and/or replacement need and underlying condition of client (administer cautiously in clients with congestive heart failure and renal failure)

    c. Refer to Table 9-3 for information about the use of crystalloid fluid therapy

    d. The physician prescribes specific blood component therapy based on client's underlying health status, current medical status, and client's own personal decision (i.e., religious beliefs) to allow transfusion therapy

B. Monitoring parameters

    1. Daily weights

    2. I&O

        a. Maintain fluid restriction or orders to increase fluids

> **b.** Properly label and time all IV solutions; run and maintain at ordered rate

        c. Measure the client's entire I&O from all sources

            1) Intake—by mouth, all IV fluids (includes IV meds), tube feedings

            2) Output—urine (urinal, bedpan, indwelling catheter, incontinence—approximate amount), nasogastric drainage, wounds, diarrhea, and emesis

> **d.** Accurately record findings and review 24-hour totals for several days to determine trends in fluid balance

        e. Use trended I&Os in conjunction with daily weights, labs, and knowledge of underlying pathophysiology to determine if client is responding appropriately to IV therapy

        f. Monitor for extremes such as fluid intake greatly exceeding output or output greatly exceeding intake (remember, however, this could be part of the resolution of the problem—i.e., client receiving diuretics for fluid volume excess may have output that greatly exceeds intake with eventual balancing of I&O; correspondingly, a client in hypovolemic shock may have intake greatly exceeding output in order to build up vascular volume)

Table 9-3 **Crystalloid Fluid Replacement Therapy**		
Hypotonic Fluids	**Isotonic Fluids**	**Hypertonic Fluids**
Indicated for cellular dehydration, hyperosmolar states (due to severe hyperglycemia), and to treat hypernatremia. Hypotonic fluids provide free water that dilutes plasma and assists with renal excretion of wastes.	Indicated for hypovolemia (ECF volume deficit) and postoperative fluid management. Isotonic fluids expand vascular compartment and lower hemoglobin and hematocrit concentrations.	Indicated for electrolyte replacement, hyponatremia, and to correct fluid shifting because this leads to cellular dehydration.
Do not give to clients with increased ICP (can increase cerebral edema), abnormal fluid shifts (third spacing), hypotension (can lower BP further), or during code situations (can worsen neurological outcome).	Do not give lactated solutions to clients with liver disease; monitor client for signs and symptoms of FVE. Cautious use in clients with CHF or RF because they are already prone to developing FVE.	Do not give to clients who are already at risk for cellular dehydration (hyperosmolar serum). Cautious use in clients with cardiac or renal failure.

        g. Correlate I&O trend with changes in client's weight; generally, weight gain occurs when intake exceeds output and weight loss occurs when output exceeds intake

        h. Notify the physician of any significant imbalance

        i. In general, high urine output indicates intravascular fluid volume excess (for example, nocturia with heart failure); low urine output with high specific gravity indicates intravascular fluid volume deficit (for example, dehydration); low urine output with low specific gravity indicates renal disease

    3. Trending of pertinent labs

        a. Review pertinent laboratory and diagnostic test results related to specific replacement therapies

        b. Look for improvement of underlying condition as evidenced by lab results and other assessment findings

        c. In general, if a client is being appropriately treated for an isotonic fluid volume deficit, the following should be seen:

           1) An increase in urinary output

           2) A decrease in urine specific gravity

           3) An increase in body weight

           4) An increase in blood pressure (if client was hypotensive)

           5) A decreased pulse rate

           6) Improved skin turgor and moist mucous membranes

           7) Decreased BUN, serum osmolality, and hematocrit

        d. If client is being appropriately treated for a fluid volume excess, the following should be seen:

           1) Improvement in breath sounds

           2) Increase in urine output (in response to diuretics), hematocrit, BUN, and serum osmolality

           3) Decreased weight

           4) Decrease in blood pressure if client's BP was elevated

           5) Decrease in or resolution of edema

C. Priority nursing diagnoses

    1. Deficient Fluid Volume

    2. Excess Fluid Volume

    3. Risk for Impaired Gas Exchange

    4. Risk for Decreased Cardiac Output

    5. Risk for Ineffective Tissue Perfusion: cerebral, renal

D. Therapeutic management

    1. Carefully evaluate client's individualized fluid and electrolyte needs

    2. Give appropriate IV fluid(s) as maintenance and/or replacement therapy

    3. Monitor client responses to therapy on a daily basis or more often in unstable clients with review of pertinent labs, daily weights, I&O, and comprehensive client physical assessments

    4. Prevent complications (fluid volume excess, dehydration)

E. Planning and implementation

    1. Assist client to maintain and/or restore adequate plasma, cellular, or intracellular volume

        a. Encourage oral fluid intake if client able to ingest liquids

        b. Place fluids that client enjoys at the bedside

        c. Infuse appropriate IV solution at ordered rate

        d. Assess client each shift or at least daily for signs and symptoms of adequate hydration (moist mucous membranes, elastic skin turgor, no complaints of thirst, vital signs within normal limits, adequate urine output, level of consciousness within normal limits)

         e. Monitor vital signs frequently

         f. Carefully record I&O from all sources and weigh client daily

         g. Review pertinent laboratory results on a daily basis; closely follow any trends and interpret their significance

         h. Administer fluid challenge if needed to help determine volume status and renal status for clients with underlying clinical conditions; note that some clients may be at risk for developing FVE due to inability to handle fluids, such as those with heart failure

    2. Support client in achieving adequate oxygen-carrying capacity and coagulation status as needed

         a. Administer compatible blood and blood products, carefully applying knowledge of transfusion principles and following agency procedure

         b. Assess the client for signs of improved oxygenation: respirations with greater ease, increased tissue perfusion, improved capillary refill, increased activity tolerance, improved oxygen saturation, and possibly increased alertness

         c. Assess the client for signs of improved coagulation status: decreased bleeding, decreased petechiae, ecchymosis, no gingival oozing, guiac-negative stool

    3. Prevent potential complications of IV therapy in client

         a. Maintain a sterile IV system when priming tubings and administering IV fluids

         b. Observe the IV insertion site regularly for signs of infection or phlebitis

         c. Be alert to signs and symptoms of fluid volume overload (pulmonary congestion, shortness of breath, elevated vital signs, edema, and weight gain)

         d. Infuse hypertonic solutions (selected crystalloids and colloids) slowly

         e. Be alert to signs and symptoms of fluid volume deficit (dry mucous membranes, thirst, weight loss, increased heart rate, decreased blood pressure, poor perfusion, orthostatic hypotension)

         f. Do not infuse hypotonic solutions (D_5W, ½NS) in clients at risk for increased intracranial pressure or third-space fluid shifts

         g. Premedicate clients as ordered prior to transfusions of blood or blood products; carefully assess for signs or symptoms of transfusion reaction and intervene accordingly

F. Client education

    1. Explain need for increased oral intake if appropriate

    2. Teach client how to follow sodium and fluid restriction if appropriate

    3. Teach client to weigh self daily

    4. Review signs and symptoms of dehydration with client

    5. Instruct client to change positions slowly if any signs of dizziness or lightheadedness occur

    6. Review signs and symptoms of overhydration with client

    7. Instruct client to report to the nurse any pain, swelling, leaking, redness, or hardness (induration) at IV site

    8. Explain rationale for blood/blood product transfusion and procedure to client

    9. Verify that client has received informed consent prior to transfusing blood

   10. Teach client to inform the nurse immediately if he or she experiences signs or symptoms of transfusion reaction (chills, fever, nausea, abdominal cramps)

G. Evaluation

    1. Client exhibits adequate hydration status demonstrated by warm dry skin, moist mucous membranes, no complaints of excessive thirst, capillary refill <3 seconds, regular strong peripheral pulses, stable weight, vital signs and urine output within normal limits, no edema, and clear lung sounds

    2. Client exhibits adequate oxygenation and coagulation status as demonstrated by: no bleeding; vital signs within normal limits; adequate perfusion with improved

capillary refill; hemoglobin, hematocrit, platelets, PT, and PTT within normal limits for client; and improved activity tolerance

3. Client experiences no significant adverse effects from transfusion of blood or blood products

Case Study

A 35-year-old female client with severe anemia, tachycardia, and shortness of breath is admitted to your unit. The physician has ordered two units of PRBCs.

1. What assessments will you make before transfusing the blood?

2. What are priority nursing diagnoses for this client?

3. What will you teach this client about the transfusion prior to beginning it?

4. What steps will you follow to administer the transfusion safely?

5. How will you evaluate the effectiveness of the transfusion for this client?

For suggested responses, see pages 205–206.

For suggested responses, see pages 205–206.

POSTTEST

1. A client with dry skin and mucous membranes is weak, has orthostatic blood pressure changes, and has decreased urine output. The client's serum osmolality, however, is normal. Which IV fluid would the nurse anticipate being prescribed for this client?

1. 5% dextrose in water
2. 0.45% sodium chloride
3. 10% dextrose in water
4. 0.9% sodium chloride

2. A client receiving a transfusion of packed RBCs suddenly sounds hoarse, begins wheezing, is diaphoretic and short of breath, and reports palpitations. Blood pressure is 76/52. What is the nurse's priority action?

1. Stop the transfusion.
2. Infuse normal saline (NS) rapidly to maintain intravascular volume.
3. Administer epinephrine and steroids.
4. Maintain the client's airway and ask a staff member to notify the physician.

3. Which of the following outcomes would the nurse anticipate after infusion of 25% albumin to a client in hypovolemic shock?

1. Increase in heart rate
2. Decrease in temperature
3. Decrease in peripheral perfusion
4. Increase in blood pressure

4. Which action should the nurse take when a client is receiving a granulocyte transfusion? Select all that apply.

1. Administer the granulocytes rapidly.
2. Premedicate with an antihistamine, a steroid, and an antipyretic.
3. Attach a microaggregate filter to the IV tubing.
4. Check lymphocyte count following the transfusion.
5. Administer the granulocytes slowly because of allergenicity.

POSTTEST

5 Which laboratory test should the nurse monitor closely in an older adult client with congestive heart failure (CHF) who is receiving IV albumin?

1. Platelet count
2. Hematocrit
3. Serum bilirubin
4. Prothrombin time (PT)

6 The nurse is conducting a class for clients with cancer who frequently receive blood products. The nurse explains that if a client becomes alloimmunized, which of the following would be the most effective way to increase the platelet count?

1. Transfuse single-donor platelet units.
2. Transfuse HLA-matched donor platelets.
3. Use a WBC filter to minimize infusion of WBCs.
4. Premedicate the client with diphenhydramine (Benadryl) and acetaminophen (Tylenol).

7 A physician has ordered dextran for a client while waiting for the results of the blood type and cross-match. The nurse anticipates that which of the following would be an advantage of using dextran for this client?

1. Contains no risk of transfusion-related illnesses
2. Has a decreased risk for anaphylaxis as compared to hetastarch or albumin
3. Promotes hydration of tissues
4. Has no effect on clotting factors

8 Which intervention should the nurse include in developing a plan of care for a client receiving Hespan?

1. Draw a specimen for type and cross-match prior to beginning Hespan infusion.
2. Monitor client for signs of hypovolemia.
3. Expect decreased urine output as body begins conserving plasma volume.
4. Monitor for transient changes in PT, PTT, and clotting times.

9 A client will receive two units of packed red blood cells (PRBCs). The nurse places highest priority on teaching the client which of the following?

1. The rationale for the transfusion
2. Overview of the procedure so the client will know what to expect
3. Signs and symptoms to report to the nurse if they should occur
4. Frequency with which vital signs will be taken so as not to alarm the client

10 A client scheduled to receive four units of packed red blood cells (PRBCs) with premedication therapy wants to know what effect premedication will have on reducing chances of a transfusion reaction. What is the best response by the nurse?

1. "Hives and airway swelling may occur due to an allergic reaction but will be prevented by the medications."
2. "You have no need to worry because your doctor has ordered medications to prevent a reaction."
3. "Chilling and fever caused by previous exposure to blood or blood products may occur but these are minimized by the medications."
4. "The premedication will prevent incompatible blood reactions that could result in shortness of breath and kidney problems."

➤ *See pages 194–196 for Answers and Rationales.*

POSTTEST

ANSWERS & RATIONALES

Pretest

1 **Answer: 3, 5** **Rationale:** A client who is hemorrhaging and in shock requires immediate restoration of oxygen-carrying capacity. With no time available for cross-matching, universal donor blood (type O, Rh-negative) is administered. Establishing an intravenous site should be done prior to transfusing blood products. Type AB, Rh-positive blood can only be given to type AB, Rh-positive recipients. Albumin has no oxygen-carrying capacity, which is essential for a trauma client. Platelets may be administered if needed, but they are not oxygen-carrying cells, which is the first priority. **Cognitive Level:** Analyzing **Client Need:** Pharmacological and Parenteral Therapies **Integrated Process:** Nursing Process: Implementation **Content Area:** Adult Health **Strategy:** Recognize that the need for the client to receive a blood replacement is secondary to the type of fluid losses to have an IV access and receive transfusions from a universal donor. **Reference:** LeMone, P., & Burke, K. (2008). *Medical surgical nursing: Critical thinking in client care* (4th ed.). Upper Saddle River, NJ: Pearson/Prentice Hall, pp. 262–263.

2 **Answer: 2** **Rationale:** Normal saline is an isotonic solution that will replace lost vascular volume and promote perfusion. In addition, when blood is available, it can be hung with the normal saline. D_5W is hypotonic in the bloodstream once dextrose is metabolized, providing free water that moves into the interstitial space and cells. Administration can cause further fluid shifting, which will not help to replace lost volume or promote perfusion. A solution of 0.45% sodium chloride is hypotonic, and an isotonic solution or a volume expander would be a better choice in order to prevent fluid from moving into the interstitium. Dextrose will cause lysis of red blood cells. **Cognitive Level:** Analyzing **Client Need:** Pharmacological and Parenteral Therapies **Integrated Process:** Nursing Process: Diagnosis **Content Area:** Adult Health **Strategy:** Recognize the need for replacement with a isotonic fluid to direct you to the correct option. **Reference:** LeMone, P., & Burke, K. (2008). *Medical surgical nursing: Critical thinking in client care* (4th ed.). Upper Saddle River, NJ: Pearson/Prentice Hall, p. 207.

3 **Answer: 1** **Rationale:** Each unit of PRBCs should raise the hemoglobin by 1 gram and hematocrit by 3%. The nurse should be aware of expected responses to therapy in order to validate that treatment has been effective. **Cognitive Level:** Applying **Client Need:** Reduction of Risk Potential **Integrated Process:** Nursing Process: Evaluation **Content Area:** Adult Health **Strategy:** Recall the expected changes that would be effected by a transfusion of PRBCs and multiply that by 2. **Reference:** LeMone, P.,

& Burke, K. (2008). *Medical surgical nursing: Critical thinking in client care* (4th ed.). Upper Saddle River, NJ: Pearson/Prentice Hall, pp. 262–263.

4 **Answer: 1, 5** **Rationale:** Coumadin depresses the synthesis of vitamin K–dependent clotting factors in the liver, resulting in a prolonged PT/INR (extrinsic coagulation pathway). FFP contains the needed clotting factors and will reverse the PT/INR. The PT/INR needs to be adjusted to the therapeutic range for the client's underlying condition. The aPTT/PTT measures the intrinsic coagulation pathway and is a guide for heparin therapy. Albumin restores protein but not clotting factors. Platelets are needed for blood clotting but they will not restore clotting factors. **Cognitive Level:** Analyzing **Client Need:** Pharmacological and Parenteral Therapies **Integrated Process:** Nursing Process: Planning **Content Area:** Adult Health **Strategy:** Recall the role of Coumadin in the clotting cascade to direct you to the correct options. **Reference:** Adams, M., & Koch, R. (2010). *Pharmacology: Connections to nursing practice.* Upper Saddle River, NJ: Pearson Education, pp. 650–652.

5 **Answer: 1** **Rationale:** Albumin is given to facilitate remobilization of third space fluids. In the case of ascites, it would pull fluid from the abdomen into the intravascular space, resulting in a decrease in abdominal girth. The increase in intravascular fluid would lead to an increase in blood pressure. The pulse may increase in compensation to the increased blood volume, but this does not reflect effectiveness of the albumin treatment. A decrease in weight would most likely be seen as the reabsorbed abdominal fluid is excreted by the kidneys. **Cognitive Level:** Applying **Client Need:** Pharmacological and Parenteral Therapies **Integrated Process:** Nursing Process: Evaluation **Content Area:** Adult Health **Strategy:** Critical words are *ascites* and *albumin*. Recall the physiology of ascites and recognize the purpose of the albumin in treatment of ascites to direct you to the correct option. **Reference:** LeMone, P., & Burke, K. (2008). *Medical surgical nursing: Critical thinking in client care* (4th ed.). Upper Saddle River, NJ: Pearson/Prentice Hall, pp. 262–263.

6 **Answer: 2** **Rationale:** The client's plasma is hypertonic (very concentrated) to begin with and thus serum osmolality, BUN, and hematocrit would be elevated from hemoconcentration. Once isotonic fluids are administered, the plasma concentration should decrease and all three laboratory test results should show a corresponding decrease. BUN and serum osmolality should not remain increased. An increase in all three parameters would be expected in a client who has not yet been treated for hypertonic dehydration. A decrease in hematocrit should occur with the administration of isotonic fluid therapy. **Cognitive Level:** Analyzing

Client Need: Reduction of Risk Potential **Integrated Process:** Nursing Process: Evaluation **Content Area:** Adult Health **Strategy:** Critical words are *isotonic fluids* and *hypertonic dehydration*. Recall the effect of isotonic fluids on serum osmolarity to choose correctly. **Reference:** LeMone, P., Burke, K., & Bauldoff, G. (2011). *Medical surgical nursing: Critical thinking in patient care* (5th ed.). Upper Saddle River, NJ: Pearson Education, pp. 194–195.

7 **Answer: 3** **Rationale:** Abrupt changes in weight are an important clue to changes in fluid status. Unusual losses—i.e., fever or diarrhea—are significant; they need to be reported and may help the client prevent a fluid volume deficit (FVD) in the future, especially because the client is taking a diuretic. Increasing salt and fluids may put the client at significant risk for fluid volume excess (FVE) considering the history of CHF. Taking a diuretic on alternate days only may put the client at risk for fluid volume excess. Drinking one glass of water a day only is grossly insufficient and can put the client at risk for fluid volume deficit. **Cognitive Level:** Analyzing **Client Need:** Physiological Adaptation **Integrated Process:** Teaching and Learning **Content Area:** Adult Health **Strategy:** Critical words are *CHF* and *isotonic dehydration*. Eliminate incorrect options because they reflect unsafe behaviors. **Reference:** LeMone, P., Burke, K., & Bauldoff, G. (2011). *Medical surgical nursing: Critical thinking in patient care* (5th ed.). Upper Saddle River, NJ: Pearson Education, p. 199.

8 **Answer: 2** **Rationale:** A client with type B blood can only receive type B (client/recipient has no anti-B antibodies) and type O (contains no antigens for recipient to react to). Because the client is Rh-negative and has been previously exposed to Rh-positive blood, the client may have antibodies to Rh-positive blood. Therefore only Rh-negative blood should be administered. The client cannot receive type O positive blood due to the identified negative Rh factor. The client has incompatibility with type AB negative blood because of the type A antigens. The client cannot receive type A blood or Rh-positive blood. **Cognitive Level:** Analyzing **Client Need:** Pharmacological and Parenteral Therapies **Integrated Process:** Teaching and Learning **Content Area:** Adult Health **Strategy:** Recognize the risk for Rh incompatibility existing in the client to direct you to the correct option. **Reference:** LeMone, P., Burke, K., & Bauldoff, G. (2011). *Medical surgical nursing: Critical thinking in patient care* (5th ed.). Upper Saddle River, NJ: Pearson Education, pp. 246–247.

9 **Answer: 3** **Rationale:** Acknowledging that the risk exists but stating it is low may help the client with decision-making. Saying all blood products are safe is not accurate and offers false reassurance to the client. Giving "medical" advice is nontherapeutic and may increase client anxiety if the nurse is offering an alternative to the treatment plan. Having family or friends donate is not helpful because it may delay treatment and there is no evidence that designated donor blood is safer. **Cognitive Level:** Analyzing **Client Need:** Pharmacological and Parenteral Therapies **Integrated Process:** Teaching and Learning **Content Area:** Adult Health **Strategy:** Critical words are *alleviate anxiety* and *disease transmission*. Eliminate options that are completely or partially inaccurate, provide false reassurance, or do not answer the client's question. **Reference:** LeMone, P., Burke, K., & Bauldoff, G. (2011). *Medical surgical nursing: Critical thinking in patient care* (5th ed.). Upper Saddle River, NJ: Pearson Education, pp. 246–247.

10 **Answer: 3** **Rationale:** FFP is derived from one unit of whole blood and contains the clotting factors that the client needs plus fibrinogen. Even though whole blood contains some clotting factors, it is deficient in others and is indicated for significant acute blood loss (which is not the client's problem). Improved oxygen-carrying capacity (rendered by the infusion of packed red cells) is something the client does not need. Hemophilia is a clotting disorder that requires clotting factor replacement. Albumin contains no clotting factors. **Cognitive Level:** Applying **Client Need:** Pharmacological and Parenteral Therapies **Integrated Process:** Nursing Process: Assessment **Content Area:** Adult Health **Strategy:** The critical word is *hemophilia*. Recall the deficiency of clotting factors associated with this illness to choose correctly. **Reference:** LeMone, P., Burke, K., & Bauldoff, G. (2011). *Medical surgical nursing: Critical thinking in patient care* (5th ed.). Upper Saddle River, NJ: Pearson Education, p. 246.

Posttest

1 **Answer: 4** **Rationale:** The client is manifesting signs and symptoms of dehydration. Because the serum remains isotonic, this is isotonic dehydration or hypovolemia. Appropriate treatment is with an isotonic fluid to replace fluid volume. Once the dextrose is metabolized, 5% dextrose in water is a hypotonic solution that would cause fluid shifting leading to cellular edema, because the client's cells are normal size and free water is not needed by them. 0.45% sodium chloride is a hypotonic solution; because the client has an isotonic dehydration, this would cause fluid shifting leading to cellular edema. 10% dextrose in water is hypertonic and could cause fluid shifting into the vascular compartment from the cells, leading to cellular dehydration. **Cognitive Level:** Analyzing **Client Need:** Pharmacological and Parenteral Therapies **Integrated Process:** Nursing Process: Diagnosis **Content Area:** Adult Health **Strategy:** Critical words are *normal osmolality*, indicating the fluid replacement will need to maintain the normal osmolality. Recognize the need to restore fluid balance with use of an isotonic solution to direct you to the correct option. **Reference:** LeMone, P., Burke, K., & Bauldoff, G. (2011). *Medical surgical nursing: Critical thinking in patient care* (5th ed.). Upper Saddle River, NJ: Pearson Education, pp. 195–196.

2 **Answer: 1 Rationale:** The client is experiencing a severe allergic/anaphylactic reaction. The nurse should first stop the infusion of any more blood. The nurse should maintain IV access by infusing NS through a clean IV tubing (one not contaminated with blood) to maintain the intravascular volume and prevent vascular collapse once the transfusion is stopped. Hospital protocol may include the administration of epinephrine and steroids. It is always critical to follow current standards of care and hospital protocols during transfusion therapy. The nurse should maintain the client's airway, administer oxygen, and have another staff member notify the physician once the cause of the reaction is terminated. **Cognitive Level:** Analyzing **Client Need:** Pharmacological and Parenteral Therapies **Integrated Process:** Nursing Process: Implementation **Content Area:** Adult Health **Strategy:** The critical word is *priority*, indicating all or some of the options are correct and may be done almost simultaneously, but one takes highest precedence. Recognize the client's symptoms represent an anaphylactic response to direct you to the correct option. **Reference:** LeMone, P., Burke, K., & Bauldoff, G. (2011). *Medical surgical nursing: Critical thinking in patient care* (5th ed.). Upper Saddle River, NJ: Pearson Education, p. 246.

3 **Answer: 4 Rationale:** 25% albumin is a hypertonic colloid solution that will expand the plasma volume. This increase in plasma volume should increase blood pressure. Because the albumin should increase the blood volume and blood pressure, the strain on the heart should be reduced, thus decreasing the heart rate. The increase in volume should not affect temperature. The increase in volume will not decrease peripheral perfusion; rather, it will have the opposite effect. **Cognitive Level:** Applying **Client Need:** Pharmacological and Parenteral Therapies **Integrated Process:** Nursing Process: Evaluation **Content Area:** Adult Health **Strategy:** Recognize that albumin is a plasma expander to direct you to the correct option. **Reference:** LeMone, P., Burke, K., & Bauldoff, G. (2011). *Medical surgical nursing: Critical thinking in patient care* (5th ed.). Upper Saddle River, NJ: Pearson Education, pp. 195–196.

4 **Answer: 2, 5 Rationale:** A client receiving granulocytes is expected to experience fever and chills due to high potential for development of allergic reactions. The client should be premedicated with medications: antihistamines, steroids, and an antipyretic. Granulocytes should be administered slowly. Granulocytes should not be administered rapidly. A microaggregate filter would trap the granulocytes and nullify the transfusion. Although lymphocytes are present in the transfusion, they are granulocytes and the neutrophil count is the appropriate laboratory value to trend. **Cognitive Level:** Analyzing **Client Need:** Pharmacological and Parenteral Therapies **Integrated Process:** Nursing Process: Implementation **Content Area:** Adult Health **Strategy:** The critical word is *granulocyte*. Recall the increased risk for reactions with this type of transfusion to direct you to the correct options. The wording of the question indicates that more than one option is correct. **Reference:** LeMone, P., Burke, K., & Bauldoff, G. (2011). *Medical surgical nursing: Critical thinking in patient care* (5th ed.). Upper Saddle River, NJ: Pearson Education, pp. 195–196.

5 **Answer: 2 Rationale:** A client with CHF has a compromised cardiac pump and therefore already has an increased risk for fluid volume excess or overload. Albumin is a hypertonic colloid solution that can cause circulatory overload. This represents a double risk, then, for a client with CHF. The hematocrit would decrease as the plasma volume increases (hemodilution). The platelet count would increase if the client had a transfusion of platelets. Serum bilirubin will be unaffected by albumin administration. The PT would not change because of an infusion of albumin. **Cognitive Level:** Analyzing **Client Need:** Pharmacological and Parenteral Therapies **Integrated Process:** Nursing Process: Assessment **Content Area:** Adult Health **Strategy:** Critical words are *older adult*, *CHF*, and *albumin*. Recall the effect of albumin on fluid balance and the underlying pathophysiology of CHF to direct you to the correct option. **Reference:** LeMone, P., Burke, K., & Bauldoff, G. (2011). *Medical surgical nursing: Critical thinking in patient care* (5th ed.). Upper Saddle River, NJ: Pearson Education, p. 246.

6 **Answer: 2 Rationale:** Clients may develop HLA antibodies in response to previous transfusions of blood that are not leukodepleted. Because platelets carry class 1 HLA antigens, the HLA antibodies will quickly destroy them. Therefore, attempting to match the donor's platelet antigens with the recipient's and then transfusing these platelets should increase the platelet count. All of the other options are incorrect because they will not reverse alloimmunization. **Cognitive Level:** Analyzing **Client Need:** Pharmacological and Parenteral Therapies **Integrated Process:** Teaching and Learning **Content Area:** Adult Health **Strategy:** The critical word is *alloimmunized*. Recall the physiology of this process to direct you to the correct option. **Reference:** LeMone, P., Burke, K., & Bauldoff, G. (2011). *Medical surgical nursing: Critical thinking in patient care* (5th ed.). Upper Saddle River, NJ: Pearson Education, p. 246.

7 **Answer: 1 Rationale:** Dextran is a glucose solution that is not extracted from human plasma and therefore presents no risk of transmission of viruses. Dextran has a higher risk for anaphylaxis as compared to hetastarch and albumin. Dextran promotes dehydration of tissues because of its hyperosmolar effect. Dextran does affect clotting factors. **Cognitive Level:** Understanding **Client Need:** Pharmacological and Parenteral Therapies **Integrated Process:** Nursing Process: Diagnosis **Content Area:** Adult Health **Strategy:** Note that dextran is being given in lieu of blood products to provide some clues to its advantages. Recall the properties of dextran to eliminate the incorrect options. **Reference:** LeMone, P., Burke, K., & Bauldoff, G. (2011). *Medical surgical nursing: Critical thinking in patient care* (5th ed.). Upper Saddle River, NJ: Pearson Education, pp. 195–196.

8 **Answer: 4** **Rationale:** Hespan can dilute clotting factors and therefore create transient changes in PT, PTT, and clotting times. Hespan will not interfere with blood typing and cross-matching. Hespan expands the plasma volume and thus can cause hypervolemia. Urine output will be increased because Hespan causes osmotic diuresis. **Cognitive Level:** Analyzing **Client Need:** Pharmacological and Parenteral Therapies **Integrated Process:** Nursing Process: Planning **Content Area:** Adult Health **Strategy:** Review the purpose of using Hespan to expand intravascular fluid volume. Recall Hespan's effect on clotting factors to choose correctly. **Reference:** LeMone, P., Burke, K., & Bauldoff, G. (2011). *Medical surgical nursing: Critical thinking in patient care* (5th ed.). Upper Saddle River, NJ: Pearson Education, p. 261.

9 **Answer: 3** **Rationale:** The nurse's highest priority is client safety; therefore, it is imperative that the client know what to report to the nurse should a reaction occur— i.e., chilling, fever, itching, shortness of breath, or back pain. All of the other options should be explained to the client to promote understanding and comfort but are not the highest priority. **Cognitive Level:** Analyzing **Client Need:** Pharmacological and Parenteral Therapies **Integrated Process:** Nursing Process: Implementation

Content Area: Adult Health **Strategy:** The critical words are *highest priority*, indicating all or some of the options are correct, but one takes more precedence. Choose the option that addresses safety. **Reference:** LeMone, P., Burke, K., & Bauldoff, G. (2011). *Medical surgical nursing: Critical thinking in patient care* (5th ed.). Upper Saddle River, NJ: Pearson Education, pp. 246–247.

10 **Answer: 3** **Rationale:** Chilling and fever are associated with a mild nonhemolytic febrile reaction, which is the most common reaction and one that may be minimized through premedication. Hives are a common occurrence, but airway swelling is not and will probably not be managed by premedication alone. Telling the client not to worry because medications have been ordered gives false reassurance and is nontherapeutic. Stating that premedication will prevent incompatible blood reactions suggests a possible hemolytic reaction that is uncommon and would not be minimized by premedication. **Cognitive Level:** Analyzing **Client Need:** Pharmacological and Parenteral Therapies **Integrated Process:** Communication and Documentation **Content Area:** Adult Health **Strategy:** Recall the purpose for giving premedication before PRBCs to direct you to the correct option. **Reference:** LeMone, P., Burke, K., & Bauldoff, G. (2011). *Medical surgical nursing: Critical thinking in patient care* (5th ed.). Upper Saddle River, NJ: Pearson Education, pp. 246–247.

References

Berman, A., & Snyder, S. (2012). *Kozier & Erb's Fundamentals of nursing: Concepts, process, and practice* (9th ed.). Upper Saddle River, NJ: Pearson Education.

Ignatavicius, D., & Workman, M. (2009). *Medical-surgical nursing: Critical thinking in collaborative care* (6th ed.). St. Louis, MO: Elsevier Saunders.

Kee, J. L. (2009). *Handbook of laboratory and diagnostic tests with nursing implications* (6th ed.). Upper Saddle River, NJ: Pearson Education.

LeMone, P., & Burke, K. (2011). *Medical-surgical nursing: Critical thinking in client care* (5th ed.). Upper Saddle River: NJ: Pearson Education.

Osborne, K. S., Wraa, C. E., & Watson, A. B. (2010). *Medical-surgical nursing: Preparation for practice.* Upper Saddle River, NJ: Pearson Education.

Smeltzer, S., Bare, B., Hinkle, J., & Cheever, K. (2010). *Brunner & Suddarth's textbook of medical-surgical nursing* (12th ed.). Philadelphia, PA: Lippincott Williams & Wilkins.

Smith, S., Duell, D., & Martin, B. (2011). *Clinical nursing skills: Basic to advanced skills* (8th ed.). Upper Saddle River, NJ: Pearson Education.

Appendix

➤ Practice to Pass Suggested Answers

Chapter 1

Page 7: *Answer*—Hypotonic fluids (D_5W, ¼NS, ½NS) are contraindicated because they provide free water that is pulled into cells. Cerebral cells absorb such water more rapidly than other cells, which would worsen cerebral edema in a client who has sustained a head injury and insult to the brain. Isotonic fluids tend to remain in the vascular system, rather than shift into tissues.

Page 11: *Answer*—Three percent saline is very hypertonic with a high concentration of sodium. It will increase serum sodium levels and draw water from the cells into the vascular space, causing hypervolemia, hypernatremia, and cellular dehydration. Only limited doses in very controlled amounts should be infused. The infusion should be controlled with an infusion pump and the client should be closely monitored for the development of circulatory overload, pulmonary edema, rising serum sodium levels, and cerebral cell dehydration. Frequent monitoring should include the following:

- Vital signs and pulse oximetry
- Neurological assessment
- Respiratory assessment with auscultation of lungs for crackles
- Hourly urine output
- Serum electrolyte levels

Page 16: *Answer*—This client's clinical manifestations are indicative of hypovolemia and impending shock. Hemorrhage from trauma is causing an isotonic fluid loss that is primarily ECF. Isotonic intravenous fluids remain in the ECF and are used to expand vascular volume. The client needs large volumes of isotonic fluids (normal saline, Ringer's solution, or lactated Ringer's) infused rapidly to increase vascular volume and prevent shock. If hemorrhage is massive, blood infusions may be needed to restore volume.

Page 18: *Answer*—This elderly client should be monitored closely for signs of hypervolemia and circulatory overload due to reduced cardiac and renal reserves consistent with the aging process. Monitoring should include (1) I&O,

(2) observing for signs of venous congestion (neck vein distention, delayed hand vein emptying), (3) peripheral edema, and (4) pulmonary congestion (tachypnea, dyspnea, moist lung crackles). Daily weights will reveal acute weight gain.

Page 19: *Answer*—Explain in simple terms that the child is losing water and minerals and needs both replaced. Suggest that she give the child small sips of a commercial oral rehydration solution (e.g., Pedialyte, Infalyte) frequently to replace the fluid and electrolytes lost through diarrhea and vomiting. Explain that this is a balanced solution that does not provide too much sugar or salt, which can make diarrhea worse. She should also be advised to continue a regular diet as soon as the child will eat food. This will help resolve the diarrhea and provide calories, protein, fluid, and electrolytes as well.

Page 22: *Answer*—The half-strength formula is a hypotonic solution that provides excess free water. If given on a regular basis, it could lead to inadequate calories, insufficient protein, hypotonic fluid volume excess, and water intoxication as the fluid is pulled into cells. This should be explained in simple terms that the mother can understand. If finances are a problem, she should be referred to a community agency that can help her obtain assistance in getting formula for the baby.

Page 23: *Answer*—This is an elderly person with a history of heart disease who is receiving intravenous fluid therapy at a fairly rapid rate. Awakening at night with dyspnea and a cough signals possible fluid overload and impending pulmonary edema. The nurse should first slow the IV rate to 10–20 mL/hour to maintain IV access without infusing much fluid. The next actions should include focused assessment of respiratory status, providing emergency supplemental oxygen, and notifying the physician. This client may need intravenous diuretics and other rapid interventions to prevent acute pulmonary edema.

Page 25: *Answer*—The fluid should be controlled with an infusion pump to prevent accidental fluid overload in this infant. An infant's small body size and immature kidneys put him or her at higher risk for fluid volume overload if fluids are infused too rapidly. Monitoring should include (1) checking the intravenous infusion frequently, (2) I&O, (3) serial weights, and (4) vital signs in an effort to prevent accidental overinfusion of fluid and early detection of clinical signs of fluid overload.

Chapter 2

Page 35: *Answer*—Because serum sodium level is the primary determinant of plasma osmolality, it is easy to get a rough estimate of a client's plasma osmolality if the serum sodium level is known. Taking the known serum sodium level and doubling that figure gives a rough estimate of plasma osmolality. This can be helpful in the clinical setting to evaluate a client's osmolar state.

Page 36: *Answer*—The chief regulation of sodium occurs in the kidneys where it is reabsorbed along with chloride. The reabsorption of these two electrolytes plays an important role in water balance. Renal regulation of sodium is influenced as a response to different volume states.

Page 37: *Answer*—Water will shift from the ECF (area of lower volume of solutes) to the ICF (area of higher volume of solutes) in an attempt to restore equilibrium. This results in a decreased circulating plasma volume and an increase in cellular swelling.

Page 40: *Answer*—The pathophysiologic effects of hyponatremia are primarily seen in the central nervous system and result in neurological depression. Muscular weakness is seen as neuromuscular involvement occurs. Nausea and other GI complaints are seen as gastrointestinal involvement occurs. These effects are due to fluid shifting between the ECF and ICF as cellular swelling occurs.

Page 41: *Answer*—A client who is NPO and on NG suctioning is at risk for hyponatremia due to restricted oral replacement and the loss of gastric secretions. Clients who are on prolonged NPO status should have their hydration level maintained via parenteral routes. In addition, the loss of gastrointestinal secretions can lead to further electrolyte and fluid losses that will require adequate replacement therapies. Monitoring and recording intake and output is essential in the care of this client. Amount, color, and consistency of NG drainage should be monitored for potential electrolyte and fluid imbalances.

In addition, bowel sounds should be assessed on this client to see if there is resumption of normal peristalsis. Client should be in a safe position with the NG tube secure so as to prevent further complications related to potential aspiration. The suction equipment should be monitored for the correct setting and the canister changed as needed. Placement and verification of the NG tube should be evaluated at least once a shift (if not more in case there is medication administration) to validate correct placement.

Page 47: *Answer*—The following measures should be instituted in taking care of a client with hypernatremia:

- Monitor neurological status, and level of consciousness (LOC), and observe for potential seizures.
- Keep the bed in the low position, side rails up, and the call bell in place.
- Assist with ambulation and mobility as needed.
- Make sure that environment is safe so as to prevent risk of falls and injury to client.

Chapter 3

Page 57: *Answer*—Potassium (K^+) in the intracellular fluid (ICF) is important for conduction of electrical impulses, which make the muscles in the body work. Too much or too little potassium can be detrimental to health by affecting neuromuscular excitability, acid–base balance, and cardiac contractility. Elevated or decreased levels can lead to the development of cardiac arrhythmias, which can be life-threatening. It is very important to have a K^+ level in the normal therapeutic range so as to avoid compromise.

Page 57: *Answer*— Clients who are hypokalemic may be weak and have muscle cramps. Clients should be assisted when ambulating in order to provide support and maintain balance. Have a call bell in reach and side rails up when the client is in bed. Assist the client to change position slowly to minimize the risk of orthostatic hypotension. Monitor the client's level of consciousness and his or her respiratory, cardiac, and GI status. Administer medications as ordered to restore normal serum levels. Monitor the client's labs accordingly to evaluate response to treatment.

Page 59: *Answer*— Because potassium never leaves the body in relative hypokalemia, it is important to monitor the client closely to ensure that rebound hyperkalemia does not occur with treatment. Remember, a serum potassium level that is low secondary to shifting does not indicate where the potassium loss has occurred. Clients who have relative hypokalemia may be at risk to develop hyperkalemia due to overaggressive treatment. It is important to adequately assess clients who may be exhibiting hypokalemia as a result of water intoxication, alkalosis states, and increased insulin secretion.

Page 63: *Answer*—When KCl is administered intravenously, it should be diluted in enough solution to deliver no more than 10 mEq/mL. No more than 40 mEq should be added to a liter of solution when using a peripheral line. If a solution contains more than 20 mEq/hr, the client should be on continuous ECG monitoring with serum levels checked every four to six hours. Potassium should be infused using an infusion pump to ensure accurate rate of administration. Close monitoring of the IV site should be done because KCl is very irritating to veins. If the site is red or infiltrated, the IV must be discontinued to prevent damage to the vessel.

Page 64: *Answer*—Foods that are high in potassium include potatoes, bananas, watermelon, yogurt, and acorn squash. These are considered good sources because they contain the most K^+ per kilocalorie. Potassium is found in whole grains, meats, milk, fruits, vegetables, grains, and legumes and is present in most foods in the Western diet. It is important for the nurse to note that ingestion of large amounts of licorice can lead to hypokalemia and the client's dietary selections should be monitored for this. In addition, it is important to note if the client is using salt substitutes because they are usually high in K^+. It is also important to assess the client for use of dietary (nutritional) supplements for their potential effects on

K⁺ levels. Collaboration with a dietitian is essential in the management of these clients.

Page 65: *Answer*—Potassium is forced out of the cells and into the extracellular spaces during massive tissue destruction. Potassium enters the vascular space and hyperkalemia develops. Cellular trauma can lead to the release of large levels of K⁺, and all clients should be monitored closely for potential problems as a result of hyperkalemia.

Chapter 4

Page 78: *Answer*—The parathyroid hormone, activated vitamin D, and calcitonin tightly control serum calcium levels. When there are alterations in any of these systems, disturbances in calcium levels can occur, leading to hypo- or hypercalcemia.

Page 83: *Answer*—Predisposing clinical conditions that can lead to calcium imbalances are related to inadequate intestinal absorption, deposition of ionized calcium into bone or soft tissue, or decreases in PTH and vitamin D levels. All of these factors can lead to decreased physiologic availability of calcium.

Page 86: *Answer*—Calcium plays an important role in determining the speed of ion fluxes through nerve and muscle membranes. The effects of too little calcium lead to an increase in nervous system irritability. This irritability is exhibited by tetany, as well as in Chvostek and Trousseau signs, and may develop into seizures.

Page 88: *Answer*—The therapeutic response to calcium gluconate therapy can be evaluated by noting resolution of dysrhythmias, tingling and paresthesias, and signs of tetany, and by noting a return of serum calcium to a level of 8.5 to 9 mg dL. Appropriate nursing interventions for a client receiving this type of therapy should include evaluating the IV site for signs of extravasation that can happen with calcium gluconate or calcium chloride, close titration of dose, and continuous ECG monitoring.

Page 90: *Answer*—Differences in the CNS as a result of hypocalcemia include clinical manifestations such as depression, anxiety, irritability, delusions, hallucinations, and convulsions. Hypercalcemia produces clinical manifestations such as lethargy, subtle personality changes, or acute changes such as psychosis, stupor, and possibly coma. Similarities in the CNS as a result of altered calcium levels (hypo- and hypercalcemia) result in clinical manifestations such as memory impairment and confusion.

Page 94: *Answer*—Foods to avoid are cheeses, milk, and other dairy products; canned salmon and sardines; rhubarb; spinach and other dark green leafy vegetables; and tofu. Calcium supplements and antacids such as Oscal and Tums should be avoided. During the nursing assessment, the client should be questioned as to food likes and dislikes and for any history of peptic ulcer disease or gastric distress because this increases the likelihood of increased use of calcium-containing antacids and calcium-rich foods.

Chapter 5

Page 104: *Answer*—Good sources of magnesium include green leafy vegetables, nuts, legumes, seafood, whole grains, bananas, oranges, cocoa, and chocolate.

Page 105: *Answer*—Because the two function together to help run the sodium-potassium pump, a change in one effects a change in the other.

Page 106: *Answer*—Maalox, Mylanta, Riopan, Gaviscon, Gelusil, and Di-Gel are common brand-name antacids that are high in magnesium.

Page 107: *Answer*—Cardiovascular symptoms include hypotension, flushing and sweating, arrhythmias, and possibly cardiac arrest.

Page 108: *Answer*—Calcium gluconate is an antagonist of magnesium and is given as an emergency treatment for severe hypermagnesemia.

Chapter 6

Page 122: *Answer*—In metabolic alkalosis, chloride is decreased because the kidneys retain bicarbonate and excrete chloride. Increased bicarbonate in the body leads to potassium and sodium depletion, which affects extracellular volume depletion, resulting in accompanying chloride loss.

Page 124: *Answer*—Hypochloremia reflects a decrease in serum chloride, <95 mEq/L. Chloride levels are usually not altered independently but rather are seen in conjunction with other electrolyte and acid–base imbalances. It is important to check serum sodium and potassium levels and assess the client's acid–base status to help establish the etiology of the chloride deficit. In addition, it is important to ascertain clinical factors that would lead to chloride deficit such as disease states, GI loss, endocrine disturbance, and volume expansion in order to more clearly describe the hypochloremic state. Depending on the serum value, the following strategies can be used for correction: (1) increase intake of foods high in chloride or (2) administer sodium chloride intravenously, or potassium chloride if potassium level is also low.

Page 124: *Answer*—A Medrol dose pack is a steroid that causes sodium and chloride retention and fluid volume excess. Lasix (furosemide) is a loop diuretic that promotes sodium, chloride, potassium, and water excretion. The Medrol dose pack would be most likely to cause an increase in serum chloride levels.

Page 124: *Answer*—The nurse should assess the client for deep, rapid, vigorous respirations. A client who is hyperchloremic should present with metabolic acidosis with a normal anion gap. In addition, to increase respiratory rate and depth, the client may also experience headache, drowsiness, and confusion. Depending on the state of acidosis, signs and symptoms will vary as the client attempts to return to normal acid–base balance by using compensatory mechanisms. The client can progress into shock states with accompanying dysrhythmias, so careful monitoring is critical to maintain client safety and establish favorable clinical outcomes.

Page 125: *Answer*—The client is likely experiencing hyperchloremia, because high fever, severe vomiting, and diarrhea would lead to a state of dehydration. Hyperchloremia is associated with dehydration states because fluid losses contribute to severe electrolyte deficiencies. The client is also likely to be suffering from both sodium and potassium losses. Remember, chloride imbalance states usually do not exist independently but rather occur together with sodium, potassium, and water imbalances. Metabolic acidosis may be associated with a high chloride also.

Chapter 7

Page 135: *Answer*—Phosphorus is abundant in fish, poultry, eggs, red meat, and organ meats, such as brain, liver, and kidney. It is also found in dairy products such as milk. Legumes, whole grains, and nuts are other rich sources of phosphorus.

Page 138: *Answer*—The client may report circumoral and fingertip/extremity numbness and tingling. The client may also exhibit muscle weakness, parasthesias, tremors, spasms, and signs of tetany.

Page 140: *Answer*—When giving potassium phosphate, use an infusion pump and do not exceed a rate of infusion greater than 10 mEq/hr; give the dose slowly over two to six hours as ordered. Watch for complications of IV administration, including tetany from hypocalcemia, hypotension from too rapid an infusion rate, and formation of calcium and phosphorus deposits in the tissues. Monitor infusion site for signs of infiltration, which may lead to tissue necrosis or sloughing.

Page 142: *Answer*—The client may exhibit any of the following manifestations:

- Metastatic calcification, including oliguria, corneal haziness, conjunctivitis, and irregular heart rate
- EKG changes and conduction disturbance, tachycardia, deposits of calcium phosphate in the cardiac tissues
- Numbness and tingling around the mouth and in the fingertips, muscle spasms, and tetany
- Decreased calcium
- Anorexia, nausea, and vomiting
- Muscle weakness, hyperreflexia, and tetany

Page 143: *Answer*—Phosphate-binding medications contain either aluminum, magnesium, or calcium as the cation that binds to the phosphate anion. Products that bind phosphate will have one of these or may have aluminum and magnesium together, because they have opposing effects on the GI tract.

Chapter 8

Page 155: *Answer*—The nurse would examine the client's ABG results. With uncompensated respiratory acidosis, the pH is less than 7.35, $PaCO_2$ is greater than 45 mm Hg, and the HCO_3^- is normal (22–26 mEq/L). In a client with respiratory acidosis, compensation would involve the kidneys retaining bicarbonate and returning it to the ECF. Compensation would reflect an increase in the bicarbonate level.

Page 156: *Answer*—As acidosis occurs, H^+ ions move into the cell and potassium moves into the ECF, elevating the serum potassium level. Hyperkalemia can cause serious cardiac conduction defects and can be fatal. When someone is acidotic, the potassium level must be monitored closely. Transcellular shifting of potassium is affected by acid–base balance. With acidosis, H^+ is excreted and K^+ is retained leading to hyperkalemia. With alkalosis, K^+ is excreted and H^+ is retained leading to hypokalemia.

Page 158: *Answer*—Clients with type 1 diabetes require insulin to control glucose levels. When there is insufficient insulin, fats are metabolized and free fatty acids accumulate, which can result in the development of diabetic ketoacidosis. Control of glucose levels with adequate insulin is the best prevention.

Page 161: *Answer*—Monitoring the amount of NG drainage and replacing the amount lost with an equal amount of an electrolyte solution can prevent excessive H^+ ion loss. It is important to account for intake and output and correlate with serum electrolyte levels. If fluids and electrolytes are being removed via suction, then the client may be at risk to develop further electrolyte imbalance, which could be complicated by acid–base disturbances.

Page 163: *Answer*—Conditions leading to the development of metabolic alkalosis result in depleted potassium levels, which can significantly affect cardiac function. Transcellular shifting of potassium is also affected by acid–base balance. Clients who are alkalotic have decreased potassium levels and are likely to become even more hypokalemic. Hypokalemia affects cardiac conduction leading to the development of dysrhythmias that can become life threatening. These clients must be monitored closely so prompt management and intervention can be implemented.

Chapter 9

Page 174: *Answer*—The client has a very hyperosmolar serum and is experiencing osmotic diuresis and dehydration. 0.9% NaCl (normal saline) will begin to replace the fluid volume that is being lost as a result of the osmotic diuresis. It also expands plasma volume to increase the glomerular filtration rate, which will protect the kidneys from the complication of acute renal failure. Serum osmolality should begin to decrease (insulin is needed, of course). Although one might expect serum sodium to be high in this dehydrated client, a good amount of sodium is being lost in the urine as a result of the osmotic diuresis. Therefore, the serum sodium is low to begin with and should increase with 0.9% NaCl IV replacement. Blood pressure should increase, heart rate should decrease, and perfusion should improve.

Page 174: *Answer*—Priority assessments include obtaining baseline and frequent vital signs and determining adequacy of organ perfusion by assessing level of consciousness (LOC), urine output, and skin color. It is important to be alert to the fact that the client may develop possible dehydration or fluid overload due to the cellular dynamic effects of the hypertonic albumin. It is equally important to monitor the client for the possibility of a febrile reaction. Priority interventions include maintaining a patent airway and providing adequate ventilation and oxygenation. Albumin should be infused as rapidly as the client will tolerate, while paying close attention to lung sounds for possible pulmonary edema and for other indications of fluid volume excess (FVE). The client may be at greater risk for fluid volume excess if there is a significant cardiac history. Even without a cardiac history, given the client's age, there may be some cardiac insufficiency due to the normal aging process. It is therefore important to place the client in a supine position with legs elevated in order to maximize organ perfusion. If the client cannot tolerate this position due to respiratory compromise, then position the client with the head elevated at 30 to 45 degrees. If the client is at risk for increased intracranial pressure (if head injury present), the head of the bed should be elevated to 30 degrees. Keep the client warm. If trauma occurred or may have occurred, observe for increased bleeding, especially as the blood pressure rises. Monitor hemoglobin, hematocrit, electrolytes, and serum albumin. Expected outcomes for this client include an increased colloidal oncotic pressure with a corresponding increase in cardiac output, increased blood pressure, decreased heart rate, decreased respiratory rate, improved organ perfusion, increased urine output, increased serum albumin, and decreased hematocrit.

Page 177: *Answer*—Stop the infusion, because the client may be experiencing an anaphylactic reaction. Maintain the client's airway and provide high flow oxygen. Enlist assistance and have one colleague bring the crash cart and another notify the physician. Administer epinephrine per hospital protocol. Quickly change the IV line at the hub and infuse 0.9% normal saline (NS) to help maintain blood volume. The client should be attached to a cardiac monitor and pulse oximetry. Heart rate, respiratory rate, and oxygen saturation are monitored continuously and blood pressure readings should be taken frequently. Additional medications such as diphenhydramine (Benadryl), methylprednisolone sodium succinate (Solumedrol), and aminophylline (Theophylline) may be ordered by the physician. The client may need to be intubated. The physician may order additional IV fluids. A vasopressor—i.e., dopamine—may be ordered if the client is unable to maintain an adequate blood pressure. Once the client has stabilized, continue to observe the client for several hours. Once it has been determined that the client is allergic

to the Hespan, the client should be advised to wear a Medic Alert bracelet indicating the allergy.

Page 181: *Answer*—An appropriate response to the client's concern would be to tell the client, "The chemotherapy that you are receiving to treat the leukemia puts you at increased risk for infection. Specially treating the blood you will receive helps to ensure that it will not be a source of infection for you while you are at increased risk."

Page 184: *Answer*—Laboratory results to review in evaluating the effectiveness of transfusion therapy for a client with DIC include hemoglobin, hematocrit, RBC count, platelet count, partial thromboplastin time (PTT), prothrombin time (PT) or International Normalized Ratio (INR), and fibrinogen level. While transfusions of PRBCs, platelets, fresh frozen plasma (FFP), and possibly cryoprecipitate will help to replenish blood components, additional blood loss may occur through the presence of this coagulopathy. The presence of DIC complicates the clinical picture because unless the underlying mechanism is identified and treated, replacement therapies are aimed at supportive management and are not curative. Therefore, lab values are bound to plunge again and again until the underlying cause is identified and treated.

Page 184: *Answer*—The nurse should first explain to the client what the transfusion is for, what to expect during the transfusion (chilling, fever, and allergic reaction), and answer any questions that the client might have. To safely administer granulocytes to this client, the nurse should begin by premedicating the client as ordered by the physician, generally with diphenhydramine (Benadryl), steroids, and an antipyretic. When hanging the unit, the nurse must verify that it is ABO and Rh compatible because it contains RBCs and is preferably HLA compatible. The nurse is also aware that the granulocytes must be administered within 24 hours after being collected and are maximally effective when given as soon as possible after collection. The nurse must use a standard inline filter (not a microaggregate filter, which will trap the WBCs) and administer the transfusion slowly, generally at a rate of 50 mL per hour for four hours. Monitor the client for expected side effects. Cover the client with a warm blanket to prevent chilling. Monitor the client for hypertension and treat it if needed. Only discontinue the transfusion if the client develops severe respiratory distress. Be aware that granulocytes are generally administered for at least four to five days, one unit a day or until the infection resolves.

Page 187: *Answer*—If the client has any difficulty swallowing as a result of a prior stroke, it is important that the home health aide assists the client to an upright position with the head and neck flexed slightly forward. Liquids should be thick or semisolid (gelatin, pudding, and milk shakes). The home health aide should offer the client fluid frequently and consider preferences when purchasing and preparing the fluids. It is also important that cold fluids are served cold and hot fluids are served hot. The client and home health aide must be aware if fluid restriction is necessary due to underlying CHF and/or renal insufficiency and maintain the limits of that restriction. The home health aide should keep a record of the client's intake and output and note the characteristics of urine output. It is important that daily weights be obtained. The aide should examine the client's skin and mucous membranes for signs of adequate hydration. The client should be instructed to report any excess thirst to the aide. All abnormal losses from fever, diaphoresis, or diarrhea, for example, should be reported to the physician. Last but not least, the client and aide should be instructed about good handwashing techniques and protecting themselves from infection.

➤ Case Study Suggested Answers

Chapter 1

1. Questions to ask the mother include the following:
   - How high has the fever been, how many times has the infant vomited, how many stools has the infant had today?
   - Has the infant been able to keep any food or fluids down?
   - When did the infant last urinate?
   - Is the infant acting "normal"? Are there any changes in behavior or activity?
   - Has there been any weight lost in the past two days?
   - Have you used any treatments or medicines at home? If so, which ones and how often? What effect did they have?
2. Serious fluid imbalance is indicated by the following:
   - Assessing infant's level of alertness, activity, interaction and response to others (lethargy, listlessness, and/or reduced activity/interaction are signs of serious dehydration).
   - Counting heart rate (tachycardia is an early sign of fluid volume deficit in infants).
   - Observing skin and mucous membranes (dry oral mucosa and tongue, furrowed tongue, and no tears when crying are all signs of fluid volume loss).
   - Palpating fontanels (sunken fontanels are a sign of significant fluid volume loss).
3. Control the fluid rate with an infusion pump to prevent infusing a volume too large for the child's size. Explain all procedures to the parents and provide emotional support. Monitor the child for signs of improvement as well as fluid overload.
4. Give the child small, frequent sips of a commercial oral rehydration solution (e.g., Pedialyte, Infalyte) to replace both fluid and electrolyte losses without giving excess sugar or salt, which can make diarrhea worse. Resume regular foods as soon as the infant will eat them. Once the infant is eating and the diarrhea is getting better, add a variety of fluids the infant likes, avoiding those with high sugar or salt content.
5. The BRAT diet is a transition diet used to assist clients when they have gastrointestinal tract alterations (nausea, vomiting, or diarrhea). It is not meant for long-term use as it does not provide adequate amounts of required nutrients and calories. Once the infant is able to keep food and fluids down, it is important to progress the client's diet back to the original pattern.

Chapter 2

1. Client's past medical history (PMH) reveals hypertension diagnosed six weeks ago with a prescription of hydrochlorothiazide and a low-sodium diet. Current findings related to history of present illness (HPI) or chief complaint reveals dizziness, nausea, weakness, abdominal cramps, and headache. Onset of symptoms three days ago with worsening by today indicates that the client's condition is becoming more acute. These findings suggest that the client might be experiencing a sodium deficit. The use of a thiazide diuretic can lead to a sodium deficit, and the increase in neurological complaints of dizziness, weakness, and headache are consistent with hyponatremia.
2. Questions that should be asked prior to performing a physical examination should include the following:
   - Are you taking your diuretic as ordered? Clarify information relative to dosage, frequency, and compliance with treatment regimen.
   - Have you ever experienced these kinds of symptoms before?
   - Are there any contributory health problems that could affect your overall condition? Do you suffer from any acute or chronic disease process?
   - Are you taking any other medications, either prescription or OTC?
   - Have you been experiencing thirst?
   - Have you had excessive perspiration or sweating in the last few days?
   - You stated that you have been dizzy. Can you explain what that means to you? Are you having blurred vision? Are you having difficulty concentrating?
   - Can you tell me where you feel your headache and describe the type of discomfort that you experience (obtain pain characteristics)?
   - Have you taken any medication today to relieve any of your symptoms?
   - Obtain an accurate intake and output record from the client for the past 24 hours.
3. Clinical findings consistent with hyponatremia are tachycardia, hypotension, dry mucous membranes, muscular weakness, and flat neck veins. This data would be consistent with physical examination findings.
4. Based on the data obtained thus far and knowledge of fluid and electrolytes, the nurse expects a Na level <135 mEq/L (which would indicate hyponatremia), a serum osmolality <275 mOsm/kg (which would indicate decreased plasma osmolality), a serum chloride level <97 mEq/L (which would indicate hypochloremia), and a specific gravity of <1.008 (which would indicate a decreased ability to concentrate urine).

5. Discharge teaching that should be included in the plan of care for this client includes the following:
   - Teach the client the signs and symptoms of hyponatremia (such as abdominal cramps, nausea, muscle weakness) so that he will be able to identify potential problems and report to his health care provider.
   - Teach the client the importance of drinking liquids containing sodium during periods of heavy sweating and/or high environmental temperatures as the client's occupation requires him to be outdoors.
   - Teach the client to comply with regularly scheduled lab/diagnostic tests to monitor sodium and other electrolyte levels while taking diuretic therapy.
   - Teach the client about low-sodium diet instructions and verify that the client is meeting dietary goals. Refer to a dietitian for follow-up if needed.
   - Teach the client the importance of safety upon ambulation as diuretic therapy and that hyponatremia can lead to hypotension. Discuss slow change of positioning and monitor BP during therapy.
   - Teach the client to keep all regularly scheduled health care appointments and report findings immediately to health care provider so that prompt recognition and treatment of symptoms can be started.

Chapter 3

1. The nurse should question this client closely about any medications that the client is taking (both prescription and over-the-counter). Particular attention should be given if the client is taking potassium supplements and/or digitalis preparations. The nurse should question this client about any acute or chronic disease process that could increase the risk for developing hypokalemia. In addition, any recent medical or surgical treatment should be explored with the client. The nurse should question this client regarding diet history. The nurse should also question the client regarding signs and symptoms of hypokalemia.
2. The client could manifest many other signs and symptoms, such as fatigue, muscle weakness, leg cramps, nausea, vomiting, paralytic ileus, paresthesias, polyuria, weak and irregular pulse, hyperglycemia, and ECG changes consistent with hypokalemia.
3. A serum chemistry panel should be drawn for this client because episodes of diarrhea are associated with potential fluid and electrolyte depletion. Magnesium levels and calcium levels should be looked at closely because hypokalemia often occurs in conjunction with losses of these two electrolytes. Arterial blood gases might be drawn to determine acid–base status, which could be influenced by loss of GI fluids leading to the development of metabolic alkalosis. ECG monitoring is indicated for this client because the client is complaining of cardiac effects. Depending on ECG baseline, additional labs might be ordered if further cardiac compromise was suspected (cardiac enzymes). If the client continues to have diarrhea, then a stool sample should be obtained for culture and sensitivity.
4. The client would be given either oral or parenteral potassium supplements depending on the baseline potassium level. If the level was low (below 3.0 mEq/L), then IV potassium would be the treatment of choice until the level reached 3.0 mEq/L; then oral supplements would be sufficient. Even at higher levels, some clients are unable to consume sufficient potassium to raise serum levels. These clients might have to remain on IV therapy with KCl in addition to oral supplements. If the diarrhea continues and the stool sample identifies a specific pathogen, then further medical treatment may be warranted by using either antibiotic therapy to treat the organism; otherwise, antidiarrheal agents may be ordered to prevent excess fluid loss.
5. Teaching for this client should include information related to the nature of the complaint. As the client's clinical presentation denotes hypokalemia, the client should be given information relative to signs and symptoms of hypokalemia and to report to the health care provider if these should occur. Client teaching should further include specifics regarding whether the client's diet therapy and/or current medications contribute to potassium balance in the body. Because the client will most likely be started on K^+ supplementation, the client should be aware of potential interactions and adequate sources of potassium in the diet in order to maintain serum levels. Regarding the most effective teaching methods for the client, it is important to individualize so that the client can have both verbal and written information. Including significant family members may be warranted in order to reinforce information and help others participate in the client's health care upon discharge. Teaching should be an ongoing process started upon admission and continuing to discharge. In addition, follow-up reinforcement should be included so that the client continues with prescribed therapy.

Chapter 4

1. These signs and symptoms are caused by hypercalcemia from osteocytic activity of malignancy.
2. The chief cause appears to be osteoclastic bone resorption, mediated by PTH or other substances secreted by the tumor. The result is that more calcium is released from the bone into the ECF.
3. Isotonic saline diuresis will lead rapidly to increased renal excretion, depending upon renal function. Biphosphonate drugs (pamidronate, Aredia) are now first-line therapy with saline diuresis because they inhibit osteoclasts from resorbing bone. Plicamycin (Mithramycin) is extraordinarily effective in clients with hypercalcemia that results from skeletal metastasis.

4. Priority nursing interventions include the following:
   - Monitor for signs of continuing hypercalcemia.
   - Monitor for signs of impending hypocalcemia from overcorrection secondary to treatment.
   - Monitor client carefully for signs of heart failure from saline diuresis.
   - Monitor for side effects of biphosphonate therapy.
   - Monitor for side effects of plicamycin.
   - Move the client with great care to avoid pain or fractures.
   - Pain management therapy should be an integral part of the treatment plan.
5. There will be an absence of the presenting clinical manifestations. Calcium and phosphorus levels will normalize. Serum creatinine will indicate effectively functioning kidneys and a urine output of two to three L/day. There are minimal side effects of medication therapy. There are no signs of heart failure. Fluid volume is stable with signs of overhydration. The client will state a reduction in pain, and the client is moved or ambulated without increased pain.

Chapter 5

1. The client has low weight for height. This leads to questions about starvation, dietary habits, anorexia, bulimia, and diabetes.
2. Data should also be gathered about alcohol use and over-the-counter medications, including diuretics, laxatives, enemas, and diet aids.
3. The client should have measurement of electrolytes, including potassium, magnesium and calcium levels, and an electrocardiogram (ECG).
4. Depending on the findings, dietary evaluation, mental health counseling, and endocrinology evaluation could be indicated.
5. Instructions would include avoiding foods high in magnesium, antacids, laxatives, enemas, and magnesium supplements if there are high magnesium levels. Instructions would further include avoiding alcohol, diuretics, hyperglycemia, and treating unresolved vomiting or diarrhea if there were low magnesium levels.

Chapter 6

1. The following questions should be posed to the client upon admission:
   - How long have you been vomiting?
   - Can you estimate the amount, color, and frequency of emesis?
   - Have you been experiencing any nausea?
   - What methods have you used to help during the time you have been experiencing GI symptoms?
   - Have you noticed any muscle tremors, twitching, or breathing problems?
   - Have you had any other symptoms such as dizziness or excessive sweating?
   - Have you been running a fever?
   - Are you being treated for any medical condition at the present time?
   - Are you taking any medications, either prescription or OTC at the present time or recently?

   This is just a partial listing of questions that could be posed to the client to provide a more accurate assessment.
2. Reported vital signs reveal a BP within normal limits but at the lower end of the normal range. It would be pertinent to obtain a height and weight on the client and to correlate BP findings with client history and physical status. Assess the client for muscle tremors and twitching and maintain safety precautions so as to prevent fall injuries if the client is feeling dizzy. Assess the client's skin turgor for evidence of dehydration and document findings.
3. Nursing diagnoses that could apply to this client include the following:
   - Alterations in Acid–Base Balance related to GI losses
   - Alterations in Fluid and Electrolyte Balance related to GI losses
   - Imbalanced Nutrition: Less Than Body Requirements related to altered intake pattern
   - Impaired Skin Integrity related to fluid losses
   - Risk for Injury related to volume and electrolyte depletion
4. Interventions to implement would be to verify physician orders with the expectation that pertinent lab/diagnostic tests, such as a serum chemistries, would be ordered for the client to establish both a baseline and to evaluate response to treatment. Because the client is dehydrated and unable to keep down solid foods, parenteral administration of fluids would be required to rehydrate the client and correct fluid and electrolyte imbalances. The client would most likely be experiencing chloride, sodium, and potassium deficits in addition to volume deficits. If the client continues to experience vomiting and/nausea, then the use of antiemetics may be indicated to prevent further fluid and electrolyte loss.
5. Discharge instructions would focus on maintaining hydration levels and electrolyte balance. Dietary instructions would include foods that are high in sodium, chloride, and potassium; these may be necessary to restore balance. The client should also receive instructions regarding the importance of early intervention in cases of severe GI symptoms so as to avoid hospitalization and to institute prompt treatment.

Chapter 7

1. Mr. G. will have hyperphosphatemia because the chronic renal failure will prevent his kidneys from eliminating excess phosphates.
2. As the kidneys fail, the nephrons (the functional units of the kidney) are not able to perform their intended functions adequately. Because the kidneys ordinarily

eliminate excess phosphorus, this substance is retained in the bloodstream, leading to high phosphorus levels.

3. Many foods are naturally rich in phosphorus, making dietary management somewhat difficult. Mr. G. should avoid foods that are especially rich in phosphorus, such as fish, poultry, eggs, red meat, organ meats, dairy products, legumes, whole grains, and nuts.

4. Hemodialysis will compensate for the lack of functioning of the kidneys and help to eliminate excess phosphates from the bloodstream.

5. Mr. G. will be receiving a phosphate-binding agent as part of his medication therapy. The active ingredient in the medication that is ordered will be either aluminum, magnesium, or calcium. Currently, calcium-based products (with calcium carbonate or Tums as an example) are popular for use in clients with renal failure because a client with this diagnosis often has concurrent hypocalcemia. Mr. G. should also be taught to read the labels of over-the-counter medications and products and avoid using those that are high in phosphorus or phosphate content.

Chapter 8

1. Due to the chronic nature of COPD, this client would most likely have ABG values consistent with chronic respiratory acidosis. Compensation would be expected because of the chronic nature of COPD, but because of the acute onset of URI, decompensation could occur depending on the client's baseline status and nature of acute exacerbation. Due to retention of acids, the pH would be low and the $PaCO_2$ would be elevated, with the HCO_3^- elevated to compensate.

2. The client with COPD should be taught ways to get rid of as much CO_2 as possible. The client should be taught purse-lipped breathing and to take bronchodilators as ordered by the physician to promote dilation of the bronchial tree. The client should also be taught the signs and symptoms of infection and to get the pneumonia and flu vaccines yearly because these two conditions could exacerbate the respiratory condition.

3. A client with COPD becomes insensitive to CO_2 elevations as a respiratory stimulus. Due to the chronic nature of this disease process, compensation has taken place and high levels of oxygen affect the respiratory center. When an oxygen concentration is too high, it will actually knock out the client's stimulus to breathe. However, it is imperative to treat acute hypoxia when needed; intubation can be done if the hypoxic drive is "knocked out."

4. Because of chronic lung disease, this client's alveoli have been unable to get rid of excess CO_2. As a result, clients with COPD show chronically high CO_2 levels on ABG results. This is considered a normal/abnormal finding in clients with chronic COPD. A client who does not have COPD retains the normal response stimulus of CO_2 for ventilatory drive. Clients without airway disease are able to ventilate and perform gas exchange using normal

mechanisms. They are able to maintain CO_2 balance by breathing patterns and are not subject to CO_2 retention.

5. Clients with COPD frequently develop cardiac problems along with their lung disease. The chronic hypoxemia leads to pulmonary vasoconstriction, which can lead to development of right heart failure. Potassium-wasting diuretics are used to treat both conditions. When potassium is lost, hydrogen ions tend to move out of the cell into the blood creating an alkalotic state. The client should be taught the signs and symptoms of hypokalemia and metabolic alkalosis and to report potential problems to the physician. Clients should eat foods high in potassium, if not already on a potassium supplement. Clients should also be taught to notify the physician immediately if severe diarrhea develops, as this might cause the development of metabolic alkalosis.

Chapter 9

1. The nurse should check baseline vital signs, heart rhythm, and lung sounds as well as assess for other signs and symptoms of anemia. It is also important for the nurse to know the type of anemia the client has, its cause, and the client's current hematocrit and hemoglobin (as well as total RBC count and RBC indices if available). The client should be asked whether she's ever had a transfusion of blood or a blood product before, when that was, and whether she had a reaction. Ensure that the client has given informed consent after speaking with the physician and that all transfusion-related questions have been answered.

2. The following are priority nursing diagnoses: Impaired Gas Exchange, Ineffective Breathing Pattern, Altered Tissue Perfusion, and Activity Intolerance. While the blood is transfusing, the client may also be at Risk for Injury. Knowledge Deficit may also be appropriate as the client needs to understand the reason for the transfusion (to improve the oxygen-carrying capacity of the blood), procedures that will be done during the transfusion process (identification of blood product, frequent vital signs, length of transfusion therapy, and signs and symptoms of transfusion reactions), and posttransfusion procedures (follow-up blood work and continued observation).

3. Prior to beginning the transfusion, it is important to determine that the client has informed consent and has signed the consent form. It is important to answer all questions regarding the administration of this blood product. If the client has additional questions or concerns that are beyond the scope of nursing practice, the physician should be notified. If there are no questions or if the client's questions have been answered to satisfaction, then the nurse should apprise the client of the steps that will be taken during the blood transfusion procedure. The client will be typed and cross-matched for two units of PRBCs by the lab. Once the type and cross-match has been completed, an IV site will be established for the transfusion. The blood unit will be brought to the floor

and two RNs will verify the original order and (at the bedside) check the client's blood bank band with the unit in order to verify information concerning the blood unit (name, unit number, type and Rh, and expiration date). The client will be monitored throughout the course of therapy with frequent vital signs and observation. If any additional medication is ordered either as a premedication or in between units, the nurse will administer it per the physician's order. Following completion of the transfusion of the units, lab work will be drawn to see how the client responded to the therapy.

4. Following hospital policy and procedure will help to maintain safe transfusion therapy, but it alone may not prevent the occurrence of a transfusion reaction. In order to maintain transfusion safety, it is important to remain with the client during the first 15 minutes of any transfusion therapy to assess for potential transfusion reactions. If the client should develop any signs or symptoms of a transfusion reaction, stop or slow the transfusion depending on type of reaction and hospital policy, attend to the client, and notify the physician and the blood bank when appropriate. Using proper equipment, monitoring parameters, and assessing the client (not merely the equipment) will promote transfusion safety in the clinical setting.

5. In order to evaluate the effectiveness of transfusion therapy, the nurse should expect a decrease in heart rate, respiratory rate, improvement of clinical symptoms (decrease in shortness of breath and increased tissue perfusion) and increased activity tolerance. Diagnostic results posttransfusion should reflect an increase of two grams in hemoglobin and a 6% increase in hematocrit.

Index

Page numbers followed by b indicate box; those followed by f indicate figure; those followed by t indicate table.

Black
tourmaline